Edited by

MARGARET B. ARBUCKLE, PhD
Associate Director
Center for Youth, Family, and Community Partnerships
University of North Carolina at Greensboro
Greensboro, North Carolina

&

CHARLOTTE A. HERRICK, PhD, RN
Professor Emeritus
Psychiatric Nursing and Case Management, School of Nursing
University of North Carolina at Greensboro
Greensboro, North Carolina

D1215155

CHILD & ADOLESCENT
MENTAL HEALTH

Interdisciplinary Systems of Care

JONES AND BARTLETT PUBLISHERS
Sudbury, Massachusetts
BOSTON   TORONTO   LONDON   SINGAPORE

World Headquarters

Jones and Bartlett
Publishers
40 Tall Pine Drive
Sudbury, MA 01776
978-443-5000
info@jbpub.com
www.jbpub.com

Jones and Bartlett
Publishers Canada
6339 Ormindale Way
Mississauga, ON L5V 1J2
CANADA

Jones and Bartlett
Publishers International
Barb House, Barb Mews
London W6 7PA
UK

Jones and Bartlett's books and products are available through most bookstores and online booksellers. To contact Jones and Bartlett Publishers directly, call 800-832-0034, fax 978-443-8000, or visit our website at www.jbpub.com.

Substantial discounts on bulk quantities of Jones and Bartlett's publications are available to corporations, professional associations, and other qualified organizations. For details and specific discount information, contact the special sales department at Jones and Bartlett via the above contact information or send an email to specialsales@jbpub.com.

Copyright © 2006 by Jones and Bartlett Publishers, Inc.

Library of Congress Cataloging-in-Publication Data
Arbuckle, Margaret B.
 Child and adolescent mental health : interdisciplinary systems of care / Margaret B. Arbuckle, Charlotte A. Herrick.
   p. ; cm.
 Includes bibliographical references.
 ISBN 0-7637-2908-6 (pbk.)
 1. Child mental health services. 2. Teenagers—Mental health services. 3. Integrated delivery of health care.
 [DNLM: 1. Delivery of Health Care, Integrated—organization & administration—Adolescent. 2. Delivery of Health Care, Integrated—organization & administration—Child. 3. Mental Health Services—organization & administration—Adolescent. 4. Mental Health Services—organization & administration—Child. 5. Adolescent Health Services—organization & administration. 6. Child Health Services—organization & administration. 7. Interprofessional Relations. 8. Professional-Family Relations.] I. Arbuckle, Margaret Bourdeaux. II. Title.
 RJ499.H536 2005
 618.92'89—dc22

                                                                                              2005004506

Production Credits
Acquisitions Editor: Kevin Sullivan
Associate Editor: Amy Sibley
Production Director: Amy Rose
Production Assistant: Kate Hennessy
Marketing Manager: Emily Ekle
Manufacturing Buyer: Therese Connell
Composition: Auburn Associates, Inc.
Cover Design: Tim Dziewit
Cover Image: © Digital Vision
Printing and Binding: Malloy Inc.
Cover Printing: Malloy Inc.

Printed in the United States of America
09 08 07 06 05   10 9 8 7 6 5 4 3 2 1

Dedication

We dedicate this book with the hope for a better future to the following:

- All of the children, adolescents, adults, and families who require complex health and mental health care with the hope that your quality of life improves because of System of Care.
- All of the professionals who are caring for families with complex needs with the hope that System of Care will guide your practice.

Acknowledgments

From Charlotte and Margaret

- To all of the contributors for the various chapters or sections within chapters of this textbook for their hard work and their dedication.
- To the authors of the chapter on "Parents' Voices", who developed a course in System of Care, Interdisciplinary Practice with us. They have presented at national meetings with us, and Frederick Douglas assisted in the development of a presentation for an international meeting.
- To Elizabeth Tournquist for her editorial support.

From Charlotte

- To Bob Herrick, my husband who was my first role model in caring for children with emotional disturbances and their families, who believed in the values and principles of System of Care long before System of Care was a national endeavor. His sacrifices during this project allowed me to see it to fruition.
- To Dean Lynne Pearcey for mentoring me when I first became a faculty member. As Dean, she has inspired me, as well as others along the path to scholarship.
- To my Psychosocial Nursing students during the Fall Semester of 2004, who were so supportive of me during the writing of this text and supportive of each other's quest for knowledge.

From Margaret

- To Howard Arbuckle, my husband and constant encourager, who continues to amaze me in the depth of his understanding about children's needs.
- To Elizabeth, Mathew, and Ada Adele, our children, who each are special in their own way and through their gifts of intelligence, character, tenacity, and humor, have succeeded in life into young adulthood with great accomplishment.
- To the members of the Guilford County Community Collaborative and my colleagues at the University of North Carolina at Greensboro whose work in implementing System of Care provided the inspiration for this book.

To Each Other

To our partnership. We have been co-authors in a joint venture. Our relationship has grown into one of mutual respect and awe. We have collaborated equally, mutually, and respectfully as partners from different disciplines. We believe we are the role models for future generations. We shared the responsibilities and were equal contributors to the project. Charlotte had the vision, while Margaret attended to the details. Both of us recruited and worked with the contributors. Both authors edited the chapters, each contributing her expertise, and some chapters were written together. We hope to convey to future generations that interdisciplinary work is rewarding and mutually beneficial.

Table of Contents

Foreword

BETH A. STROUL

Mental health problems in children and adolescents have created a public health crisis in this country. These problems affect a growing number of youth. They impact these children and their families in all spheres of their lives, and their consequences are costly and often tragic. Recent studies indicate an alarmingly high prevalence rate, with approximately 1 in 5 children having a diagnosable mental disorder and 1 in 10 youth having a serious emotional or behavioral disorder that is severe enough to cause substantial impairment in functioning at home, at school, or in the community (Friedman, Katz-Leavy, Manderscheid, & Sondheimer, 1996). The National Institute of Mental Health (NIMH) National Advisory Mental Health Council's Workgroup on Child and Adolescent Mental Health concluded that "no other illnesses damage so many children so seriously" (National Advisory Mental Health Council, 2001, p. 1).

In conjunction with this prevalence rate, there is an extremely high level of unmet need. It is estimated that up to 80% of children with emotional and behavioral disorders do not receive mental health services (Ringel & Sturm, 2001). Former Surgeon General David Satcher, at his National Conference on Children's Mental Health, stated that "growing numbers of children are suffering needlessly because their emotional, behavioral, and developmental needs are not being met by those very institutions which were explicitly created to take care of them" (Satcher, 2000, p. 1). Despite these levels of prevalence and unmet need and the serious impact of mental health problems on the functioning of our children, our nation has failed to develop a comprehensive, systematic approach to this crisis in children's mental health.

The inadequacy of the children's mental health system has been repeatedly documented for many years. The Joint Commission on Mental Health of Children (1969) concluded that only a fraction of children in need were actually receiving mental health services and that the services that were provided were largely ineffective. Subsequent policy studies documented similar conclusions, indicating that children were not getting needed mental health services. Those served were often in excessively restrictive settings; services were limited to outpatient, inpatient, and residential treatment with few intermediate care, community-based options available, and the coordination between child-serving systems responsible for mental health needs was weak (Knitzer, 1982; President's Commission on Mental Health, 1978; US Congress, Office of Technology Assessment, 1986). These various reports served as a catalyst for federal attention to children's mental health. The Child and Adolescent Service System Program was launched by the NIMH in 1984 with the objective of helping states and communities build their capacity to develop Systems of Care particularly targeted for children with serious and complex needs (children with "serious emotional disturbances") who were involved with multiple service sectors, for example, mental health, special education, child welfare, and juvenile justice. An early accomplishment of Child and Adolescent Service System Program was the refining of the concept of a System of Care to serve as a framework for reform (Stroul & Friedman, 1986, 1996). A System of Care was defined as "a comprehensive spectrum of mental health and other services and supports organized into a coordinated network to meet the complex and changing needs of children and their families" (Stroul & Friedman, 1986, p. 3). It included a set of core values and principles to guide service delivery to children and families. The core values specify that services should be *community-based, child-centered and family-focused*, and *culturally appropriate*. Key principles specify that services should be *comprehensive with a broad array of services and supports; individualized* to each child and family; provided in the *least restrictive, appropriate setting; coordinated* at both the system and service delivery levels; include *early intervention* efforts; and engage *families and youth* as full partners. The System of Care framework is based on eight overlapping areas of need, with children and families at the center, in recognition that no one system can meet the diverse and multiple needs of children with serious emotional disturbances and their families. Thus, the framework includes the mental health, social, educational, health, substance abuse, vocational, recreational, and operational dimensions—all functions that need to be accounted for in order to support children and families adequately.

This System of Care approach helped to seed other federal and foundation initiatives geared to developing more comprehensive, integrated systems of community-based services and supports for children. The largest of these programs, the federal Comprehensive Community Mental Health Services for Children and Their Families Program, authorized by Congress in 1992, has a current budget of over $100 million and, to date, has provided 96 grants to states, communities, territories, and Indian tribes and tribal organizations to improve Systems of Care to meet the needs of youth with emotional problems and their families (US Department of Health and Human Services, 2002). A national evaluation of this program shows a reduction in mental health problems and costly out-of-state residential placements and an increase in behavioral and emotional strengths. Residential stability and school attendance and performance improved, and contacts with law enforcement and substance use decreased (Center for Mental Health Services, in press).

Despite progress in improving Systems of Care for children with emotional disorders and their families, recent examinations have highlighted areas that need improvement and that represent significant challenges. The landmark report *Mental Health: A Report of the Surgeon General* (US Department of Health and Human Services, 1999) underscored the need for a developmental perspective for understanding and treating mental disorders in children and synthesized the evidence base for services. The goal of providing care for children with mental health needs in their homes and communities was further supported in 1999 by the US Supreme Court's ground-breaking Olmstead decision, which specified that the institutionalization of persons with disabilities who, given appropriate supports, could live in the community is a form of discrimination. The intent of the Olmstead decision for children with serious emotional disorders is consistent with the System of Care philosophy—avoiding out-of-home placements to the extent possible and returning children to their home communities in a timely way with appropriate services and supports in place (Lezak & Macbeth, 2002). In 2000, the US Surgeon General convened a national conference on children's mental health that resulted in a national action agenda that set forth children's mental health as a national priority and delineated action steps to organize and coordinate services in the child's cultural and community context (US Public Health Service, 2000). This movement toward comprehensive, community-based care culminated most recently in President Bush's New Freedom Initiative, which included proposals to eliminate barriers for people with disabilities. As part of this initiative, the president issued an executive order to create a presidential commission on mental health, with a specific mandate to study the existing mental health service delivery system and make recommendations for improvements that will enable adults with serious mental illness and children with serious emotional disorders to live, work, learn, and fully function in their homes and communities. In July 2003, the President's New Freedom Commission on Mental Health issued its report, *Achieving the Promise: Transforming Mental Health Care in America*. The report presented recommendations that, in aggregate, would begin to change how mental health care is organized, financed, and delivered in order to achieve the goal of recovery and resilience and a thriving life in the community. Given the complex needs of children with mental health problems, the New Freedom Commission on Mental Health created a subcommittee on children and families to study the existing service delivery system for children and their families. The subcommittee crafted a vision for children's mental health that is based on the System of Care approach and that calls for a broad array of services and supports to be provided in the child's community, in partnership with the family, and in congruence with the culture, values, and preferences of the child and family. The vision goes beyond the focus on children with serious emotional disturbances and also focuses on using more of a public health model to prevent mental health problems and create conditions that promote positive socioemotional health for children.

Achieving this vision will require a significant transformation of the current service delivery system: its organization, financing, and clinical services and supports. Transformation and strategies to achieve this were proposed by the subcommittee in the following areas:

- Developing comprehensive home and community-based services and supports
- Developing family partnerships and family support
- Providing culturally competent care and reducing unmet need and disparities in access to services
- Individualizing care
- Implementing evidence-based practices
- Coordinating services, responsibility, and funding to reduce fragmentation

- Increasing prevention, early identification, and early intervention
- Strengthening early childhood intervention
- Expanding mental health services in schools
- Strengthening accountability and quality improvement

These transformations comprise a blueprint for change in children's mental health, with the hope of improving services and supports and, of course, outcomes for children and their families.

A critical challenge for the field is creating an adequate workforce, with both the numbers of professionals and the values and competencies needed, to accompany a comprehensive and transformed approach to children's mental health. Although curricula are slow to change, the nature of pre-service training must be shifted to the new philosophy underlying service delivery, based on the inclusion of families as partners in service delivery, the shift from an almost exclusive focus on office and clinic-based practice to a greater emphasis on an individualized home and community-based service approach, and the role of interdisciplinary collaboration in service planning and intervention. Training must include strengths-based approaches, individualized care, and the clinical advances embedded in evidence-based and promising practices (Friedman, 1993; Morris & Hanley, 2001). For providers working with children and families across all disciplines, a transformed service delivery system would require expanded roles and approaches to care. In order to fulfill these roles, training is needed that goes beyond the clinical treatment of disorders and also develops an ability to harness the strengths of the child, to partner with families in treatment planning and decision making, and to consult and collaborate with providers in other child serving systems. Given the stalled movement toward parity and the shrinking funds in the specialty mental health system, providers must be prepared to work in nonmental health settings, such as schools, juvenile justice, primary care, and child welfare, where there is a high prevalence of mental health problems. Training in evidence-based practices is increasingly important as consumers, families, and payers are committed to getting "services that work" based on science or best clinical consensus. With the growing disparities in access, quality, and outcomes of services for diverse ethnic and racial populations, providers must become better trained to work with culturally diverse children and their families. Training must enhance cultural competence, and the field must create specific incentives and strategies to recruit and train culturally and linguistically diverse practitioners. A great need and opportunity exists as well for professionals who are trained to work effectively with preschool children and their families.

Child and Adolescent Mental Health: Interdisciplinary Systems of Care tackles the challenge of workforce development by creating one of the few texts focused on undergraduate and graduate students across disciplines in the helping professions. Various chapters address the perspectives of psychologists, nurses, psychiatrists, social workers, educators, recreation specialists, families, and others and discuss the integration of the System of Care philosophy and approach in schools, the juvenile justice system, substance abuse treatment, and more. It makes a substantial contribution to the transformation process and will serve as model for other institutions of higher education to work collaboratively across disciplines toward the common goal of "achieving the promise" in children's mental health.

References

Center for Mental Health Services (In press). *Annual report to Congress on the evaluation of the comprehensive community mental health services for children and their families program, 2001.* Atlanta, GA: ORC Macro.

Friedman, R. M. (1993). Preparation of students to work with children and families: Is it meeting the need? *Administration and Policy in Mental Health, 20,* 297–310.

Friedman, R., Katz-Leavy, J., Manderscheid, R., & Sondheimer, D. (1996). Prevalence of serious emotional disturbance in children and adolescents. In R. W. Manderscheid & M. A. Sonnenschein (Eds.), *Mental Health, United States, 1996* (pp. 71–88). Rockville, MD: Center for Mental Health Services.

Joint Commission on the Mental Health of Children. (1969). *Crisis in child mental health.* New York: Harper & Row.

Knitzer, J. (1982). *Unclaimed children: The failure of public responsibility to children and adolescents in need of mental health services.* Washington, DC: Children's Defense Fund.

Lezak, A., & Macbeth, G. (Eds.). (2002). *Overcoming barriers to serving our children in the community.* Rockville, MD: US Department of Health and Human Services.

Morris, J. A., & Hanley, J. H. (2001). Human resource development: A critical gap in child mental health reform. *Administration and Policy in Mental Health, 28*(3), 219–227.

National Advisory Mental Health Council Workgroup on Child and Adolescent Mental Health Intervention Development and Deployment. (2001). *Blueprint for change: Research on child and adolescent mental health.* Rockville, MD: National Institute of Mental Health.

New Freedom Commission on Mental Health. (2003). *Achieving the promise: Transforming mental health care in America: Final report.* Rockville, MD: US Department of Health and Human Services, Pub. No. SMA-03-3832.

President's Commission on Mental Health. (1978). *Report of the sub-task panel on infants, children, and adolescents.* Washington, DC: Author.

Ringel, J., & Sturm, R. (2001). National estimates of mental health utilization and expenditure for children in 1998. *Journal of Behavioral Health Services and Research, 28*(3), 319–332.

Satcher, D. (2000). *Foreword: Report of the Surgeon General's conference on children's mental health: A national action agenda.* Washington, DC: US Public Health Service.

Stroul, B., & Friedman, R. (1986). *A system of care for children and youth with severe emotional disturbances.* Washington, DC: Georgetown University Child Development Center, National Technical Assistance Center for Children's Mental Health.

Stroul, B., & Friedman, R. (1996). The system of care concept and philosophy. In B. Stroul (Ed.), *Children's mental health: Creating systems of care in a changing society.* Baltimore: Paul Brookes Publishing.

US Congress, Office of Technology Assessment. (1986). *Children's mental health: Problems and services: A background paper.* Washington, DC: Author.

US Department of Health and Human Services. (1999). *Mental health: A report of the Surgeon General.* Rockville, MD: US Public Health Service.

US Department of Health and Human Services, SAMHSA, CMHS. (2002). *Cooperative agreements for the comprehensive community mental health services for children and their families program* (No. SM-02-002).

US Public Health Service. (2000). *Report of the Surgeon General's conference on children's mental health: A national action agenda.* Washington, DC: US Public Health Service.

Preface

MARGARET B. ARBUCKLE & CHARLOTTE A. HERRICK

Child and Adolescent Mental Health: Interdisciplinary Systems of Care is a resource to families and professionals, both those in training and those in the service delivery sector, who share the authors' concern that we must do a better job of addressing the serious needs of children, adolescents, and families in today's society. Opening the morning paper or tuning in to the evening news exposes one to stories of youth whose life experiences are horrendous because of the economic circumstances of their families, their own behavioral challenges resulting in illegal drug use, gang activity, and poor school performance, or infractions of the law resulting in incarceration. Of course, not every story is negative. Most children grow successfully into adolescence and move from high school into higher education or employment. However, the focus of *Child and Adolescent Mental Health* is on those whose lives are troubled.

Although the range of normal development varies widely, many children and adolescents have emotional problems that are more severe than the usual mood swings experienced by most during childhood. Twenty percent of children have mild to moderate functional impairments, whereas 5% to 9% suffer from a severe emotional disturbance. Their ability to function "socially, academically, or emotionally" is significantly impaired by this severe emotional disturbance (U.S. Department of Health & Human Services: Fundamentals of Mental Health and Mental Illness , 1999, p. 46).

Today, substantial evidence suggests that mental illness is influenced through multiple factors—including biological and environmental factors. The Surgeon General's Report (1999) identified specific risk factors, which indicated that some children are more vulnerable than others. We know that prevention programs have shown that early interventions can reduce the impact of risk factors, thereby improving the healthy development of children.

The risk factors among children are as follows (U.S. Department of Health and Human Services: Fundamentals of Mental Health and Mental Illness,1999):

- Physical problems
- Intellectual problems, such as mental retardation and learning disabilities
- Low birth weight
- A family history of mental illness or substance abuse
- Multigenerational poverty
- Caregiver separation or abuse or neglect

Access to care for children who are emotionally disturbed is not as readily available as access to care for an adult suffering from heart disease or cancer. "There are serious resource limitations . . . that [prevent access to] needed mental health services" for children and their families (Athey, 1999, p. 556). Often, emergency service personnel do not have the time to address the family's issues during their child's medical or mental health crisis, even if the emergency admission has to do with self-destructive behavior. It is estimated that only 24% of the hospitals across the country will arrange for children's mental health services (U.S. Department of Health & Human Services: Fundamentals of Mental Health and Mental Illness, 1999 and U.S. Department of Health & Human Services: Health Resources and Services Administration, 1999).

These problems are compounded by the societal obstacles preventing access to services for those with mental illness. As reported in the Executive Summary of the President's New Freedom Commission on Mental Health (Hogan, 2003), "Stigma surrounding mental illness, unfair treatment limitations and financial requirements placed on mental health benefits in private health insurance, and the fragmented mental health service delivery system" interfere with appropriate access to services for all citizens with mental illnesses. These issues are compounded for children and youth. There are challenges in diagnosis of mental health issues for youth. The youth are dependent on their families for access to payment for medical care, and the availability of services designed for youth to meet their specific needs is scarce.

Child and Adolescent Mental Health is the result of collaborative work that the authors completed with other faculty members at the

University of North Carolina at Greensboro and faculty colleagues around the country. Family members in the community also share their experiences of living with children with serious emotional disturbance and describe their interactions with service providers from deeply committed community agencies who connect youth to appropriate services but at times experience frustration in facilitating access to the services for the reasons enumerated previously here.

Ideas described as System of Care are those that can be applied to other children and adults with life challenges, whether educational, physical, or emotional. However, the stimulus for writing *Child and Adolescent Mental Health* is the deep hope that readers are motivated to work with imagination and commitment to address the needs of youth and families whose lives are impacted by mental illness. It is through this work that we ensure a bright and successful future for these children.

References

Athey, J.L. (1999) Emergency Medical Services for Children. In H. M. Wallace, G. Green, K. J. Jaros, L. L. Paine, M. Story (Ed.), *Health and Welfare for Families in the 21st Century* (pp. 547–550). Boston: Jones and Bartlett Publishers.

Hogan, M.F. (2003). Letter to President Bush, as Chairman of the President's New Freedom Commission on Mental Health. *Achieving the promise: Transforming mental health care in America, executive summary*. Rockville, MD: The Department of Health and Human Services (DHHS Publication No. SMA-0303831). Available at http://www.mentalhealthcommission.gov/reports/reports.htm. Accessed July 7, 2005.

U.S. Department of Health and Human Services: Fundamentals of Mental Health and Mental Illness (1999). *Mental health: A report of the Surgeon General* (pp. 31–116). Rockville, Md.: U.S. Department of Health and Human Services, Substance Abuse and Mental Health Services Administration, Center for Mental Health Services. National Institutes of Health. National Institute of Mental Illness.

U.S. Department of Health and Human Services: Health Resources and Services Administration (1999). *Maternal Child Health Bureau*. Available at http://www.mchb.hrsa.gov/. Accessed June 22, 2005.

Contributors

Margaret B. Arbuckle, PhD
Associate Director
Center for Youth, Family, and
   Community Partnerships
University of North Carolina at
   Greensboro
Greensboro, North Carolina

T. Robin Bartlett, PhD, RN, BC
Assistant Professor
School of Nursing
University of North Carolina at
   Greensboro
Greensboro, North Carolina

Paula Brooke
Graduate Assistant
Department of Recreation, Parks and
   Tourism
University of North Carolina at
   Greensboro
Greensboro, North Carolina

Joy Cherry, RN, BSN
Master's Student
School of Nursing
University of North Carolina at
   Greensboro
Greensboro, North Carolina

Jacalyn A. Claes, PhD, LCSW
Associate Professor
Department of Social Work
University of North Carolina at
   Greensboro
Greensboro, North Carolina

Grey Cockerham
Self Advocate
University of North Carolina at
   Greensboro
Greensboro, North Carolina

Jewell E. Cooper, PhD, MS, BA
Assistant Professor
Department of Curriculum and
   Instruction
University of North Carolina at
   Greensboro
Greensboro, North Carolina

Elizabeth Dobyns, BSN
Former Site Director System of Care Grant
Guilford Center
Mental Health Consultant
Reidsville, North Carolina

Reverend Frederick Douglas
Co-Teacher and Parent Advocate
System of Care Interdisciplinary Course
Parent of Member of Vulnerable
   Population
Greensboro, North Carolina

Jacqueline Etemad, MD
Clinical Professor of Psychiatry
University of California, San Francisco
San Francisco, California

Maria E. Fernandez, PhD
Research Director
North Carolina System of Care
   Demonstration Projects
Division of Mental Health,
   Developmental Disabilities and
   Substance Abuse
North Carolina Department of Human
   Resources
Raleigh, North Carolina

Terri Grant, MPPM
Project Director
North Carolina System of Care
Division of Mental Health, Develop-
   mental Disabilities and Substance
   Abuse
North Carolina Department of Human
   Resources
Raleigh, North Carolina

Charlotte A. Herrick, PhD, RN
Professor Emeritus
Psychiatric Nursing and Case
   Management
School of Nursing
University of North Carolina at
   Greensboro
Greensboro, North Carolina

Libby Jones
Parent Advocate and Co-Teacher
Parent of Member of Vulnerable
   Population
SUCCESS, Parent Organization
Greensboro, North Carolina

Randy Kohlenberg, PhD
Professor
School of Music
University of North Carolina at
   Greensboro
Greensboro, North Carolina

Stephanie Kurtts, PhD, MAED, BS
Assistant Professor
Department of Specialized Education
   Services
University of North Carolina at
   Greensboro
Greensboro, North Carolina

Kimberly D. Miller, MS, CTRS
Project Coordinator
Department of Recreation, Parks and
   Tourism
University of North Carolina at
   Greensboro
Greensboro, North Carolina

Mark O'Donnell, MPH
*Local Management Team Technical
   Assistance Advisor*
Division of Mental Health,
   Developmental Disabilities and
   Substance Abuse
North Carolina Department of Human
   Resources
Raleigh, North Carolina

Geraldine S. Pearson, PhD, APRN
*Assistant Professor and Director Home
   Care Program*
School of Medicine
Department of Psychiatry
University of Connecticut Health Center
Farmington, Connecticut

Gerald Ponder, PhD
Professor
Department of Curriculum and
   Instruction
School of Education
University of North Carolina at
   Greensboro
Greensboro, North Carolina

Stuart J. Schleien, PhD
Professor and Department Head
Department of Recreation, Parks, and
    Tourism
University of North Carolina at
    Greensboro
Greensboro, North Carolina

Carolyn Schmidt, RN, BSN
Nurse Case Manager
Guilford Department of Social Services
Liaison
Department of Public Health, Child
    Division
Clinical Preceptor
Nursing Case Management Course
University of North Carolina at
    Greensboro
Greensboro, North Carolina

Terri Lisabeth Shelton, PhD
Professor of Psychology
Director, Center for Youth, Family,
    and Community Partnerships
University of North Carolina at
    Greensboro
Greensboro, North Carolina

Sarah Moore Shoffner, PhD
Associate Professor and Director,
    Internship Program
Department of Human Development
    and Family Studies
University of North Carolina at
    Greensboro
Greensboro, North Carolina

Susan M. Taccheri, MD
Psychiatrist
Former Director of Psychiatric Medical
    Services
Guilford Center
Currently Oaklawn Psychiatric Center
Elkhurst, Indiana

About the Authors

Margaret Bourdeaux Arbuckle, PhD

Dr. Margaret Bourdeaux Arbuckle graduated from Salem College and received her PhD and Masters of Education at the University of North Carolina at Greensboro in Human Development and Family Studies. She has been a practitioner in early childhood education having taught preschoolers and served as director of a demonstration childcare center. She has provided leadership in advocating for improved quality in childcare and in provision of state funds to support pre-kindergarten programs. Dr. Arbuckle has provided state and local advocacy leadership in the development of programs and public policy addressing education, child welfare, juvenile justice, and health and mental health needs of children and families. She has chaired numerous community/ state agency boards, such as the Guilford County Partnership for Children (Smart Start) and the North Carolina Child Advocacy Institute Board. She served as a Guilford County Commissioner and in this capacity facilitated the development of the County Children's Cabinet.

Presently, Dr. Arbuckle is the Executive Director of Guilford Education Alliance, a local advocacy organization to promote and support education. Prior to this appointment, she was an Associate Director of the Center for Youth, Family and Community Partnerships at UNCG. In this capacity, she provided leadership in implementation of the Comprehensive Community Mental Health Services for Children and their Families Program grant in Guilford County giving leadership at the university and community level in training in System of Care values, principles, and implementation, with particular emphasis on partnerships among professionals and parents and implementing cultural competency in services to meet the needs of families and children. She has overseen Housing and Urban Development grants, a Youth Build program and a Community Outreach Partnership Center, and a project addressing the application of System of Care into the Juvenile Justice System serving adjudicated youth. Additionally, Dr. Arbuckle has developed grants for development of services to address preschoolers in childcare settings who have mental health needs and the support of programs to train service providers in cultural competence. Dr. Arbuckle's research interests have focused on community development, children's mental health, implementation of System of Care, family-centered service delivery, and cultural competence.

Dr. Arbuckle has made numerous presentations on her work at national and state conferences and co-authored "Teaching Interprofessional Practice: A Course on a System of Care for Children with Severe Emotional Disturbance and Their Families," published in the *Journal of Family Nursing*, "A Community Responds: On the Way toward Cultural Competence" published in *Focal Point,* and "Modeling Empowerment in Teaching Future Social Workers" in the *Journal of Baccalaureate Social Work Educators.*

Dr. Arbuckle is married to Howard B. Arbuckle III and they have three children, Elizabeth, Mathew, and Ada Adele.

CHARLOTTE A. HERRICK, PhD, RN

Charlotte A. Herrick is currently teaching psychiatric nursing and case management at the University of North Carolina at Greensboro School of Nursing. She is currently a Visiting Professor and as a retiree, she is a professor emeritus.

In her previous role as chairman of Community Practice, she became involved in a grant to infuse System of Care principles into nursing courses, particularly those in her department, which included psychosocial nursing and community health nursing. As a faculty member, she participated in the development of a course, System of Care: Interdisciplinary Practice, sponsored by several university departments.

Prior to academia, Charlotte was a nurse and therapist at a mental health center. She worked with children with severe emotional disturbances and their families and adults who were persistently and chronically mentally ill. She has also worked with children who were autistic or multiply handicapped and their parents in a school for special children. The school was involved in one of the first Children and

Adolescent Service System Program (CASSP) grants. Dr. Herrick has numerous publications in nursing journals and has presented at workshops and nursing conferences nationally and internationally.

Currently, Charlotte lives with her husband, a child psychiatrist and former academician, who works with children in a local mental health center. Her greatest joy is to travel around the USA and Europe visiting friends and family. She has 5 sons and 11 grandchildren, who live on or between the two coasts, and one son in Paris, France.

I

System of Care for Children Who Are Severely Emotionally Disturbed: An Interdisciplinary Case Management Approach to the Delivery of Care to Children and Families with Complex Needs

System of Care Principles and Practice: Implementing Family-Centered Care for Families and Children with Complex Needs

MARGARET BOURDEAUX ARBUCKLE

Objectives

- Discuss the historical background that has led to the development of the System of Care philosophy.
- Discuss the need for interdisciplinary care coordination.
- Identify the reasons for the development of interdisciplinary family-centered care.
- Explain the core values and principles of System of Care.
- Define the method for care coordination, that is, wraparound services.
- Incorporate values and principles into discussions about the delivery of services for all persons with complex needs.
- Discuss the achievement of cultural competence as essential to family-centered care.

The Reasons for System of Care: Why Interdisciplinary, Family-Centered, Culturally Competent, Strength-Based Service Delivery?

Since the 1980s, professionals in the mental health, health, and medical professions and in education have become increasingly aware that the traditional service delivery model with "clients" as recipients of services is no longer effective. Professionals and leaders in federal and state governments have begun to recognize that to address the complex needs and issues of youth and families services must be delivered that are comprehensive across the continuum of care. The development of the System of Care philosophy of service delivery, including the values and principles of family-centered, community-based, and culturally competent care, has been the focus of many program developers and researchers in the health, mental health, social service, and education fields.

This chapter describes the history of the System of Care developments, examines initiatives at the federal level as these values were incorporated into mental health services for children and youth, and sets the stage for in-depth discussion about implementing these values into service systems for children, youth, and families whose needs are complex. Application of these values and principles to the care of all populations with complex health, social, and educational needs is explored.

The Need for System of Care: The Story of Mary

Mary is a 14-year-old biracial girl (she has a black mother and a white father) living in a small town outside of a larger city, in a neighborhood that is primarily apartments and low-income housing. She lives with her mother, who is divorced from her father, and with her mother's companion, a man who drinks heavily and is sometimes physically abusive to Mary's mother. Mary's mother works part time in a neighborhood store, and because of the family's income, the family is eligible for Medicaid and food stamps. Mary has a younger brother in the fifth grade and an older sister who is living independently with her boyfriend, and who is working at a fast-food restaurant. Her father has moved to another city and has only occasional contact with Mary, as his present wife, who is pregnant, is not comfortable around Mary.

Mary suffers from epilepsy and had several serious seizures beginning as she entered puberty. The Health Department physician has prescribed medication that controls the seizures if taken daily. Mary is in denial about this medical condition and will sometimes not take her medication voluntarily.

The Department of Social Services removed Mary from the home when her mother was noncompliant with a court order that alleged abuse and neglect during the time of the divorce 2 years ago. After being sent to a foster home, Mary ran away and appeared at the home of one of her friends. The allegations were substantiated, and as a result, Mary's mother is very angry with "the system" and is fearful that there may be further investigations because of her present live-in boyfriend's outbursts of anger. The Department of Social Services returned Mary to her mother when the mother convinced the social worker that she could protect and care for Mary now that the divorce was settled. Mary's mother works as a receptionist for a small beauty parlor in the neighborhood. She does not have a car and walks to and from work every day.

Mary has a history of stealing items from other students at school and occasionally has been questioned by the owner of the convenience store down the street when he suspected that she was stealing candy. When Mary was 13 years old, she was arrested for shoplifting and was under court supervision with the Department of Juvenile Justice. She is now on probation, and her juvenile court counselor checks in on Mary monthly either at school or at home.

Mary is a special education student with a learning disability and an IQ of 70. She is in danger of failing the eighth grade and struggles with reading. At school she has displayed outbursts of anger—never assaulting anyone but turning over desks in the classroom and throwing things. The guidance counselor at school has befriended Mary and when meeting with her individually finds that she has a "sweet side." Mary has several friends at school that she pals around with, and they always eat lunch together in the cafeteria.

Over a year and a half ago, the school referred Mary to the community mental health center because of her outbursts in the classroom and her verbal threats to the teacher. She received a psychological assessment and now receives individual therapy weekly at the center.

Mary is not unique.

This description of Mary could describe any one of the approximately

- 20% of the children living in the United States who have a mental health disorder (www.surgeongeneral.gov/library/mentalhealth/chapter6/sec1.html)

- half-million children who are in out-of-home care in the child welfare system (http://ndas.cwla.org)
- 6 million children who have special education needs (http://www.ed.gov/about/reports/annual/osep/2002/appendix-a-pt1.pdf)
- 2.3 million children in the juvenile justice system (http://www.ojjjdp.ncjrs.org/ojstatbb/cirp /)
- 20 million children living with a chronic health problem (http://www.ahrq.gov/news/focus/chchild.htm)

Many children are "lucky" and have only one of these issues that must be addressed daily in their lives. Too often, however, children have multiple problems and issues, and their needs require that they interact with professionals from multiple service systems.

United States citizens are fortunate that over time human service systems and special education programs have been developed to address the specific needs of children and families. Although many children and families can be on waiting lists for services, multiple services and many service systems are available. We have special education programs in the public schools to assist teachers and parents in addressing the educational needs of children with learning disabilities. We have child welfare to protect children from abuse and neglect. We have a juvenile justice system that addresses specific law enforcement issues of children. We have health care for children with chronic illnesses, and we have mental health systems to address behavioral and social/emotional disorders of children. However, many children's needs overlap service systems, and thus, the need exists for a coordinated and comprehensive system of care that incorporates values and principles of mutual respect *among* professionals and *with* family members and professionals.

Assuming that all children are enrolled in school (unfortunately, because of mental health and/or behavioral issues, children with problems often are suspended or expelled from school), children who require professional attention outside of their educational need must interact with both the educational system and another service system designated to meet the other needs. Health care services may be "routine," such as regular doctor's checkups, even for a child with a chronic health problem. However, if the child's and family's financial situation makes them eligible for public services, such as the Department of Social Services, the Department of Mental Health and Developmental Disabilities, the Department of Juvenile Justice, or the Department of Public Health, the children's and family's lives become more complicated!

Mary is an example of a child with multiple needs who is eligible for public services because of the family's economic circumstances. Mary is involved with the Department of Social Services and has a child protective services worker; she receives health care through the Department of Public Health, Child, and Adolescent Health Services Division. Mary is also supervised by a juvenile court counselor from the juvenile justice system and has a therapist from the Department of Mental Health Services. She attends public school, where she receives supplemental services for her learning disability and her behavioral challenges. In addition to the regular classroom teachers, at least five professionals are involved in planning services for Mary and her family!

In Mary's story, the mother is very angry with the Department of Social Services because of their accusations about abuse and neglect. She is suspicious of the social worker's motives and feels that she is interfering in her family's life. Mary's mother resents the visits of the social worker, who is providing follow-up child protective services visits to the family, and her hurt and anger may spill over to interactions with the other professionals in Mary's life. In addition, the family must rely on public transportation, and because they live in a suburban community, public transportation is likely to be limited. This creates challenges, if not barriers, in getting the necessary services located in the city. Because of Mary's parents' divorce and their poor economic situation, the family is isolated from social supports such as friends, neighbors, faith-based organizations, work-related friends, and parents of their children's friends. Families such as Mary's who have multiple issues to address become so consumed by their troubles that they become increasingly isolated from the regular channels of social support.

The story of Mary and her family is not unique. Many children and families have complex needs. In particular, children with mental health needs, both those with a formal diagnosis and those whose social and emotional development is such that their behavior is inappropriate in the school setting, interface with many professionals. The System of Care philosophy and movement emerged to address the needs of children with a serious emotional disturbance. Over time, it has become recognized that the values and principles appropriate for these special children should also be incorporated into services for children who have learning differences, complex health needs, and child welfare and safety issues and for those within the juvenile justice system. This same philosophical approach can also be applied to other populations of persons who have complex special needs.

Too often, services are provided to children and families in isolation, without coordination of their care. The human service delivery system is fragmented and difficult for families to negotiate. Teachers do not talk with the social workers from the Department of System of Social Services. Juvenile court counselors do not confer with the teachers, and the therapist interacts only with the child and family and thus is not aware of behavioral issues in the school classroom unless the child or parent tells him or her.

In traditional service delivery, families are not included in the development of a plan of care for their child because the professional assumes the role of decision maker. Professionals may dictate to the family the plan of care, as well as the services that will be provided. In traditional case management, a professional case manager will meet with the family, question them about their needs, and then write a plan of services for them. When the family and child do not adhere to the professionals' recommendations, they are deemed noncompliant and may be dismissed from the service system.

However, the human service and educational service sectors are changing. Children and families present complex, overlapping issues, and professionals have begun to recognize the need for interdisciplinary, collaborative planning and service delivery to meet their needs (Brandon & Knapp, 1999; Edwards & Smith, 1998; Forbes & Fitzsimons, 1993). Additionally, budgetary pressure, at the federal, state, and local levels, has mandated that the human service professions develop more efficient and effective service delivery systems. An additional influence has been the family advocacy movement, which has led to families demanding more timely and appropriate services for their children.

An understanding of the complexity of service delivery systems for children, particularly children with mental health needs, provides a background for examining the historical context for the development of a system of care, which is a seamless service delivery system that is family centered, interdisciplinary, collaborative, culturally competent, and community based, and that builds on the child's and family's strengths rather than focusing on only the problems.

Historical Background: The Development of a System of Care

Community Mental Health

Since the late 1800s, child guidance clinics have served children and families in the community. Child guidance clinics initially addressed the needs of children whose lives were severely impacted by poverty and/or mental retardation and focused on children who broke the law. Interventions were about punishment, not treatment. However, one of the major advances within the child guidance movement was a "shift from punishment to correction: we should fix troubled children, not further harm them" (Lourie, 2003, p. 2).

It was not until the 1930s that the child guidance movement began service delivery to middle- and upper-class children; at this point, it was acknowledged that in any socio-economic class children's behavior could get them into trouble. As a result of the work conducted during the child guidance movement, we began to understand that children's life circumstances and societal forces could impact their development and behavior. Although the child guidance clinics were community based, they evolved over time into a private practice model for the field of child mental health, thus isolating mental health care from other children's services (Lourie, 2003).

In the 1960s, a major shift in mental health service delivery occurred. The Community Mental Health Centers Construction Act of 1963 (P.L. 88-164) funded states and communities across the country to establish Community Mental Health Centers to meet the needs of the mentally ill (Lourie, 2003). However, because of limited funding and complicated reimbursement and payment systems, few centers provided services for children and their families with complex needs.

In 1972, thanks to child advocates, Congress passed an amendment to the Community Mental Health Act to provide funds for special children's programs. This legislation paved the way for a 1974 ruling that all federally funded Community Mental Health programs must include services for children and adolescents (P.L. 96-398). However, the mandate was insufficiently funded and consequently poorly implemented. In 1978, the President's Commission on Mental Health identified target populations that were underserved by community mental health centers, including children and adolescents with a severe emotional disturbance. Unfortunately, however, children's services remained underfunded. The President's Commission on Mental Health, under the Carter administration in 1980, put forth the Mental Health System Act (P.L. 96-398I), but because of the passage of the Omnibus Budget Reconciliation Act of 1981 (P.L. 79-35), under the Reagan administration, it was never funded. Federal monies for Community Mental Health were rescinded, and eventually, all direct funding for the mentally ill was replaced by federal block grants to states (Lourie, 2003).

However, with the initiation of the Child and Adolescent Service System Program (CASSP) in 1984 within the National Institutes of Mental Health, increased attention was given to define the need for a systematic approach to meeting the mental health needs of children and adolescents. Since CASSP was established, the focus of Community Mental Health legislation has continued to include children. The State Comprehensive Mental Health Services Plan Act (P.L. 99-660) in 1986 required states to build mental health services that are community based. In 1989, the law was amended. Community Mental Health Centers were mandated to establish programs for children and adolescents. However, these services continued to be delivered by individual agencies, with little coordination or cooperation among other community agencies. Consequently, the mental health and health care service delivery system for children and adolescents remained both fragmented and costly, leaving families to negotiate a complex care system in which they frequently get lost in the maze of fragmented services (Hodges, Nesman, & Hernandez, 1998; Lourie, 2003).

In summary, funding for mental health was originally state-supported with patients' mental health needs addressed in large state institutions, focused primarily on mentally ill adults and children who were mentally retarded. During the 1960s, funding for mental health care was federalized, as adults with mental illness and children with mental retardation were moved out of state hospitals and back to their communities to be served by community agencies. After the Omnibus Budget Reconciliation Act of 1981 was passed, mental health funding again became the responsibility of the states. Mental health services for children and adolescents remained inadequate, primarily because of a lack of funds to support children's programs.

System of Care

Under the leadership of First Lady Rosalynn Carter with her interest in mental health, the President's Commission on Mental Health was convened and published a report in 1978. Although this was a landmark report on mental health issues, the section on the needs of children was only an appendix to the final report. Not until years later, with the publication of *Unclaimed Children* by Jane Knitzer (1982) of the child advocacy organization the Children's Defense Fund, was attention given to the needs of children with serious emotional disturbances.

This report documented the terrible state of services for children in need of mental health services and created a cry of outrage from families and service providers, resulting in a new surge of child advocacy for children's mental health services (Lourie, 2003).

The report of the President's commission and the response to *Unclaimed Children* resulted in funding in 1984 that established the Child and Adolescent Service System Program in the National Institute of Mental Health. The goals were to assist states and communities to establish system of care programs for children with serious emotional problems. CASSP funded three research centers on children and adolescent mental health to study needed improvements in children's mental health care. These centers are the National Technical Assistance Center for Children's Mental Health at Georgetown University, the Research and Training Center for Children's Mental Health at the University of South Florida, and the Research and Training Center on Family Support and Children's Mental Health at Portland State University (Stroul, 1996).

All three universities have continued to serve as national centers for training and research based on a philosophy of care that incorporates the values and principles of a system of care based on core values and principles. Various groups who advocate for children's mental health care have lobbied for federal funding, which has provided grant monies to states across the country to establish system of care programs for children's mental health.

Advocacy organizations, whose members include families, professionals, and private citizens that have influenced federal and state legislation, include the American Mental Health Association, the Children's Defense Fund, the Federation of Families for Children's Mental Health, and the National Alliance for the Mentally Ill Child and Adolescent Network (Stroul, 1996). The latter two were established in the 1980s during the push for mental health services for children and adolescents. Both of these advocacy organizations devote their attention to children with emotional disturbances and their families and have become a respected public voice on behalf of children. Both organizations include a wide constituency of parents, professionals, and child advocates (Allen & Petr, 1998; Huffine & Anderson, 2003).

Over the years, since the Joint Commission on the Mental Health of Children report written in 1969, numerous efforts have been made to define how best to deliver mental health services to children. In the past, children were isolated from their families and were institutionalized. However, the coming together of professional knowledge and the family advocacy movement resulted in the development of the System of Care philosophy and the definition of appropriate service delivery through CASSP.

It was recognized that children with serious emotional disturbance and their families need more than a continuum of services operating in isolation. A continuum of care refers to services that could be appropriate for children at different points in time—from restrictive ones such as hospitalization to less restrictive ones that offer in-home or in-school interventions. However, it was recognized that these children also need a system of service that includes the continuum of care but also includes a way for the professionals in the service systems to interact with each other so that services are coordinated. Roles for family members are as important in caring for these children as are service providers and "normalized" connections with community services, such as those in recreational settings and religious organizations that families without children with special needs "normally" access. All of this should be within the context of the family's culture and individual needs. Recognition by professionals in the research centers, combined with the strong advocacy of family members for a support system to provide services so that their children with emotional and behavioral challenges could function successfully within the home, school, and community, led to the definition of a system of care for children with serious emotional disturbances. It is as follows:

> A comprehensive spectrum of mental health and other necessary services which are organized into a coordinated network to meet the multiple and changing needs of children and adolescents with severe emotional disturbances and their families (Stroul & Friedman, 1986, p. 3).

The Values and Principles of System of Care

The research efforts of the three universities that are centers for training and research on a philosophy of care that incorporates the values of system of care and other researchers across the country led to the development of a *philosophy* of care for children with serious emotional disturbances. Although service system configurations may differ between states or even among communities within states, CASSP defined a set of values and principles around which the service system should be organized in order to meet the needs of the children with complex needs who are served by multiple service systems. These values and principles were developed with input and participation of parents, service providers, administrators, policymakers, researchers, and advocates (Stroul, 1996).

Stroul and Friedman (1986) developed the system of care philosophy as a framework for the delivery of mental health services for children and adolescents with serious emotional disturbances and their families (Stroul, 1996; Stroul & Friedman, 1986). In 1992, the CASSP concepts became codified into law when Congress ratified the Comprehensive Community Mental Health Services for Children and Their Families Act (P.L. 102-321).

System of Care Values and Principles

Core Values

1. The System of Care should be *child centered and family focused*, with the needs of the child and family dictating the types and mix of services provided.
2. The System of Care should be *community based*, with the locus of services as well as the management and decision-making responsibility resting at the community level.
3. The System of Care should be *culturally competent*, with agencies, programs, and services that are responsive to cultural, racial, and ethnic differences of the populations they serve.

Guiding Principles

1. Children with emotional disturbances should have access to a comprehensive array of services that address the child's physical, emotional, and educational needs.

2. Children with emotional disturbances should receive individualized services in accordance with the unique needs and potentials of each child and should be guided by an individualized service plan.

3. Children with emotional disturbances should receive services within the least restrictive, most normative environment that is clinically appropriate.

4. The families and surrogate families of children with emotional disturbances should be full participants in all aspects of the planning and delivery of services.

5. Children with emotional disturbances should receive services that are integrated, with linkages between child-serving agencies and programs and mechanisms for planning, developing, and coordinating services.

6. Children with emotional disturbances should be provided with case management or similar mechanisms to ensure that multiple services are delivered in a coordinated and therapeutic manner and that children can move through the system of services in accordance with their changing needs.

7. The system of care should promote early identification and intervention for children with emotional disturbances in order to enhance the likelihood of positive outcomes.

8. Children with emotional disturbances should be ensured smooth transitions to the adult services system as they reach maturity.

9. The rights of children with emotional disturbances should be protected, and effective advocacy efforts for children and youth with emotional disturbances should be promoted.

10. Children with emotional disturbances should receive services without regard to race, religion, national origin, sex, physical disability, or other characteristics, and services should be sensitive and responsive to cultural differences and special needs.

What Do the Core Values Mean?

The first core value of System of Care, which is central to the paradigm shift from traditional service delivery to adopting the System of Care philosophical approach to working with families and children with serious emotional disturbances, is that the service system will be *child centered and family focused.* In traditional service delivery, families are offered choices from an array of pre-existing services, and the recipients are expected to conform to the expectations of the service system. In Mary's example, this would mean that she and her family would be expected to "fit" into an existing service most likely offered within an agency setting during "normal" work hours. If the family did not adhere to professionals' expectations, they would be considered difficult and nonconforming and would probably be dismissed from the agency because of noncompliance.

In a service system that adheres to the core value of child-centered and family-focused care, service providers and the family agree to the services and the setting that are most convenient. Implicit in this value is respect for the individual dignity of the child and family and the expectation that the child's needs will be met within the context of the family. In traditional mental health services, the child is often hospitalized for long periods of time or removed from the family and placed in an institutional setting. However, this core value includes the commitment to preserve the family unit, and this means determining how to meet the needs of the family as well as the child so that the integrity of the family is preserved (Stroul, 1996).

The second core value of System of Care service delivery is that services will be offered in the community and that decisions about the service array will be made in the community. As mentioned previously, historically, children with serious emotional disturbance have been removed from their homes and institutionalized. A core value of System of Care is a commitment to serve children within the community and to determine an array of services that provide for the child remaining in the home and having appropriate supports within the community to be successful living at home, participating in school, and living in the community. There is flexibility to the service array, the accessibility of the services, and the actual delivery of the services so that needs can be met within the local setting. For example, for Mary and her family, this could mean that instead of Mary being expected to receive therapeutic intervention in the therapist's office, the therapist would meet Mary at home, perhaps working with the family unit as a whole in the home setting.

The third core value of System of Care—cultural competence within the service system—has gained importance over time as the System of Care philosophy has been put into practice and there has been a deepened understanding of family-centered, community-based service delivery. Each family has its unique culture, traditions, practices, and beliefs. Also inherent in this are the influence of the ethnic group, the religious beliefs, the educational level, the economic status, and the life experiences of the family members. Culture, ethnicity, and personal beliefs about mental health and illness influence behavior that is considered appropriate for both the individual and family interactions. The cultural competence of the service system can influence how, where, and why services are accessed by a family and its receptivity to services. It is most important that service providers work within the community and the cultural influence of its citizens to determine appropriate policies and practices that are culturally sensitive and responsive to the unique needs of the population served (Stroul, 1996).

What About the Guiding Principles?

For each of the guiding principles of System of Care, key words warrant discussion (Pumariega & Winters, 2003).

1. *Comprehensive*: The service array should include services that are needed to meet the person's specific mental health needs/health needs/educational needs but that also should include other services that are supportive. For example, in Mary's situation, the family needs assistance with transportation in addition to appropriate therapeutic intervention for Mary.

2. *Individualized*: Rather than expecting the child and family to conform to a prescribed set of services, the service array is based on the individual needs and preferences of the child and family. Additionally, an important concept in individualization is recognizing the child's and family's strengths and using these as the basis for planning services. For example, Mary has a special friend with whom she felt safe enough to turn to when she was placed in out-of-home care. This unique relationship and Mary's capacity to have this relationship are among Mary's strengths and could be used to tailor her support services to meet her individual needs.

3. *Most normative environment*: All efforts should be made to support the child and family to live and receive services in the way that is most typical for a child of the same age. Children with special needs sometimes need hospitalization or special interventions that are intensive, and they may need much supervision; however, services should be designed so that the child and family function within the home, school, and community in a way that reflects what is normal for children and families within that community. Thus, Mary should remain in her home and should have the recommended therapy as a part of her normal life. The therapist can meet with her at home or conduct therapy sessions by playing games with Mary or taking her on outings that allow for time for discussion and interaction.

4. *Family participation*: "Nothing about us without us!" This adage that describes the way that families want to participate in planning and intervention is a core principle in this philosophical framework. As the plan of care is comprehensive, family centered, and child focused, it cannot be developed and implemented without full participation of the family and child, if developmentally appropriate. Families must be a part of the planning for services and participate fully in service delivery.

5. *Service integration*: Children and families have complex needs and interact with multiple service systems. It is imperative that the array of services provided is coordinated and integrated so that there are no conflicting expectations for the child and family and so that the services are interwoven and coordinated in a complementary fashion. In Mary's situation, this would mean that all of the professionals would meet together to coordinate the plans for Mary, exchange information about Mary's needs, and plan cooperatively with Mary and her family for the services that will be provided.

6. *Case management*: This describes the coordination role of a professional and/or parent on the team of professionals and support persons working with the child and family. In order to facilitate the coordination of services, one person needs to be in charge who can assess the changing needs of the child and family and make adjustments to the plans as necessary. As System of Care philosophy has developed over the years and the family voice has become stronger, many families have requested that the term "case management" be changed to "care coordination." Families do not like to be referred to as "cases." Instead, we can acknowledge that everyone needs care, sometimes from multiple sources. Thus, it is important that the care be coordinated!

7. *Early identification and early intervention*: Time is critical in the life of a child, and the sooner appropriate services are provided to address a child's needs, the less likely it is that the need will become pervasive and long term. Early intervention is a term that is used to address the needs of children with developmental disabilities during infancy and early childhood in order to prevent more complications over time. This same concept can apply to children with social/emotional needs or children identified with educational needs or learning differences. The sooner appropriate

intervention begins, the more likely the concern is to be addressed. In Mary's situation, it would have been best to recognize her learning difference early in her schooling and to provide tutorial support in order to avoid the likelihood of her failing a grade later.

8. *Smooth transitions*: We have created our service system by categories of disability and by ages. Children with learning differences and/or mental health/health problems need continuing services and supports, often throughout their lifetime. As a child ages from one service system to another, professionals and family members have a responsibility to plan for this so that there are no lapses in service delivery and needs are addressed continuously. For example, in Mary's situation, the teachers and mental health therapist need to be planning with Mary and her mother on her transition from middle to high school so that her support system goes with her from one setting to the other.

9. *Protection of individual rights and advocacy*: Over time, through statutory actions, children have been provided services and protection. The individual right to an education, no matter the individual's learning differences or health needs, and the right to live in a safe environment are examples of children's rights. Service systems should also advocate meeting children's needs through individual advocacy or case advocacy or class advocacy (advocacy for a group of children with similar needs). Just as parents have the right to advocate for their children, professionals have the right and the duty to advocate for the children in their service to ensure that they are served optimally.

10. *Nondiscrimination*: Children have the right to services without regard to their race, economic status, disability, religious beliefs, and so forth. Services should be provided to all children and families. As we work to be culturally competent in our service delivery, we must become more informed about cultural differences and, most importantly, have interpreters available to facilitate communication between service providers and family members.

Putting System of Care into Practice

We have seen from our example of Mary that a child and family can be involved with multiple service systems at the same time. Also, we have explored the development of a System of Care philosophical approach to meet the needs of children and families with complex needs through a service system that is family centered, community based, and culturally competent, and that includes individualized, strength-based service delivery. How has this service system been put into practice?

An interdisciplinary/interagency service system is termed "Wraparound Service Delivery," and it incorporates the values and principles of the system of care philosophy. First used by Dr. Lenore Behar, a leader in North Carolina and the nation in children's mental health, the term "wraparound" describes the process of surrounding a child and family with services and supports that provide coordinated care to meet the individual needs of the child and family and to provide the opportunity for the child to be successful at home, at school, and in the community.

Wraparound

The Evolution of the Wraparound Process

The wraparound process has evolved over the last 40 years—starting first in Canada in the 1960s and then being used during the 1970s in Chicago in a program called Kaleidoscope. Kaleidoscope was established by Karl Dennis, who based his program on the philosophical framework similar to System of Care. He later expanded wraparound to include in-home family support services, therapeutic foster care, and other community support services. He found that these interventions prevented out-of-home placements (VanDenBerg, 1999).

In the 1980s, Alaska developed the "Alaska Youth Initiative" using the wraparound process (VanDenBerg & Grealish, 1996). Alaskan mental health authorities concluded that this effort was highly successful, as indicated by the number of children successfully treated in their communities after returning to Alaska from residential institutions outside of the state. Vermont initiated a community-based project in a small town of 10,000, and the program was so successful that later it was expanded statewide. Funding for the statewide program combined state, federal, and local monies and a grant from the Robert Wood Johnson Foundation (Clarke, Schaefer, Burchard, & Welkowitz, 1992; Yoe et al., 1996). In the 1990s, a System of Care project was developed in Pitt, Edgecombe, and Nash counties in North Carolina and was funded as one of the System of Care demonstration grants by the Center for Mental Health Services. As a collaborative effort by the State Department of Mental Health, Developmental Disabilities, and Substance Abuse and East Carolina University, this became the prototype for the development of System of Care programs throughout North Carolina. These services were implemented as an alternative to institutionalization of youth, as part of the settlement of the "Willie M. lawsuit," which stipulated that the state had to provide individualized, community-based services for severely mentally ill children who were also violent (VanDenBerg, 1999).

The most recent legislation to affect System of Care was the federal Olmstead decision (2001), which supported the rights of children to community-based services instead of institutionalization because of a lack of available community-based resources. In response, states across the nation have developed plans using the wraparound process as the "cornerstone of their compliance" (VanDenBerg, Bruns, & Burchard, 2003, p. 7). The wraparound process calls for flexible and comprehensive community-based services to help children stay in their communities and remain out of more restrictive residential institutions.

By 1995, the number of sites using variations of the wraparound process had grown rapidly. The Center for Mental Health Services had funded 31 demonstration grants across the country (VanDenBerg, 1999). The implementation of System of Care programs for children and families with complex health care and mental health needs has grown nationwide. Outcome data retrieved from 22 sites has pointed to the effectiveness of wraparound as a framework for implementing System of Care to achieve an improved mental health delivery system for children and families with complex needs (Center for Mental Health Services, 1999). (For further discussion on outcome data, see Chapter 15.)

A Paradigm Shift from Individually Centered Care to Family-Centered Care
Core Values: Families, Ethnicity, and Culture

Family-Centered Care

Implementing System of Care into the delivery of services using wraparound services is a philosophy to guide policies and practices. Wraparound demands flexibility in order to adapt services to the unique needs of each family and community. The Executive Committee of the National Resource Network for Child and Family Mental Health Services (1999), who compiled the findings from 22 of the 1997 Center for Mental Health Services System of Care grantees, concluded that families must be involved in the beginning of the development of a System of Care program and that they should serve on many system levels. Family members can play key roles as trainers, data collectors, advocates, and service providers. The numerous wraparound programs across the country have developed uniquely to meet the needs and build on the resources of individual communities, and all attest to the need for family involvement in order to provide culturally competent family-centered care.

Freud, along with the rapid development of medical and pharmaceutical technologies, greatly influenced mental health care in the 20th century. The focus was on the pathology of the individual or family system rather than on individual or family strengths. Consequently, families were frequently blamed for their loved one's illness or were not considered at all in the therapeutic regime. There was even a time when families of emotionally disturbed children were "the pariahs of their communities" (Huffine & Anderson, 2003, p. 35). The application of systems theory to understanding family dynamics has contributed to changing the focus to families as partners, or "family-centered care." CASSP further fostered the involvement of families' participation in all areas of service planning and delivery (Allen & Petr, 1998). As early as 1977, the Surgeon General called for the establishment of a national agenda to develop a coordinated system of care for children that was family centered and community based. Today, viewing the family as the client and involving family members in the care of their physically or mentally ill children or adults are considered best practice (Allen & Petr).

In their review of the literature across health care disciplines, Allen and Petr (1998) defined family-centered service delivery as the recognition of "the centrality of the family in the lives of individuals. It is guided by fully informed choices made by the family and focused on the family's strength and capabilities" (p. 9). The key System of Care elements of family-centered care are (1) the family as the unit of care, (2) informed family choice, and (3) a focus on strengths. Hopefully, this approach will reverse the tradition of blaming parents and disempowering families. Developing health care delivery systems based on System of Care principles for all vulnerable populations is the challenge for health care professionals of the future.

Cultural Competence

In order to truly incorporate family-centered care into the service delivery model, cultural competence must be central. Each family brings its own personal culture, traditions, and beliefs, with the broader framework of the family's ethnic origin, religious practices, and geographic origin.

The population of the United States is a mix of people from different cultures, races, and ethnic groups, and this mix continues to change rapidly. This trend of increased diversity is predicted to continue throughout the century. Effective service delivery requires that health care providers recognize these changes and respond to the cultural complexity and rich diversity of Americans. Health care agencies and schools must recruit and retain health care providers and teachers from culturally diverse groups to serve more ethnic and culturally diverse clientele (Spector, 2004). The education, health care, and mental health care systems must respond to demographic changes by developing culturally competent policies and practices.

Definitions

- *Culture* is the sum total of socially inherited characteristics of a human group.
- *Ethnicity* pertains to a social group within a cultural and social system—a group of people who share common and distinctive racial, national, religious, linguistic, and/or cultural heritage.
- *Cultural competence* is the ability of educators, service providers, health care providers, and organizations to understand and respond effectively to the unique cultural and linguistic needs of various populations who are not part of the American mainstream. Cultural competence implies that the provider understands and is in tune with the total context of the client, family, and their situation (adapted from Isaacs-Shockley, Cross, Bazron, Dennis, & Benjamin, 1996; Spector, 2004, pp. 5, 11).

Ethnicity and Culture

Cultural and ethnic differences, which result from influences of the past, including history, religion, and family traditions, affect the structure and functioning of a family. For example it is generally accepted that historically, African Americans tend to have a matriarchal structure in which the mother or maternal grandmother is the head of the household, and involving the mother in decision making is vitally important. In contrast, Hispanic families tend to be patriarchal, and thus, involving the father or the paternal grandfather is necessary. Societal developments have also changed the family structure and functioning in mainstream America. Variability among family structures will most likely continue to change during the next millennium. The white middle-class family of four with mother as the homemaker and dad working as the breadwinner is the traditional family structure of the past, but it is not the structure today. Understanding family structures paves the way to cultural competence.

Cultural Competence Model: A Definition

As noted in Table 1-1, cultural competence is "a set of congruent behaviors, attitudes, and policies that are found in a system, agency, or group of professionals that enables them to work effectively in a context of cultural differences" (Pumariega, 2003, pp. 87–88).

Barriers to Cultural Competence

The ways in which educators and health care providers relate to family members depend on their understanding of the needs of the family within the context of the family's culture, ethnicity, structure, and functioning, as well as the family's support systems within the community and the community's values. Unfortunately, a number of barriers to mental health care exist for populations who are not in the American mainstream. These barriers to culturally appropriate mental health care include a lack of minority practitioners, a lack of culturally competent services, and a lack of knowledge and skills among health care providers (Pumariega, 2003; Spector, 2000).

Many health care programs and services have not addressed the barriers as listed in Table 1-2 that inhibit access to health care because of cultural differences and thus are unresponsive to cultural, racial, and ethnic differences. Consequently, families have become disappointed, frustrated, and angry at the lack of sensitivity to their values and beliefs. In order to provide family-centered care, health care providers must be culturally sensitive, and system of care agencies must educate and support staff to become culturally competent (Stroul, 1996).

The Road Map to Cultural Competence

The development of cultural competence involves an ongoing process that requires patience and flexibility. The professional must be open to change. Achieving cultural competence should be a goal for agencies as well as service providers. The first step on the road is self-

Table 1-1	Qualities of Cultural Competence and a Culturally Competent Agency

Culturally competent professionals exhibit the following qualities:
- An awareness and acceptance of cultural differences
- The ability to articulate information about their own culture and biases
- An understanding of the dynamics of working across cultures
- An acquired knowledge about the cultures residing in their own community
- The ability to adapt practice skills to fit the cultural needs of the client
- Advocacy on behalf of children and families from various cultural origins

A culturally competent agency or organization should
- Value and adapt to the cultural diversity and the needs of the community
- Conduct an ongoing self-assessment of cultural attitudes, values, professional skills, and abilities to meet the needs of consumers
- Develop services that are culturally appropriate
- Mandate culturally competent practices and policies
- Understand and manage the dynamics of cultural differences
- Institutionalize cultural knowledge through training and experience with cultural encounters
- Provide linguistic support
- Redesign services to better accommodate the needs of diverse groups of clients and families
- Work with natural and informal support systems within the ethnic community, such as churches, spiritual healers, and community leaders
- Use paraprofessionals and others from the ethnic community as consultants and as staff
- Analyze data from information systems to plan and develop new services that are culturally appropriate and to improve existing services

Adapted from Benjamin and Isaacs-Shockley (1996) and Pumariega (2003).

awareness. Understanding one's heritage is important in order to identify one's own values, including biases. Knowledge of the demographics of the local community will assist in understanding the needs of the community (Campinha-Bacote, 1997). Understanding one's

Table 1-2	Barriers to Cultural Competence

- A lack of self-awareness
- Ethnocentrism, which is the belief that one's own culture, belief system, or life style is superior to others
- Racism and other *isms*, such as sexism, classism, ageism
- Prejudice, that is, negative expectations based on judgments that are a result of a lack of knowledge or understanding of a person's heritage
- Discrimination that occurs when a person's rights are denied because of prejudice
- Stereotyping, which is making generalizations by comparing an individual to a group of people with similar characteristics, or assuming that all individuals from a particular group are alike
- Negative bias, for example, ignoring strengths
- Cultural blindness—the belief that culture does not matter
- A lack of motivation to become culturally competent
- Resistance to change because of too many demands and time constraints
- No funds to train or educate staff
- Insufficient leadership or leadership that is culturally unaware
- A lack of political support
- Xenophobia, which is a morbid fear of strangers or foreigners

Adapted from Kavanagh (1999); Isaacs-Shockley, Cross, Bazron, Dennis, and Benjamin (1996); and Spector (2000, 2004).

own beliefs about education/health/illness before working with a family helps to provide culturally competent care. In order to develop appropriate treatment and intervention plans that the family will agree and adhere to, the service provider must understand the family's perceptions of health and wellness and then identify the treatments that are a good match with their cultural traditions (Isaacs-Shockley et al., 1996; Spector, 2004). Taking advantage of opportunities to participate with people from other cultures will enhance the service provider's cultural sensitivity (Campinha-Bacote, 1997). Integrating knowledge about various cultures leads to becoming a culturally competent professional.

As the United States becomes more culturally diverse, it is critically important for educators, service providers, and health care professionals to pursue cultural competence in order to provide culturally competent care and to develop Systems of Care that honor the family's beliefs, values, and traditions. We must build a service system that is "available, accessible, affordable, acceptable, appropriate and adaptable" (Campinha-Bacote, 1997, p. 87) to meet the needs of all people requiring health care and social services.

Summary

We have learned through the influence of the family advocacy movement, the lessons gleaned from national and state efforts to provide coordinated services for children and families with complex needs, and the movement from the traditional medical model of service delivery to one that is family centered and culturally competent requires a response and support system that acknowledges persons' unique strengths and preferences, their unique characteristics and issues, and their unique capacity to receive services within the context of the community. Children and families whose needs are met within an educational and service system that respects and supports these values and principles can be successful living in the community, can be successful living within their homes, and can be successful at school.

Activities to Extend Your Learning

Family-Centered Service Delivery

■ Investigate whether your community has adopted family-centered, culturally competent, community-based services as the framework for your Department of Mental Health or your Department of Social Services. Develop a list of questions that determines whether the services meet these criteria. Call the department and request an appointment with the director or assistant director and interview the person to make your determination.

Cultural Competence

■ Read the *National Standards for Culturally and Linguistically Appropriate Services in Health care: Final Report* (2001) (gpacheco@ osophs,dhhs.gov).

The Road to Cultural Competence

The following steps may be taken to embark on the road to cultural competence.

1. Self-awareness: Examine your own cultural background and your history, ritual, and traditions.

2. Cultural awareness: Examine the demographic changes that are occurring in the United States. Identify the populations that your agency is serving. Conduct an agency assessment of the mechanisms that are in place to meet the needs of diverse populations. Examine the board of directors, the staff, and the volunteers. Do ethnic and cultural backgrounds reflect the clientele that the agency serves? Conduct a community assessment. Do minorities in your community have appropriate access to health and mental health care resources?

3. Acquire cultural knowledge. Read about the cultures that you are serving. Ask questions and listen to people talk about their beliefs, values, traditions, and likes and dislikes related to their cultural backgrounds. What are their beliefs about health, mental health/illness, and mental illness? Learn as much as you can about the cultures of the people whom you serve.

4. Cultural encounters include taking advantage of opportunities to participate socially with people from other cultures and travel to other countries, eating their foods, and participating in their rituals and traditions.

5. Cultural skills include the application of cultural knowledge to the skills used to care for clients and families and the ability to design and implement individual care plans for care that meet the needs of clients and family's values and beliefs (adapted from Boyd, 1999; Campinha-Bacote, 1997; Benjamin & Isaacs-Shockley, 1996; Isaacs-Shockley et al., 1996; Spector, 2000, 2004).

Suggested Reading

Fadiman, A. (1997). *The spirit catches you and you fall down.* New York: Farrar, Straus, Giroux.

National Data Analysis System. Child Welfare League of America [webpage]. Washington, DC: Child Welfare League of America, 2003. Available at http://ndas.cwla.org. Accessed September 11, 2004.

National Standards for Culturally and Linguistically Appropriate Services in Health Care: Final Report. (2001, March). Washington, DC: Office of Minority Health, Office of Public Health and Science, and Rockville, MD: U.S. Department of Health and Human Services.

U.S. Department of Health and Human Services. (1999). *Mental health: A report of the surgeon general.* Rockville, MD: U.S. Department of Health and Human Services, Substance Abuse and Mental Health Services Administration, Center for Mental Services, National Institutes of Health, National Institutes of Mental Health.

References

Allen, R.I., & Petr, C.G. (1998). Re-thinking family-centered practice. *The American Journal of Orthopsychiatry, 68,* 4–15.

Benjamin, M.P., & Isaacs-Shockley, M. (1996). Culturally competent service approaches. In B. Stroul (Ed.), *Children's mental health: Creating systems of care in a changing society* (pp. 475–491). Baltimore: Paul H. Brookes Publishing Co.

Boyd, M.A. (1999). Cultural issues related to mental health care. In M.A. Boyd & M.A. Nihart (Eds.), *Psychiatric nursing: contemporary practice.* Philadelphia: Lippincott.

Brandon, R.N., & Knapp, M.S. (1999). Interprofessional education and training: Transforming professional preparation to transform human services. *The American Behavioral Scientist, 42,* 876–891.

Campinha-Bacote, J. (1997). Understanding the influence of culture. In J. Haber, B. Kranovice-Miller, J.L. McMahon, & P. Price Hoskins (Eds.), *Comprehensive psychiatric nursing* (5th ed., pp. 76–90), St. Louis: C.V. Mosby.

Center for Mental Health Services, U.S. Department of Health and Human Services. Executive Summary. (1999). *Systems of care, promising practices in children's mental health:* 1998 series, Vol. VII, pp. 9–16.

Clarke, R.T., Schaefer, M., Burchard. J.D., & Welkowitz, J.W. (1992). Wrapping community-based mental health services around children with a severe behavioral disorder: An evaluation of a project wraparound. *Journal of Child and Family Studies, 1*(3), 241–261.

Edwards, J., & Smith, P. (1998). Impact of interdisciplinary education in underserved areas: Health professions collaboration in Tennessee. *Journal of Professional Nursing, 14*(3), 144–149.

Forbes, E.J., & Fitzsimons, V. (1993). Education: The key for holistic interdisciplinary collaboration. *Holistic Nursing Practice, 7*(4), 1–10.

Hodges, S., Nesman, T., & Hernandez, M. (1998). Promising practices: Building collaboration of systems of care. *Systems of care: Promising practices in children's mental health* (1998 series, Vol. VI). Washington, DC: Center for Effective Collaboration and Practice, American Institutes for Research.

Huffine, C., & Anderson, D. (2003). Family advocacy development in systems of care. In A.J. Pumariega & N.C. Winters (Eds.), *The handbook of child and adolescent systems of care: The new community psychiatry* (pp. 35–64). San Francisco: Jossey-Bass.

Isaacs-Shockley, M., Cross, T., Bazron, B.J., Dennis, K., & Benjamin, M.P. (1996). Framework for a culturally competent system of care. In Stroul's (Ed.), *Children's Mental Health. Creating System of Care in a changing society.* (pp. 23–39). Baltimore: Paul H. Brookes Publishing Co.

Kavanagh, K.H. (1999). Transcultural perspectives in mental health. In M.M. Andrews and J.S. Boyle, *Transcultural concepts in nursing care.* (3rd ed, pp. 223–261). Philadelphia: Lippincott.

Knitzer, J. (1982). *Unclaimed children: The failure of public responsibility to children and adolescents in need of mental health services.* Washington, DC: Children's Defense Fund.

Lourie, I.S. (2003). A history of community child mental health. In A.J. Pumariega & N.C. Winters (Eds.), *The handbook of child and adolescent system of care: The new community psychiatry* (pp. 1–16). San Francisco: Jossey-Bass.

National Resource Network for Child and Family Mental Health, *Executive Committee Report.* Washington, DC: 1999.

Pumariega, A.J. (2003). Cultural competence in systems of care for children's mental health. In A.J. Pumariega & N.C. Winters (Eds.), *The handbook of child and adolescent systems of care: The new community psychiatry* (pp. 82–104). San Francisco: Jossey-Bass.

Pumariega, A.J., & Winters, N.C. (Eds.) (2003). *The handbook of child and adolescent systems of care: The new community psychiatry* (pp. 20–25). San Francisco: Jossey-Bass.

Spector, R.E. (2000). *Cultural diversity in health and illness.* (5th ed). Upper Saddle River, NJ: Prentice Hall.

Spector, R.E. (2004). Cultural heritage and history. *Cultural diversity in health and illness* (6th ed). Upper Saddle River, NJ: Prentice Hall.

Stroul, B.A. (1996). *Children's mental health. Creating systems of care in a changing society.* Baltimore: Paul H. Brookes Publishing Co.

Stroul, B.A., & Friedman R.M. (1986). *A system of care for children and youth with severe emotional disturbances* (rev. ed). Washington, DC: Georgetown University Child Development Center, National Technical Assistance Center for Children's Mental Health.

U.S. Department of Justice. Office of Juvenile Justice and Delinquency Prevention. Statistical Briefing Book [webpage]. Washington, DC: OJJDP, 2001. Available at http://www.ojjdp.ncjrs.org/ojstatbb/cirp/. Accessed September 11, 2004.

VanDenBerg, J.E. (1999). History of the wraparound process. In B.J. Burns & S.K. Goldman (Eds.), Promising practices in wraparound for children with serious emotional disturbance and their families. *Systems of care: Promising practices in children's mental health* (1998 Series, Vol. IV, pp. 19–26). Washington, DC: Center for Effective Collaboration and Practice, American Institutes for Research.

VanDenBerg, J.E., Bruns, E., & Burchard, J. (2003). History of the wrap-around process. *Focal point: Quality and fidelity of wraparound* (Vol. 17, pp. 4–7). Portland, OR: Research and Training Center on Family Support and Children's Mental Health.

VanDenBerg, J.E., & Grealish, E.M. (1996). Individualized services and sup-ports through the wraparound process. Philosophy and procedures. *Journal of Child & Family Studies, 5*(1) 7–21.

Yoe, J.T., Santarcangelo, S., Atkins, M., & Burchard, J.D. (1996). Wraparound care in Vermont: Program development, implementation, and evaluation of a statewide system of individualized services. *Journal of Child and Family Studies, 5*(1), 23–39.

Chapter 2

Building Collaborative Relationships: A Paradigm Shift to Family-Centered, Interprofessional Partnerships

CHARLOTTE A. HERRICK

Relationships are the glue that holds a team together.

(Maxwell, 2003, p. 1)

Relationships are built on respect, shared experiences, trust, reciprocity and mutual enjoyments with the desire to place value on other people.

(Maxwell, 2003)

People don't care how much you know until they know how much you care.

(Maxwell, 2003, p. 7)

Objectives

- Compare the characteristics of collaborative interdisciplinary teams with the characteristics of multidisciplinary teams.
- List the benefits, challenges, and barriers to building collaborative relationships.
- Describe the characteristics of high-performing collaborative teams.
- Identify the skills needed for team membership on the part of families and professionals.
- Define wraparound.
- Identify the core elements of wraparound.
- Discuss lessons learned in the development of System of Care programs.
- Describe what you see in the future for children's mental health and health care and how you can fit into the future health care delivery system.

An interdisciplinary collaborative practice has evolved as a paradigm from client-centered professional/client relationships to family-centered professional partnerships. As health care systems have become more complex and care has becomes more fragmented, there is a greater need for families to participate actively in a child's or adult's health and mental health care. Systems of Care have been developed to improve care across the health care continuum.

Nationally, there has been a concern that the complex health care needs of children with severe emotional disturbances (SEDs) and their families, as well as clients with complex social, educational, health, and mental health care concerns, have not been adequately addressed. Collective action is needed to address the complex health and mental health needs of all people and their families. A growing awareness exists among health care professionals that no one discipline, no single approach, and no one specific intervention can provide the comprehensive services that are needed to promote the recovery of children who are suffering from serious emotional disturbances. One system of health or mental health care cannot meet the overwhelming needs of families. Chenven and Brady (2003) aptly stated, "Helping troubled youth not only takes a village, but it takes an exceptional village, one that works together focused on the goal of helping its children and families achieve their optimal potential" (p. 66). The same can be said regarding other people with multiple needs for social, educational, health, and mental health care who have chronic conditions and their families with complex needs, including the fragile older population.

Today, families are experiencing extraordinary changes because of the impact of social, demographic, and economic influences, leading to family instability. Our society must provide opportunities for families to promote their children's health and welfare, as well as their own (Allen & Petr, 1998).

The purpose of developing system of care was to acquire a seamless mental health delivery system that is interdisciplinary, family centered, culturally competent, and community based and that uses a comprehensive approach to improve the quality of mental health care for children suffering from serious emotional disturbances. System of Care is applicable, as a conceptual framework, to care for other populations with multiple needs. System of Care addresses the challenges recommended by the Institute of Medicine in their *Quality Chasm Report*, which includes the need to (1) redesign the health care system to improve the quality of care, (2) promote the coordination of care, (3) require collaborative relationships among health care professionals by changing the way that they are educated, (4) involve patients in shared decision making with providers, and (5) be more attentive to patient's values, preferences, and cultural backgrounds (Greiner & Knebel, 2003). System of Care is a paradigm that represents a shift from individually centered care delivered by a professional in the context of a patient/professional relationship to family-centered care within the context of a collaborative interdisciplinary partnership. By building a network of collaborative partnerships in the community, the client and family have a safety net when they face a health or mental health crisis. People with chronic health conditions may experience long periods of remission, but they most certainly will face crises from time to time.

Benefits and barriers exist to building interagency and interprofessional/interfamily relationships. The benefits to team members, including the child or client, family, and health care provider, outweigh the barriers. Building partnerships provides opportunities to improve the health care delivery system. Participating on an interdisciplinary team of family members and professionals fosters creativity, which enhances everyone's self-esteem—clients, family members, and professionals. Overcoming the barriers by educating the next generation of professionals and teaching those who are already service providers are some of the challenges that must be addressed to provide quality care to people with complex needs. A paradigm shift, changing the way of thinking about the delivery of health care and educational and social services, will be difficult for those who do not want to move out of their comfort zone. The challenge of building an effective team and overcoming the barriers will excite others. Building collaborative partnerships among professionals and families may be a daunting task— but worth the effort.

The Evolution of Collaborative Interdisciplinary Relationships in Health and Mental Health Care

Family Members as Collaborative Partners

The evolution of family involvement in their children's care, both in health care and mental health, progressed slowly. It started with the family therapy movement in the 1960s and 1970s, when families and psychotherapists recognized the importance of the family in the recovery of their loved one. Until then, health care delivery systems were patriarchal. Families were blamed and ignored (Allen & Petr, 1998). During the 1980s and 1990s families found their voices. They participated with professionals in advocacy groups, such as the National Alliance for the Mentally Ill and the Federation for Families. Professionals and family members joined forces to advocate for parity of mental health care with health care to obtain quality mental health care. Through their efforts, federal legislation provided the means to develop System of Care programs across the country to care for children who suffered from a serious emotional disturbance.

By the 1990s, System of Care programs developed across the nation as a collaborative approach for offering family-centered care (Simpson, Koroloff, Friesen, & Gac, 1999; Stroul, 1996; Stroul, 2003). Family–provider collaboration is defined as a team in which all members have "special skills and knowledge that can contribute to the job of improving programs and services which will benefit the child" (cited in Osher, deFur, Nava, Spencer, & Toth-Dennis, 1999, p. 15). Family members have served as collaborators, as well as mentors, advocates, System of Care program facilitators, respite care coordinators, researchers, and faculty co-teachers (Herrick, Arbuckle, & Claes, 2002; Huffine & Anderson, 2003). Family members have collaborated in all aspects of program development, implementation, and evaluation (Osher et al., 1999).

Professionals as Collaborative Partners

Mental health providers, psychiatrists, psychologists, socials workers, nurses, and others have traditionally worked collaboratively within the medical and mental health service systems to serve the mental health needs of children. The blurring of roles started when community mental health centers were established during the 1960s. However, family members were not included. Boundaries were not crossed, and thus, no relationships existed with other agencies across the service care continuum, such as child welfare, education, and juvenile justice. The multidisciplinary team approach has been a model for providing psychiatric services in acute care settings but failed to include families and professionals from other agencies. According to Chenven and Brady (2003), collaborative efforts "routinely failed to integrate the mental health system fully with other child-serving agencies" (p. 66).

Collaborative Partnerships and Interdisciplinary Teams

The term *multidisciplinary team* is often used synonymously with interdisciplinary team. However, it is important to distinguish between the two. The following definitions provide a comparison between a traditional multidisciplinary team and an interdisciplinary team. System of Care experts believe that an interdisciplinary team is essential for providing services to children with a serious emotional disturbance.

- A *team* includes a group of two or more people who share a sense of purpose. Interactions with each other enable team members to accomplish more than each alone would be able to accomplish (Bronstein, 2003; Platt, 1994). Bronstein insisted that effective team relationships must be reciprocal with clear avenues for communication.
- A *multidisciplinary team* is made up of people from different disciplines who work with clients independently and share with each other information about the client and their work with him or her.
- An *interdisciplinary team* requires a deeper level of collaboration so that the "processes are done jointly." Professionals of different disciplines and families share their knowledge and resources in an "interdependent manner" (Sorrells-Jones, 1997, p. 26). By functioning interdependently, "synergistic solutions" are found (Gage, 1998). These solutions tend to be of higher quality than those made independently.
- *Interdependence* means that team members depend on each other to reach an agreed-upon goal and to complete a task. Interactions include formal and informal communication and the ability to convey respect about a colleague's opinions and input about how to reach identified goals (Bronstein, 2003).

The following definitions clarify concepts regarding building collaborative partnerships.

Definitions of Collaboration

- Interdisciplinary collaboration means members of different disciplines contribute toward a common goal (Bronstein, 2003).
- Collaboration is a process whereby individuals work together to achieve a common goal. They share power, information, and resources; participate in joint decision making; and take collective responsibility for decisions and the outcomes. Collaboration requires incentives that will ensure that people will work together collaboratively, for example, administrative support, time, and pay for the time necessary to collaborate (DeChillo, Koren, & Mezera, 1996; Grossman & Bautista, 2002; Huber, 1996; Liedka & Whitten, 1997, cited in Koenig, 2001; Simpson et al., 1999).
- "Collaborative case management teams can provide higher quality solutions than any one individual working alone or in traditional multidisciplinary relationships" (Koenig, 2001, p. 74).
- The term *professionals* refers to people who have had specific training in one of the disciplines that contributes to the delivery of health, mental health, or other services (Simpson et al., 1999).
- A family member is the person who has ongoing responsibilities for a child or client. This person may include biological or foster parents, aunts, uncles, grandparents, siblings, or other members of the extended family who have a substantial commitment to care for the child or the client (Simpson et al., 1999).
- A partnership is described by DeChillo et al. (1996) as the family/professional relationship, which is collaborative. Collaboration, reciprocity, and equality are the distinguishing features of a partnership.

  Family–provider collaboration is the collaborative process in which participants of the interdisciplinary team, including family members, professionals, and other stakeholders, work together to improve services for clients, children, and their families (Hodges, Nesman, & Hernandez, 1999; Simpson et al., 1999). All team members, including family members, are treated as equals.
- Empowerment is the process of providing the means, including the proper tools, resources, and environments, to develop an individual's and/or a group's abilities to set and reach goals effectively (Hawks, 1992). Blanchard, Carlos, and Randolph (1996) stated that "empowerment means you have freedom to act; it also

means you are accountable for results" (p. 90). The collaborative relationship enhances the strengths of the team members, empowering them to act on behalf of others, as well as advocating for themselves.

Hodges et al. (1999) distinguished collaboration in the System of Care conceptual framework from previously established coalitions or partnerships. They claimed that earlier partnerships were temporary entities to solve a problem. However, collaboration in System of Care requires a more permanent, long-term commitment to join forces, to pool information, and "to share risks, resources, responsibilities and rewards" (p. 24). System of Care collaborative partnerships include "an interdependent system with formal roles and responsibilities" (Hodges et al., 1999, p. 24). Formerly, interagency coalitions or partnerships worked together to provide services while maintaining a separate identity. Agency structures and agendas remained the same, without changing the usual way of providing services. In the System of Care paradigm, an interagency collaboration means that the usual way of doing business is altered to meet collaborative responsibilities. Organizations must be empowered to alter their practices to meet collaborative goals.

Organizational empowerment consists of the following essential elements described by Tebbitt (1993):

1. Cultural changes occur in an organization.
2. Values are redefined, and those that still hold true are reaffirmed.
3. A paradigm shift occurs when beliefs are challenged and some are altered.
4. There is a commitment to employees and the clients that they serve.
5. Systems are redesigned to better meet the needs of all stakeholders.

Empowered teams, supported by agency leaders, will provide better care because of their ability to function at a higher level. Platt (1994) claimed that professionals cannot address the complexity of today's health care problems in isolation: "He or she needs to be working in partnership with other workers in and from the community, as well as with the client and his or her family" (p. 7). Individuals and agencies must be empowered to redesign organizations in order to build bridges across boundaries.

High Performing Teams

Collaborative partnerships are essentially high-performing interdisciplinary teams. Blanchard, Carew, and Parisi-Carew (2000) described (Table 2-1) the "characteristics of high perform-

---

Table 2-1   **The Characteristics of a High-Performing Team**

P = purpose and values shared
E = empowerment
R = relationships and communication
F = flexibility
O = optimal performance
R = recognition and appreciation
M = morale

Purpose and values: There is a commitment to common values, a vision, and a common purpose to strive for identified goals. The strategies and individual roles and responsibilities to achieve the agreed-upon goals are clear.

Empowerment: Initiative, involvement, and creativity are fostered. Problem-solving skills are enhanced. The team is supportive and committed to each other and to the continuing growth and development of its members.

Relationships and communication: All ideas, opinions, and feelings are listened to without judgment. Ground rules exist for managing conflict. Cultural differences are valued and respected. Honest and caring feedback is provided. Individual strengths are recognized, and weaknesses are reframed as strengths. Relationships are reciprocal, with give and take. Communication is two-way, open, and honest.

Flexibility: Team members share responsibility for successes and failures. Mistakes are seen as opportunities. Members are open and adaptable to change and are able to compromise to meet team goals.

Optimal performance: There is a commitment to high standards. Consequently, the chances for success are enhanced.

Recognition and appreciation: Each member's contributions are valued and accomplishments are celebrated, as are successes.

Morale: Hard work and fun are valued, and thus, there is satisfaction, pride, and enthusiasm for the work done, which leads to a sense of team spirit.

Adapted from Blanchard et al. (2000, pp. 12–13).

Table 2-2	Other Characteristics of High-Performing Teams

- There are newly created activities.
- There is a blurring of roles.
- Role equality—no hierarchy. Roles are determined by training and expertise, the needs of the organization, the situation, team members, the needs of the client, and family, and the professionals.
- Personal goals are set aside in order to reach the goals of the group.
- Roles are assigned according to a good match of talents and skills with the needs of the system, organization, or the need for specific services.
- A good balance exists between task accomplishments and group cohesion.

Adapted from the System of Care literature: Bronstein (2003); DeChillo et al. (1996); and Grossman and Bautista (2002).

ing teams" (p. 11). A brief explanation of each of these characteristics provides guidelines for the development of effective collaborative relationships.

The System of Care literature also provided guidelines (Table 2-2) that characterize the effective team.

Personal skills (Table 2-3) need to be developed in order to be an effective team member. Training programs that improve collaboration skills are recommended for all team members. It is essential that each team participant conveys respect and communicates clearly to each other that everyone's efforts are valued. Previously in this chapter, Maxwell (2003) was quoted as follows: "People don't care how much you know until they know how much you care" (p. 7).

The Benefits, Challenges, and Barriers to Developing Collaborative Relationships

Collaborative relationships among various disciplines from different agencies, with family members' participation, produce undeniable benefits to children and families. Benefits or positive outcomes for children and their families were identified by an outcome study conducted by a System of Care program in Guilford County, North Carolina, which included the following (Rogers, 2001):

Table 2-3   **Personal Characteristics of Team Members**

The team member must
- Have good interpersonal skills, including communication and listening skills
- Be flexible and willing to compromise
- Have a commitment to the overall good of the group
- Be able to provide emotional support to others
- Be self-aware, recognizing one's own biases
- Value inclusion
- Understand roles and expectations clearly
- Have a strength-based perspective

The team member must be able to convey
- Trust
- Mutual respect
- A vision for the future
- A positive and caring attitude
- Genuineness
- Nonjudgmental acceptance
- A nonblaming attitude
- Sensitivity
- The importance of collaboration
- A positive, caring attitude
- Empathy
- An understanding of hope for a better future and another person's plight

Adapted from Bronstein (2003) and Pickens (1998).

1. An improvement in school attendance, performance, and school behavior
2. Reduced incidents of criminal behavior, resulting in fewer youth accused or convicted of a crime; fewer adolescents in detention or jail
3. An increase in the level of functioning across a variety of life domains
4. A decrease in the degree of caregiver strain, as reported by 54.2% of parental respondents
5. More stable living arrangements, with more adolescents living at home and in the community

Despite the benefits, team members must be ready to meet the challenges and to overcome the barriers. Doing so takes patience, time, energy, and a commitment to providing quality mental health and health care. Attention must be paid to the group process in order to foster a team spirit (Simpson et al., 1999). The benefits, challenges, and barriers are listed in Table 2-4.

Table 2-4	Benefits, Challenges, and Barriers to Building Collaborative Relationships

Benefits from collaboration are as follows:

1. Maximized creativity
2. Improved family/professional relationships
3. An increased relevance of mental health services to better meet the needs of children and families
4. Decreased overlapping and fragmentation of services to improve the continuity of care
5. Flexible boundaries, which ease transitions from one service provider to another
6. Improved client, family, and professional satisfaction
7. Supportive relationships develop, which occur as the team becomes cohesive
8. Decreased costs
9. Greater access to funding sources for program development
10. Increased hope for the client, the child, and the family
11. Increased quality and efficiency
12. Improved quality of life for clients, children, and families

Challenges to building effective partnerships are:

1. The process is difficult and time consuming. It takes a commitment on every level; i.e., at the personal, team, and organizational/administrative levels.
2. Having people from diverse backgrounds working toward a common goal requires administrators, providers, and families coming together as equal partners to facilitate the process.
3. Socialization of team members to develop skills for collaborative teamwork.
4. Providing a clear understanding of each member's role.
5. Setting realistic goals that build on each team member's strengths.
6. Maintaining an ongoing dialogue that is open and honest.
7. Building consensus.
8. Overcoming turf issues.
9. Identifying strategies to reach goals and then assigning responsibilities.

continues

Table 2-4   Continued

Barriers to collaborative relationships:
1. American norms and values that support competition
2. Unclear mission
3. Interprofessional and interpersonal conflicts
4. Insufficient time for negotiations
5. Excessive workload
6. Inflexibility
7. Resistance to change
8. Poor negotiation skills
9. Poor group skills
10. Fear of breaching confidentiality
11. Racial and cultural polarization
12. A lack of financial resources to contribute to the collaborative
13. Miscommunication leading to misunderstandings
14. Leaving out important stakeholders
15. Bureaucratic red tape

Adapted from Bope & Jost, 1994; Bronstein, 2003; Hodges, Nesman, & Hernandez, 1999; Osher, deFur, Nava, Spencer, & Toth-Dennis, 1999; Pickens, 1998; Simpson, Koroloff, Friesen, & Gac, 1999).

Interagency Collaboration

Interagency collaboration is the result of linking agencies across the health and mental health care continuum in order to build a network of services. The intent of System of Care is to develop an integrated and seamless health/mental health system for children and families. "The process of agencies joining together for the purpose of interdependent problem solving . . . represents a fundamental reform in the way services are provided" (Hodges et al., 1999, p. 17). The agencies who have been active participants in System of Care programs include the Department of Social Services, juvenile justice, public schools, public health and child health departments, mental health, and other community agencies, identified by a collaborative case management team as important to the care of the client, the child, and the family. Other agencies that have been involved—sometimes called informal or natural support systems—are the Department of Parks and Recreation and the Boys Clubs of America, representatives of the faith community, non-profit organizations, and family support organizations. System of Care programs must be accountable to the community and to the clients whom they serve. Community support is a basic ingredient to establishing System of

Care programs and to "the evolution of the wraparound process as communities learn to 'take care of their own' " (Burns & Goldman, 1999, p. 21).

Specific factors are essential to the success of an interagency collaboration; these are listed in Table 2-5.

True Collaboration

"The emergence of families as full partners in System of Care is the key to true and lasting collaboration" (Hodges et al., 1999, p. 14). The authors claimed that true collaboration is the result of a process that occurs in developmental stages and that finally results in well-established collaborative relationships that are interagency, interprofessional, and family/professional relationships. Interagency collaborative partners network to provide community services across the health care continuum that wrap around the family to ensure that they do not get lost in the maize of potential providers and services.

Wraparound as a Philosophy of Care

Wraparound: A Philosophical Framework for Health and Mental Health Care

Wraparound is a "philosophy of care, that includes a definable planning process involving the child and family," which implements a delivery

Table 2-5	Key Factors Necessary for Interagency Collaboration

Agencies must
- Have a common purpose: promote the continuity of care across the service and health care continuum
- Have open channels of communication across agencies
- Establish interagency collaborative work teams
- Communicate frequently and have an ongoing dialogue about their vision and goals
- Develop access points along the health care continuum from prevention and primary care to long-term and chronic care
- Have flexible boundaries
- Be willing to share resources
- Provide opportunities for cross-training
- Be willing to place professionals across agencies
- Share consultation services

Adapted from Chenven and Brady (2003) and Hodges et al. (1999).

system that "results in a unique set of community services and natural supports, individualized for that child and family to achieve a positive set of outcomes" (Burns & Goldman, 1999, p. 13). Rogers (2003) defined wraparound as a method for delivering coordinated and collaborative mental health services in order to address the complex needs of children and families with multiple problems who require the services of multiple agencies. Services are coordinated and integrated across the health care continuum. These services may include crisis intervention, educational advocacy, individual and family therapy, psychological evaluation, medication evaluation and management, social service interventions, and home and respite care. The goal is to prevent admissions to more restrictive levels of care (Rogers, 2003; VanDenBerg, 1999).

Individualized care plans are developed by a collaborative interdisciplinary team and are customized to meet the needs of a specific child and family. Interventions are selected from a comprehensive array of services across the service care continuum, resulting in more positive outcomes (Winters & Terrell, 2003). As a quality care model, the wraparound/System of Care approach to delivering health care services is cost-effective. The System of Care philosophical framework is adaptable to care for all populations who have complex health and mental health care needs and/or social and educational needs.

In 1998, System of Care experts from across the country met at Duke University to identify and define the core elements of wraparound, which resulted in ten basic components that are listed in Table 2-6.

Table 2-6	Wraparound Core Elements	
Core Elements	**Description**
Community based	Services must be community based with the goal of keeping the child or adolescent in the home and community and out of residential care.
Individualized and strength based	Services and support must be individualized, built on strengths to meet the needs of children and families across all life domains in order to promote, success, safety, and permanency in the home, school, and community. Services must not be driven by service priorities.

Core Elements	Description
Culturally competent	The process must be culturally competent, building on the unique values, preferences, and beliefs of the child and family, as well as considering the racial, ethnic, and social characteristics of the child and family and their communities.
Voice and choice	Families must be fully active partners of the wrap-around process to include participating at every level, including assessment, planning, implementation, and evaluation.
Interdisciplinary, interagency, family planning, with the community ultimately owning the plan	The wraparound approach must be a team-driven process involving the family, child, natural supports, agencies, and community services, working together to develop, implement, and evaluate the individual service plan. The individual care plan should be developed and implemented based on an interagency, interdisciplinary collaborative process to include the family.
Flexible resources	Wraparound teams must have the ability to implement flexible approaches, using adequate and flexible "non-categorical" funding.
Continuation of care	The agencies and teams must make an unconditional commitment to serving children and families. If the needs of the child and family change, the services must not be discontinued, nor the family rejected; instead, the services must change to meet their new needs.
Collaboration	A service support plan should be developed by an interdisciplinary team to include the family and implemented based on an interagency, community–neighborhood collaborative process. Decisions are made by consensus.
A balanced support system	The team plan should include a balance of formal services and informal community and family resources. The team should comprise family and community support persons, with less than one-half of the team being professionals.
Outcomes-based services for best practice	Outcomes must be determined and measured for each goal established in the individualized service plan, as well as the goals established at the program and system levels. Outcomes are measured on empirical and scientific bases and are used to determine the best strategies for building the quality of the service delivery system for children with serious emotional disturbances and their families that is cost effective.

Adapted from Clarke, Schaefer, Burchard, and Welkowitz (1992); Friesen and Winters (2003); Goldman (1999); Rogers (2003); VanDenBerg (1999); VanDenBerg, Bruns, and Burchard (2003); and VanDenBerg and Grealish (1996).

Case Study Illustrating Wraparound

Wrapping Services Around a Child and Family

Andy was an 8-year-old African American boy who was referred to the mental health center by the school for violent and aggressive behavior. The principal had dismissed him from school because of his lack of control over aggressive behaviors. His father was in prison for killing an uncle, and Andy had witnessed this. Andy's mother, Jane, was a single parent of eight children. Attendance at the wraparound meeting included Jane, a care coordinator from the Department of Children and Family Services, Andy's teacher, the school principal, the family therapist, and the psychiatrist. The team decided that mother and child should be seen by the therapist weekly and that the child should be homeschooled until he could control his aggressive behaviors enough to re-enter school. Jane would be seen by the therapist to provide emotional support and to assist her with parenting skills, especially limit setting. Because the family had no transportation, Child and Family Services was responsible for their transportation to the mental health center and for coordinating all of the family's other needs. The psychiatrist prescribed an antidepressant to modify the aggressive behavior, which enhanced the child's ability to articulate his thoughts and feelings during the therapy sessions.

In working with the child in individual therapy, it quickly became apparent that he loved basketball and played it well (a strength). The child and family team met monthly or more often if any member had a concern that needed to be addressed. The goal was re-entry into school. The motivation for Andy to re-enter school was to play basketball. This wish was nurtured so that changing behavior became important to the child. Although the child responded well to individual therapy, usually playing nerf basketball as he talked to the therapist, it became clear that he needed more opportunities to play with peers. Consequently, he was placed in a play group with other children who were diagnosed with a serious emotional disturbance and who were also his age. On the first day, he immediately attacked one of the children. He misunderstood cues from other children and interpreted their behaviors as personal attacks and consequently was aggressive toward them. His aggression toward another child, as well as other observations, was discussed in individual therapy, and his thoughts and feelings at the time of the aggressive act were explored. The therapist pointed out that he could not return to school to play basketball until he could control the aggressive behavior.

In time, the aggressive behavior subsided during group play, and the Child and Family Services care coordinator was asked to contact the Boys

Club, a natural community support system, so that Andy could play basketball with children his own age. When he successfully managed to participate without fighting, he was ready to return to school. The school was willing to take him back—but not full time. His school days were increased incrementally by 3 hours at a time. After several months he was back at school full time.

This example illustrates many of the essential elements of wraparound. Because of the medical director's foresight, this child benefited from a seamless System of Care which some professionals at the mental health center labeled the "Cadillac Model." The interdisciplinary team from several agencies, which included Jane, Andy's mother, designed the individual service plan. The wraparound services that this child and family received were educational services—both special education and homeschooling—individual therapy, therapeutic group play, basketball at the Boys Club, medication management, and case management from the Department of Children and Family Services. The interdisciplinary team reflected the cultural mix of a midwestern town where whites were in the majority and blacks were a minority. Few of the residents were from other ethnic groups. The team consisted of the teacher and the principal, who were both white. However, the homeschool teacher was black. The therapist and psychiatrist were both white, and the case manager and the basketball coach at the Boys Club were black. The team addressed the cultural needs as they became apparent to the overall care of this child and family. Most of these issues concerned poverty and the lack of transportation to needed services. Access to care was enabled by the case manager, also known as the care coordinator, at the Department of Child and Family Services, who facilitated implementation of the overall plan of care.

Families and Professionals as Collaborators and Partners in System of Care

All members of the team, including family members, respect each other as equal and valuable contributors. Training for establishing new relationships is necessary for both families and professionals. Sustaining these relationships requires a belief and a commitment to the idea that long-term, collaborative partnerships improve the quality of care for children and families. The factors listed in Table 2-7 are essential to establishing a System of Care for people who are in need of multiple services. These factors are crucial to building effective collaborative relationships among professionals and family members.

Table 2-7   **The Contributions of Parents and Professionals to System of Care Teams**

Parents or family members contribute the following:

- Their own strengths, talents, and skills to the collaborative work
- Knowledge of the child's or client's history, growth, and development, and the onset of the current health or mental health condition
- Information about the client's and family's strengths and assets
- Knowledge about the child's or client's preferences and idiosyncrasies
- Information about past experiences with other systems, i.e., what interventions have and have not worked
- Assistance with planning, implementation, and evaluation
- Information about the child's or client's progress, contributing to the planning process
- Emotional support and knowledge about System of Care to other family members

Professionals contribute the following:

- Knowledge about the child's or client's current health or mental health condition
- Information about resources and proposed service options, plus assistance for families in examining the benefits and risks related to each option
- Professional skills to care for the client and family

Professionals are as follows:

- Change agents to facilitate a coordinated System of Care
- Motivators, helping clients, children, and families toward healthy lifestyles

The Qualities of Successful Parent/Professional Partnerships include the following:

- The professionals are committed to the inclusion of families and work well with diverse groups, and are able to build bridges across class and cultural boundaries.
- A safe environment to develop collegial relationships.
- Trust and mutual respect develops over time.
- Consensus is achieved about goals and strategies to reach the goals.

Adapted from Adam (1997). Cited in Osher et al. (1999).

Truly interprofessional/family relationships include "qualities of role clarity for families and service providers, interdependence and shared responsibility among collaborative partners, striving for vision-driven solutions, and a focus on the whole child in the context of the child's family and community" (Hodges et al., 1999, p. 102).

Outcome Data Provide Lessons for the Development of Future System of Care Programs

Lessons are continually learned from gathering data from programs across the country. In communities where System of Care programs have been established, outcome data point to lessons learned that provide guidelines for the development of new System of Care programs. Some of these lessons are listed in Table 2-8.

Maintaining quality requires ongoing assessment. Results of the data analysis should be shared with families and other stakeholders (Friesen & Winters, 2003). Outcome data are used to evaluate the effectiveness of a program, according to the criteria that are determined by those who are responsible for program development. Criteria for measurement may include (1) a reduction in symptoms (e.g. anxiety and aggression), (2) improved functioning, such as school performance or attendance, (3) environmental stability, including family and social supports, and (4) consumer perspectives,

---

Table 2-8   **Outcome Data and Lessons Learned**

- Family members should be involved in all stages of program development.
- Collaboration requires effort to maintain relationships, manage conflicts, and keep everyone focused on the identified goals. Ongoing dialogue is essential.
- To integrate family members successfully, an orientation period and training must be available for both family members and professionals. Periodic training needs to be conducted that is interactive and experiential, dealing with the here and now.
- Payment for family members' services on community advisory committee and other services is strongly suggested.
- Overcoming interagency concerns about confidentiality and responsibilities needs to be continually addressed by interagency work teams.
- The program personnel should reflect the cultural mix of the community.
- System of Care programs should be adapted to the unique characteristics of the community to meet the needs of the population that is the focus of care. "System of Care should be folded into the community's existing governance and infrastructure" (National Resource Network, 1999, p. 12).

Adapted from the National Resource Network (1999) and Simpson et al. (1999).

such as child and family satisfaction and quality of life. Finally, outcome measures may include the characteristics of systems, including services, interagency relationships, and costs. Outcomes may determine program modifications. After data analysis, one program decided that it needed to provide more in-home and respite services, as well as short-term foster care (VanDenBerg & Grealish, 1996). A California program examined the integration of System of Care into managed care. The authors admitted that merging System of Care values with the need to contain costs in a managed care environment was a challenge, but that cost savings were possible because of fewer out-of-home placements and reductions in admissions and lengths of stay in acute care or residential settings (Griffin, 1999). Outcomes should address both service delivery and service integration, as well as the impact on quality, costs, policies, and funding for health care and mental health care.

Summary

Since the passage of the Child and Adolescent Service System Program, the needs of children suffering from serious emotional disturbance and their families have been addressed. The development of System of Care as a framework for practice has inculcated humanitarian values into children's mental health care. This framework is holistic, flexible, and adaptable to various communities and to different populations.

Recently, there has been a call for culturally competent, family-centered health care that is practiced by an interdisciplinary team. Issues regarding quality mental health and physical health care have been addressed by the U.S. Surgeon General, the Pew Commission, the Institute of Medicine, and most recently by *Healthy People 2010*, which called for the elimination of health disparities for ethnic groups and minorities (Greiner & Knebel, 2003; Kestenbaum, 2003, who quoted the Surgeon General, p. xiii; the Pew Health Professions Commission, 1995; Spector, 2004, who addressed *Healthy People 2010*).

System of Care is not a model but a philosophical or conceptual framework for quality care, requiring a paradigm shift from a focus on the client and his or her problems to a focus on the family and its strengths—from a client-centered/professional relationship to a family-centered collaborative interdisciplinary partnership. Systematic documentation has substantiated that System of Care programs meet today's requirements for quality mental health care for children and their families. Documenting System of Care outcomes is "critically important to shape the future patterns of service delivery for this underserved and vulnerable population" (Stroul, McCormack, & Zaro, 1996, p. 333). The goal is quality care that is comprehensive and cost-effective. System of Care has been developed, implemented, and evaluated across the country.

Activities to Extend Your Learning

Suggested Activities

How do you see yourself in the future as a human service or health professional helping people who are vulnerable and fragile and their families reach their potential for a maximum level of wellness?

- What will your role be in the future? Advocate, lobbyist, program developer, or care provider?
- Identify your goals.
- What will you have to do to reach your goals?
- Develop short- and long-term plans.
- Describe your vision of the future of the mental health and the health care delivery systems. Will it be an integrated, seamless System of Care?
- Identify some strategies that may be developed to provide quality care that is cost-effective for all of our citizens.
- Describe what you might do as a community leader to advocate for the most vulnerable in our society, and to improve services for children, families, and other populations who are chronically ill.

Identify the characteristics of a "high-performing team."

- Compare two work teams in any setting; however, if possible use two work teams in the same setting.
- From what you observed, were they multidisciplinary or interdisciplinary teams?
- Ask the team members to describe the benefits, challenges, and barriers that were encountered as the teams were being developed. What are the current challenges?
- Evaluate their performances.
- Identify the characteristics of the best performing team.

What are the necessary skills to be an effective team member?

■ Examine your own skills to ascertain your potential effectiveness as a team member.

■ Is there a match between the necessary skills and your skills?

■ Do you need to improve some skills in order to be a more effective team member?

■ Identify the strategies that you might use to improve your skills.

Describe what wraparound is and include the core elements.

■ Attend an individual educational plan meeting at a public school, or a team meeting at a local mental health center or an acute care facility.

■ How does the team develop the individual educational plan or the family service plan, or how does a health care team develop a care plan or a discharge plan?

■ What is the focus, who are the professionals, and what is the involvement of the family and other disciplines from other agencies?

■ Who is responsible for implementing the plan?

■ Whose responsibility is it to do the follow-up evaluation and to collect the data regarding the outcomes?

■ How active were the participants in contributing to the plan of care?

■ Do you believe that you observed a truly collaborative team where every one was equally involved?

■ Was there evidence of flexible boundaries across agencies?

Suggested Reading

Team Building

Blanchard, K., Carew, D., & Parisi-Carew E. (2000). *The one minute manager builds high performing teams.* New York: William Morrow & Co.

Blanchard, K., Carlos, J.P., & Randolph, A. (1996). *Empowerment takes more than a minute.* New York: MFJ Books.

Interprofessional Collaboration

Casto, R.M., & Julie, M.C. (1994). *Interprofessional care and collaborative practice: The Commission on Interprofessional Education and Practice.* Pacific Grove, CA: Brooks Cole Publishing.

Pew Health Professional Commission, California Primary Care Consortium. (1995). *Interdisciplinary collaborative teams in primary care: A model curriculum and resource guide.* San Francisco: Author.

Zlotnic, J.L., McCroskey, J., Jordan-Marsh, M., Lind, J., Gibaja, M.G., Dinwiddie, S., et al. (1998). *Myths and opportunities: An examination of the impact of discipline-specific accreditation on interprofessional education: Executive summary.* Available from: http://www.cswe.org.

Systems of Care

Pumariega, A.J. (2003). *The handbook of child and adolescent system of care: The new community psychiatry.* San Francisco: Jossey-Bass.

Stroul, B.A., & Friedman, R.M. (1986). *System of care for children and youth with severe emotional disturbances* (rev. ed). Washington, DC: Georgetown University Child Development Center, National Technical Assistance Center for Children's Mental Health.

Stroul, B.A. (1996). *Children's mental health: Creating systems of care in a changing society.* Baltimore: Paul H. Brookes Publishing Co.

References

Adams, J., Biss, C., Burrell-Mohammad, V., Meyers, J., & Staton, E. (November 14, 1997). *Family/professional relationships: moving forward together,* National Peer Technical Assistance Network.

Allen, R.I., & Petr, C.G. (1998). Re-thinking family-centered practice. *The American Journal of Orthopsychiatry, 68,* 4–15.

Blanchard, K., Carew, D., & Parisi-Carew, E. (2000). *The one minute manager builds high performing teams.* New York: William Morrow & Co.

Blanchard, K., Carlos, J.P., & Randolph, A. (1996). *Empowerment takes more than a minute.* New York: MFJ Books.

Bope, E.T., & Jost, T.S. (1994). Interprofessional collaboration: Factors that affect form, function and structure. In R.M. Casto & M.C. Julie (Eds.), *Interprofessional care and collaborative practice: The commission on interprofessional education and practice.* (pp. 61–69). Pacific Grove, CA: Brooks Cole Publishing.

Bronstein, L.R. (2003). A model for interdisciplinary collaboration. *Social Work, 48,* 297–306.

Burns, B.J., & Goldman, S.K. (Eds.). (1999). Executive summary: Promising practices in wraparound for children with serious emotional disturbance and their families. *Systems of Care: Promising Practices in Children's Mental Health* (1998 Series, Vol. IV, pp. 11–18). Washington, DC: Center for Effective Collaboration and Practice, American Institutes for Research.

Chenven, M., & Brady, B. (2003). Collaboration across disciplines and among agencies within system of care. In A.J. Pumariega & N.C. Winters (Eds.), *The handbook of child and adolescent systems of care: The new community psychiatry* (pp. 66–81). San Francisco: Jossey-Bass.

Clarke, R.T., Schaefer, M., Burchard, J.D., & Welkowitz, J.W. (1992). Wrapping community-based mental health services around children with a severe behavioral disorder: An evaluation of a project wraparound. *Journal of Child and Family Studies, 1,* 241–261.

DeChillo, N., Koren, P.E., & Mezera, M. (1996). Families and professionals partnership. In B.A. Stroul (Ed.), *Children's mental health: Creating systems of care in a changing society* (pp. 389–407). Baltimore: Paul H. Brookes Publishing Co.

Friesen, B., & Winters, N.C. (2003). The role of outcomes in systems of care: Quality improvement and program evaluation. In A.J. Pumariega & N.C. Winters (Eds.), *The handbook of child and adolescent systems of care: The new community psychiatry* (pp. 459–486). San Francisco: Jossey-Bass.

Gage, M. (1998). From independence to interdependence: Creating synergistic health care teams. *Journal of Nursing Administration, 28,*17–26.

Goldman, S.K. (1999). The conceptual framework for wraparound: Definition, values, essential elements, and requirements for practice. In B.J. Burns & S.K. Goldman (Eds.), *Promising practices in wraparound for children with serious emotional disturbance and their families: System of care: Promising practice in children's mental health* (1998 Series, Vol. IV, pp. 27–34). Washington, DC: Center for Effective Collaboration and Practice, American Institutes for Research.

Greiner, A.C., & Knebel, E. (2003). *Health professions education: A bridge to quality. Executive Summary.* Washington, DC: Institute of Medicine of the National Academies, The National Academies Press.

Griffin, M. (1999). Implementing systems of care in a managed care environment. *A compilation of lessons learned.* Comprehensive Community Mental Health Services for Children and Their Families Program. *Promising practices in children's mental health, Systems of Care* (1998 Series, Vol. VII, pp. 17–19). Washington, DC: Center for Effective Collaboration and Practice, American Institutes for Research.

Grossman, S., & Bautista, C. (2002). Collaboration yields cost-effective, evidence-based nursing protocols. *Orthopaedic Nursing, 21,*30–36.

Hawks, J.H. (1992). Empowerment in nursing education: Concept analysis and application to philosophy, learning, and instruction. *Journal of Advanced Nursing, 17,* 609–618.

Herrick, C.A., Arbuckle, M.B., & Claes, J.A. (2002). Teaching inter-professional practice: A course on system of care for children with severe emotional disturbance and their families. *Journal of Family Nursing, 8,* 264–281.

Hodges, S., Nesman, T., & Hernandez, M. (1999). *Promising practices: Building collaboration of systems of care: Systems of care: Promising practices in children's mental health* (1998 series, Vol. VI). Washington, DC: Center for Effective Collaboration and Practice, American Institutes for Research.

Huber, D. (1996). *Leadership and nursing care management.* Philadelphia: W.B. Saunders.

Huffine, C., & Anderson, D. (2003). Family advocacy development in systems of care. In A.J. Pumariega & N.C. Winters (Eds.), *The handbook of child and adolescent systems of care: The new community psychiatry* (pp. 35–64). San Francisco: Jossey-Bass.

Kestenbaum, C.L. (2003). Foreword. In A.J. Pumariega and N.C. Winters (Eds.), *The handbook of child and adolescent systems of care: The new community psychiatry* (pp. xii–ix). San Francisco: Jossey-Bass.

Koenig, E. (2001). Collaborative models of case management. In E.L. Cohen & T.G. Cesta, *Nursing case management: From essentials to advanced practice applications* (3rd ed., pp. 73–80).St. Louis: Mosby.

Maxwell, J.C. (2003). *Relationships 101*. Nashville, TN: Thomas Nelson.

National Resource Network for Child and Family Mental Health Services at the Washington Business Group on Health (Ed.). (1999). A compilation of lessons learned from 22 grantees of the 1997 Comprehensive Community Mental Health Services for Children and Their Families Program. *Systems of care: Promising practices in children's mental health* (1998 Series, Vol. VII). Washington, DC: Center for Effective Collaboration and Practice, American Institutes for Research.

Osher, T., deFur, E., Nava, C., Spencer, S., & Toth-Dennis, D. (1999). New roles for families in systems of care. *Systems of care: Promising practices in children's mental health* (1998 Series, Vol. I). Washington, DC: Center for Collaboration and Practice, American Institutes for Research.

Pew Health Professions Commission. (1995). *Critical challenges: Revitalizing the health professions for the twenty-first century.* San Francisco: UCSF Center for the Health Professions.

Pickens, J. (1998). Formal and informal care of people with psychiatric disorders: Historical perspectives and current trends. *Journal of Psychosocial Nursing, 36,* 37–43.

Platt, L.J. (1994). Why bother with teams? An overview. In R.M. Casto & M.C. Julia (Eds.), *Professional care and collaborative practice* (pp. 3–10). Pacific Grove, CA: Brooks/Cole Publishing.

Rogers, K.C. (2001). Outcomes report to the community collaborative Guilford County system of care. Greensboro, NC: University of North Carolina at Greensboro.

Rogers, K. (2003). Evidence-based community-based interventions. In A.J. Pumariega & N.C. Winters (Eds.), *The handbook of child and adolescent systems of care: The new community psychiatry* (pp. 149–166). San Francisco: Jossey-Bass.

Simpson, J.S., Koroloff, N., Friesen, B.F., & Gac, J. (1999). Promising practices in family-provider collaboration. *Systems of care: Promising practices in children's mental health* (1998 Series, Vol. II). Washington, DC: Center for Effective Collaboration and Practice, American Institutes for Research.

Sorrells-Jones, J. (1997). Challenge of making it real: Interdisciplinary practice in a "seamless" organization. *Nursing Administration Quarterly, 21*(2), 20–30.

Spector, R.E. (2004). Cultural heritage and history. *Cultural diversity in health and illness* (6th ed., pp. 3–28). Upper Saddle River, NJ: Prentice-Hall.

Stroul, B.A. (1996). *Children's mental health: Creating systems of care in a changing society.* Baltimore, MD: Paul H. Brookes Publishing Co.

Stroul, B.A. (2003). Systems of care: A framework for children's mental health care. In A.J. Pumariega & N.C. Winters (Eds.), *The handbook of child and adolescent systems of care: The new community psychiatry* (pp. 17–34). San Francisco: Jossey-Bass.

Stroul, B.A., McCormack, M., & Zaro, S.M. (1996). Measuring outcomes in systems of care. In B.A. Stroul (Ed.), *Children's mental health: Creating systems of care in a changing society* (pp. 313–336). Baltimore: Paul H. Brookes Publishing Co.

Tebbitt, B.V. (1993). Demystifying organizational empowerment. *Journal of Nursing Administration, 23,* 18–23.

VanDenBerg, J.E. (1999). History of the wraparound process. In B.J. Burns & S.K. Goldman (Eds.), *Promising practices in wraparound for children with serious emotional disturbance and their families: Systems of care: Promising practices in children's mental health* (1998 Series, Vol. IV, pp. 19–26). Washington, DC: Center for Effective Collaboration and Practice, American Institutes for Research.

VanDenBerg, J.E., Bruns, E., & Burchard, J. (2003). History of the wraparound process. *Focal point: Quality and fidelity of wraparound* (Vol. 17, pp. 4–7). Portland, OR: Research and Training Center on Family Support and Children's Mental Health.

VanDenBerg, J.E., & Grealish, E.M. (1996). Individualized services and supports through the wraparound process: Philosophy and procedures. *Journal of Child and Family Studies, 5,* 7–21.

Winters, N.C. & Terrell, E. (2003) Case management, the linchpin of community based systems of care. In A.J. Pumariega & N.C. Winters (Eds.) *The Handbook of Child and Adolescent System of Care: The New Community Psychiatry.* San Francisco: Jossey-Bass.

Chapter 3

A Community's Journey: System of Care Implementation

ELIZABETH DOBYNS

Objectives

- Describe the grant goals of a federal System of Care grant for a local community.
- Explain the experiences of implementation of grant expectations into a local service system.
- Describe how the System of Care core values and guiding principles are implemented into county human service systems.
- Describe the importance of cultural change within the workplace that is necessary to implement the values and principles of System of Care.
- Describe a community's history, journey, and accomplishments in implementing System of Care into its human service system.
- Identify the lessons that are learned in a community's System of Care implementation.
- List the key points to remember in order to approach System of Care implementation.

Approximately 10 years ago (1994) in Guilford County, North Carolina, a few key professionals and political leaders began to question why the children with serious emotional disturbances continued to be placed out of their homes for services, as this was an exorbitant cost to the county. Increasing numbers of children were requiring out-of-county placement, and after their return to the community, they were often in even more serious need than before the intervention. Over time, this became a heated political issue as the costs increased. The responsibility for the children was shared between the Department of Social Services, which had custody, and the Department of Mental Health, which had responsibility for the intervention; however, neither department assumed "full" responsibility, thus creating frustration among the political leaders and friction between the two departments.

A few people began to brainstorm ideas to figure out how the situation could be addressed. Leadership in the Mental Health Department had learned of the Child and Adolescent Service System Program (CASSP) values and principles and knew that in another section of the state a federal grant from the U.S. Department of Health and Human Services Center for Mental Health Services had been implemented to facilitate adoption of these values and principles to address the complex needs of children with serious emotional disturbance. A strong component of the federal grant was developing a collaborative service system. Previously, the county had implemented collaborative structures that reached across child-serving agencies to serve children better, but each effort attempted had been unsuccessful or nonsustainable thus far.

This group of professionals began a conversation with the state of North Carolina's Department of Mental Health, Developmental Disabilities, and Substance Abuse Services, and there was agreement that the state would apply for another federal grant from the U.S. Center for Mental Health Services. If awarded, a portion would be allocated to Guilford County. Some months later, the North Carolina Division of Mental Health, Developmental Disabilities, and Substance Abuse Services was awarded a grant entitled North Carolina: Families and Communities Equal Success (NC FACES)—thus began Guilford County's community journey in October 1997.

The agencies involved were the primary child-serving agencies in the county and included the Department of Social Services, the county public schools, the Department of Juvenile Justice and Delinquency Prevention, the Department of Mental Health, Developmental Disabilities and Substance Abuse Services, and an interdisciplinary center at the University of North Carolina at Greensboro. Each agency brought its own culture of service delivery and its own history to the process, but all had the same interest—to ensure that children with serious emotional disturbances and their families were better served in their home community so that they could reach their highest potential and become productive members of society.

Each agency had its own mandate and mission, which made it challenging to integrate System of Care across agencies. However, the influence of adopting the System of Care core values and guiding principles into their work with families and children had much impact on the day-to-day work, and as a result, each of these agencies' mission statements changed as a result of the collaborative work of implementing the grant.

Here is each agency's mission at the end of the grant period, as listed on their websites.

Agency Missions

- *Department of Social Services Mission:* Using a holistic approach to assure safety, promote self-sufficiency and permanency in the lives of adults, children, and families through collaboration and partnership within the community.
- *Guilford County Public Schools Mission:* To graduate students as responsible citizens prepared to succeed in higher education or the career of their choice.
- *Juvenile Justice Mission:* To promote public safety and juvenile delinquency prevention, intervention, and treatment through the operation of a seamless, comprehensive juvenile justice system.
- *The Area Mental Health Mission:* To work in partnership to provide family-centered services that make a measurable difference in the lives of people with or at risk of developing mental illnesses, developmental disabilities, or substance abuse problems.
- *University Center for Youth, Family, and Community Partnerships Mission:* To engage faculty, administrators, and students from across the campus, as well as individuals and organizations from throughout the community in collaborative partnerships that support the healthy development of children of all ages.

Lesson learned: It is much easier to write what one intends to do than to "practice what one preaches." Each agency had to struggle and grow throughout the 6-year process in order to work collaboratively.

The County Community: Where They Started

This section explains the process of moving from serious political problems and interagency disagreements about how to serve children with serious emotional disturbance to a community collaborative that is committed to meeting the needs of children in a culturally competent manner in the community.

After receipt of the North Carolina: Families and Communities Equal Success grant, it became evident that putting these theories, goals, and principles into practice was not easy, especially when the consumers of services may not trust those who were now responsible for implementing the grant goals. In the beginning, each of these key agencies had "reputations" in the community, and there were immediate barriers to overcome if successful implementation of the grant was to occur.

- Department of Social Services reputation: In order to protect children, as is required by statute, the DSS takes children from parents and often inhibits family connections that could enhance their children's thriving and growing into confident, productive adults. The DSS had a history of judging families and not involving them quickly enough in the development of unification plans for children and their families.
- Public school reputation: Children are suspended from school if they cannot conform to all rules and if a child has serious behavior problems. The preparation of youth for higher education or a productive career may no longer be a priority if someone is a problem student.
- Department of Juvenile Justice and Delinquency Prevention reputation: Children should go to group homes if they have legal problems in the community. Court counselors will place youth in secured detention centers until group home beds are available. Youth are often sent out of county to get them away from their peers.
- Mental health reputation: Therapists and doctors decide what is best for a child without including the family. Often the therapeutic remedy includes separation of children from their parents, often blaming parents for their child's mental illness. The wait was far too long to get any mental health services for the child.
- University reputation: The university is interested in competing with larger universities, often overlooking their own community's strengths. The university "talks" community involvement but

often does not keep the best interests of the community in mind when making decisions.

However, even with these reputations, the reality was that several agencies had been awarded a grant that *required* collaboration and community involvement. The consumer community did not trust these agencies, families had had bad experiences with them, and employees practiced the way their agency trained them, which did not reflect System of Care principles.

Because of the agencies' reputations among community members and the lack of trust among the agencies, the original visionaries who had worked with the state to acquire this grant decided to begin with the university assuming the responsibility for implementation of the grant. It would handle the fiscal decisions, develop all training, and manage and deliver the services required for the grant implementation. This appeared to be the best plan because the university did not have a negative reputation related to providing mental health services for children and families. Theoretically, the university was more neutral and could start System of Care implementation with a clean slate. It was thought that families would come for services and that the university could provide the necessary leadership to collaborate with the other agencies to change the system to respond better to the families they served.

Lesson learned: Theory does not easily translate into practice.

Beginning to Put the Grant Goals into Practice

The grant goals had been developed by the State Division of Mental Health, with some consultation with the county service agencies and the university. The goals and expectations were as follows:

Goal 1: Ensure access to community-based, individualized, strengths- and family-driven services, which are provided unconditionally and reflect sensitivity to and understanding of the cultural and ethnic characteristics of consumers and families.

- Expectations: Develop a process to implement child and family team meetings as the process to develop treatment plans collaboratively with a team of providers and family members; develop a process for reviewing these plans regularly to ensure that they are working and are culturally appropriate in service delivery.

Goal 2: Develop and sustain a full partnership with families and surrogate families in developing the System of Care.

- Expectations: Include families in the treatment planning process; ensure an avenue for parent support and advocacy; include parents at system level decision making, both public agency policy and University of North Carolina at Greensboro curriculum training development.

Goal 3: Develop a governance structure for local, community-based, family-driven, fully integrated System of Care and support its development and functioning through state-level policy coordination and advocacy.

- Expectations: Develop a community collaborative that would oversee the grant goals and ensure collaboration at the system level to address barriers to serving emotionally disturbed children and their families.

Goal 4: Integrate local public and private child-serving agencies into the System of Care.

- Expectations: Involve all agencies in the implementation of System of Care principles and practice.

Goal 5: Establish a multitiered total quality improvement and outcomes system to promote state and local practice and policy that sustain and promote the System of Care.

- Expectations: Collect data on families enrolled in the grant efforts and gather quality improvement data on those delivering services to ensure practice change is resulting in better outcomes.

Goal 6: Provide state-of-the-art training and technical assistance activities to university students, community stakeholders, families, and service providers through regional public–academic liaisons to support and sustain the System of Care initiative.

- Expectations: Develop training plans at both the preservice (System of Care curricula development) and in-service levels (training to agency employees, families, and community members). Interns would be placed in agencies to experience System of Care practices and be familiar with System of Care when ready to enter the workforce.

During the first year of the grant, the university methodically worked toward meeting the goals of the grant. First, they hired several case managers. One of the core functions of a System of Care is to have case management available to coordinate planning for children and families in the service system (see principle number 6 in Chapter 1).

Criteria for a child to be "enrolled" into the grant included a severe mental health diagnosis according to DSM-IV-TR, multiagency involvement (two or more agencies), being at risk of removal or already removed from his or her home, and a high score on the Child and Adolescent Functioning Scale and level 1 on the level of eligibility. These two scoring instruments were already used for any new admission of a child or youth into the mental health system. Once a child was deemed eligible for services, a case manager was assigned to the child and his or her family.

Case management is defined as the process of assessment/ reassessment, arranging, informing, assisting, and monitoring as it pertains to the child's diagnosis and relates to the development of a treatment plan, coordination, and implementation of service delivery (adapted from the *Medicaid Service Guidelines*, 1999).

Many activities are used to create this case management process, but for System of Care, there is what is referred to as a "child and family team" process. This process has several nonnegotiable criteria: (1) no meeting should be held without the parent and primary caregiver present; (2) no meeting should be held without the youth present, unless clinically advised otherwise or developmentally inappropriate; (3) a strengths assessment of the child, family, and system should be conducted before the meeting and reviewed at every meeting; (4) key members of the team, jointly selected by the family members and the case manager to include informal, nonpaid members as well as professionals from agencies, should be present for the meeting; and (5) the plan should be developed with input from everyone, especially the family, based on the strengths and individualized needs of the family (grant goal 1).

The university contracted with the mental health association, a nonprofit organization advocating for mental health services, to hire a family advocate (grant goal 2). The university convened a group that was named the Guilford County Community Collaborative (GCCC), with representatives from the Mental Health Department, the Department of

Social Services, the Public Health Department, the Public Schools, the Department of Juvenile Justice and Delinquency Prevention, the university, private nonprofit organizations, and family members (grant goals 3 and 4). As part of the grant, the community had to agree to participate in the national evaluation of implementation of System of Care, and therefore, a data director was hired who set up a system for collecting data on families enrolled in the System of Care—basically any family who had been assigned one of the case managers (grant goal 5). Finally, intense training began, prioritizing training for the case managers to learn the new child and family team planning process (grant goal 6).

The university worked hard to implement the goals, but within one year, there were many problems in the implementation of System of Care in the community:

- The community collaborative had the right people at the table, but people were not discussing the issues. Rather, the meetings were spent giving updates, but no one responded or asked any questions. Trust had not been established, and thus frank discussion could not occur.
- A case manager was placed at each agency to "infuse" the practice into the agency, but there was little if any planning within the agency as to coordination of these case managers with the agency's routine practice. Also, these case managers' caseloads were very low compared with their agency peers, and resentment began to build.
- Referrals were not coming to the grant case managers. The mental health agency case managers were getting the referrals because families entered the mental health service system through that agency. Furthermore, the mental health agency needed Medicaid as well as state mental health allocations to fund the mental health agency, and unless the mental health center case managers had a full load, they could not afford to refer a case to the university case managers.
- The few referrals the university case managers did receive were often the children with very complex needs. This was very challenging for the inexperienced case managers and for the children and families who entered the system at the most critical point of need for treatment for the child and family.
- The university was challenged to access funding streams without a more integrated case management system, and families were not accessing wraparound services that were needed. The result

was that the university case management unit was remaining isolated as opposed to being integrated into the community agencies.

- The family advocate was feeling isolated as well, and felt driven
  by the university's goals as opposed to trying to meet the individual family's goals.
- Case management training was being provided, but combining academic knowledge with practice knowledge was not yet occurring.
- Intern placements were being requested by the university; nevertheless, none of the agencies had made changes in their practice. Thus, the experience for a student was not that of System
  of Care, but was the same historically fragmented public child-
  serving system experience.

To the university's credit, the leadership was concerned about the
success of the grant over time and recognized that what was occurring
was not the best way to approach implementation of System of Care
values and principles and meet the grant goals.

After much internal discussion, the university approached the mental health agency to move the fiscal and case management responsibilities to that agency. It was agreed that the mental health agency
would hire a site director and try implementation of the grant for a year.
The university would continue the data collection and training por-
tions of the grant and the mental health association would continue to
contract for the family advocate position. The State Division of Mental
Health/Developmental Disabilities/Substance Abuse Services agreed
that it was a good plan. However, these decisions were made by the
leadership of the university center and the director of the mental health
agency. Thus, this was a good plan but a poor decision-making process.

---

*Lesson learned: Never make decisions that impact a collaborative group
without all of the members at the table.*

Although those making these decisions had in mind the best interests of the grant implementation and the children and families served,
once the announcement was made to the community collaborative
that a few members had made this decision in isolation, the members
of the collaborative finally showed that they had a voice!

At the community collaborative meeting after the decision was
made, family members were appalled that case management would
now be provided by the mental health center. One parent told the new
site director, "I went to the university with my child to avoid the men-

tal health agency—I don't like the aroma over there. How can I trust it won't be business as usual?"

Lesson learned: One should not say that he or she will do collaborative work that involves the parents of the children served but in reality make decisions without involving them.

That very question was the challenge to the mental health agency to prove its system would not conduct "business as usual."

Historically, mental health centers had been primarily run as out-patient clinical services. Physicians prescribed medications. Nurses consulted with families, and then relayed information to the physicians; therapists decided who received additional services beyond that. Child case management was not a service in the general mental health arena until the early 1990s, and a child and family received case management services only if a therapist saw it as necessary. The case management coordination function, as defined by the management team of the county mental health agency, was limited to accessing community services and completion of applications for services.

The case management service definition did not allow nonclinical activities to be billed and required separate billing for the development of a clinical plan for a child and family. This meant that the family had to meet with multiple providers to develop separate plans with each provider, thus increasing the risk of inconsistent implementation and complicated monitoring of the "total" plan with the family.

The final complexity of the case management model at the mental health center was the fact that if a youth came into therapy and did not choose to talk or did not benefit from therapy in a reasonable time, the case was closed. Once a case was closed, the youth had no access to case management or other community-based services. Many youths, especially adolescents, do not respond to individual therapy in traditional settings, but as this system was structured, no other alternatives existed.

However, according to the local changes in grant expectations, case management services were now to be provided by the mental health center. This agency clearly had its challenges ahead, but the center also realized that it would not have to make changes alone—there would be consultation with the community collaborative.

The Journey Begins

How do agencies go about changing their reputations in order to better serve the population of children and their families needing their services? How does a group of people begin to truly collaborate and make group decisions?

Lesson learned: Keep your eye on the ball. (In other words, focus on the principles of System of Care and the families that you serve to drive decisions— not agency positions, or professional or personal stakes in the decision.)

Again, although the grant goals seemed clear and the System of Care values and principles seemed simple and sound, to begin implementation of this project through true collaboration proved to be incredibly difficult. From a system and programmatic perspective, implementing concepts and principles into daily practice at an agency can be very challenging. Furthermore, getting family members' input into crucial changes in the system is not easy.

The long journey began with the same original individuals serving on the community collaborative agreeing to participate in a retreat. Before the community of agencies and families could come together and promote change, everyone needed to agree on some basic definitions. *What does family involvement and partnership really mean to us? How do the previously mentioned values and principles translate into practice? How is everyone defining "System of Care"?*

The new site director began her task by interviewing every community collaborative member to determine the details of the agenda for the retreat. She found that each member described family involvement differently, defined System of Care differently, and had a different vision for integration of System of Care into their agency operations. Among family members, they, too, voiced differing responses to these questions. Thus, the agenda was clear—all community collaborative members must agree on the definitions of these concepts and how they should be implemented into practice.

Lesson learned: No one can keep their eye on the ball if they do not know what the ball looks like.

The Retreat

The retreat was an intensive two days of hard work. The Guilford County Community Collaborative agreed on the agenda, and an outside facilitator was hired. He had been given the Collaborative's history that included the first year's struggles at the university in incorporating case management into the agencies, the grant goals, and the System of Care core values and guiding principles. Although the meeting was intense, everyone spoke, no matter how much they disagreed. Members aired their frustrations about the first year, primarily those decisions that had been made without them. Family members spoke up, showing that they, too, had a voice that needed to be heard. The greatest benefit of the retreat was that everyone agreed to continue to meet. There was consensus on the definitions of the grant goals, and although serious conflicts arose, the entire group worked through them. Several agreements were made for future ground rules: (1) no meetings can be held before the meeting—everything gets discussed at the community collaborative table, (2) only one person may talk at a time, (3) the next agenda item would not be discussed until everyone clearly understood the current item, and (4) meetings would be held at times that could include all members, not just a time convenient for the professionals. The group was now well on its way to meeting grant goal 3 of the grant.

Implementing System of Care:
The Child and Family Team Process (Grant Goal 1)

Once the mental health center began incorporating the grant goals into its services, several steps occurred over the course of the next five years. Along the way, the steps had to be evaluated and adjusted accordingly. In grant goal 1, one of the first expectations was to ensure that treatment plans were developed collaboratively for children and their families based on their strengths. This meant that all case management staff had to be trained in an entirely new way of doing business because historically, plans had been developed to address problems or deficits instead of focusing on child/family/system strengths. Immediately, a consultant/trainer was recruited and diligent training began. Several training needs were identified:

- The child and family team model required strong group facilitation skills; however, many case managers had few facilitation skills.
- Formal training would only introduce case managers to the philosophy of System of Care, but staff needed ongoing practice to integrate the values and principles into their daily work with children and families.
- Different training methods were necessary to ensure ongoing skill development, such as mock child and family team meetings and sample case reviews.

- Supervision of case managers would be key to ongoing success.
- Reviewing plans and routinely observing child and family team meetings was a way to know practice was changing; however, some case managers were not accustomed to being observed and could become defensive when being watched.

Lesson learned: Do not teach the case managers new skills before you teach their supervisors.

As this model was integrated into the child and family unit at the mental health center, it became obvious that the ideal way to promote practice change was to engage the entire unit as opposed to training "selected" case managers. It was also important to prepare the case management supervisors to be their staff's coach, mentor, and teacher.

Over time, the mental health center management mandated that System of Care be implemented by all staff, which led to several more significant changes. All employee job descriptions were rewritten to reflect System of Care implementation expectations. Furthermore, agency performance/work plans were aligned with the job descriptions that reflected System of Care concepts. The agency changed its recruitment standards and advertised vacant positions with the expectation that applicants would have System of Care experience. Finally, cultural issues came to the surface, which led to (1) translated materials for families, (2) special efforts to recruit people of different races, and (3) cultural awareness training. Referrals to family advocacy groups were an expectation and families were informed about them during the intake process. Based on System of Care principles, informal supports became a much greater expectation, and case managers asked families regularly who else—friend, family member, preacher—they might wish to add to their child and family team.

Cultural Competency (All Grant Goals)

Cultural competence was difficult because not only was it a topic that created defensiveness among people, but also because it is so complex that it is not easily or quickly evident in the day-to-day work of an organization. Customarily, things are done "as usual" no matter the cultural needs or expectations of the customer. The expectation of the agency professionals is that the consumer should "fit" into the service, rather than acknowledging that a person's culture can impact on their acceptance of the service.

An initial effort to address the new awareness of the necessity to address cultural issues was the forming of a cultural competence task force. This group represented the public agencies, family members, and private providers. Outside consultation was necessary because much of the leadership among the agencies was white, whereas the population served was primarily African American and Hispanic.

Lesson learned: Do not have white people be the cultural competency leaders.

No matter how committed a person may be to a culturally diverse issue and cultural competency, no one can fully understand the issues that relate to a culture that is different from his or her own. One may have awareness, and one may have experienced some of the cultural traditions or rituals; however, as an individual, one will never know what it is like to be another race or another cultural group. A major issue became addressing how the system could represent the population served when the directors and management teams among the child-serving agencies were primarily white.

Outside consultation assisted the cultural competence task force. The first priority was for leadership within this task force to begin the conversation about cultural competence and diversity. It would take time for the complexions of the directors and management teams of Guilford County's agencies to change, but the conversation could start in order to accomplish the following: (1) discuss tough cultural issues that are evident from data collection of the children and families served, such as the overrepresentation of African Americans in the juvenile justice system, (2) be honest and open about the leadership and management challenges and how to ensure that over time there was commitment to be more diverse, and (3) create an environment and agency culture conducive to and knowledgeable about diverse populations so that the child-serving agencies can respond appropriately to meet the needs of the people.

This task force produced two important deliverables to the community. One was conducting cultural competency assessments within the human service agencies, and the second was the development of an assessment tool called *The Kaleidoscope, Cultural Diversity in Guilford County.* This assessment tool served two purposes: (1) to have completion of a cultural awareness assessment in itself raises an individual's awareness of their community and the agency's practice related to diversity, and (2) to serve as a baseline of knowledge to prepare educational, training, and public awareness information throughout the community.

The Kaleidoscope is a resource notebook that was developed to serve as a reference guide for several different cultural groups living in the county. It was first written as a "reference guide" to various cultural groups, and the first research was gleaned from encyclopedias and websites about each culture's country of origin. However, the final production team recognized that this information was shallow and did not address the specific experiences of the persons living in our community. Therefore, there was a change of strategy, and in addition to background material on the cultures and countries from traditional sources, the final resource book contained much information that was collected through interviews with representatives of the specific cultural groups and visits to local stores and community sites representative of the cultural groups. It provided an overview of cultural practices generally considered common to people from particular geographic locations throughout the world, and it also contained information pertinent to the cultural groups *living in our community*.

It was the hope of the cultural competence task force that these descriptions would give the reader an insight into the cultures, traditions, and practices of particular groups of people from around the world who have found themselves living in the county community. The notebooks were distributed to participating agencies, all public agencies, all community collaborative participants, and those who requested the product. The notebook came with a CD-ROM so that agencies or individuals could download it to their computers, and so that others could easily copy it.

Family Involvement (Grant Goal 2)

Lesson learned: The development of family organizations deserves the same time expectations that any other organization's development receives.

This section begins with a lesson learned because it became very evident as the grant progressed that no one knew quite what to do in this arena. Individuals become skilled professionals in their careers through numerous stages of development. After receiving professional training in a discipline, one moves from an entry-level position into a higher-level position through mentoring, supervision, and professional training in related areas such as management, program development, and leadership. However, when the development of a family organization became a grant goal, those same professionals simply hired a "parent" at a much lower rate of pay and expected development to occur.

Again, although intentions were good, the reality was that the parent representatives were rarely supervised, and were trained in System of Care but not in management, business practices, organizational development, or leadership until well into the grant implementation. Parents are naturals at developing advocacy supports for each other. They have been in the trenches, through exhausting efforts to learn the child-serving system where their child has received services, and have learned to speak out about issues related to their children. Thus, developing an advocacy network was not difficult, but that became their only focus. Meanwhile, no plan to sustain this advocacy process for others in the future was developed, nor was an organizational foundation built so that families could become independent providers for other families needing similar support and guidance.

As the grant moved forward, it became evident to both the parents and the providers that they were falling short in meeting the goal and that time was rapidly passing. As a result, locally and through a statewide effort, independent consultant contracts provided training in organizational development to the group of parents, specifically how to become a federally designated tax-exempt 501C-3 nonprofit organization. In addition, the parents received leadership training and advocacy skill development.

Partnering with parents was not easy at first, mainly because parents were not happy with the current child-serving system. Obviously, the current system was not in good shape or this grant would not have been necessary. Thus, when parents were expected to partner with the very providers that they were not happy with, who were resistant to change, many of the families showed their anger.

Lesson learned: Sometimes the pendulum must swing before partnerships can truly be formed.

Trust is built through evidence of change, and change shows that professionals mean what they say. "Lip service" had been going on for far too long, and thus, the development of relationships between professionals and parents would take time. Eventually, it did develop, and folks began to build trust among each other. Parents and professionals were working together in partnership.

SUCCESS (Supporting and Understanding Children's Challenges Expecting Satisfaction and Success), a family organization that supported families of children with serious emotional disturbance, was formed. This organization developed a "Parent Mentoring" course that included both training in mentoring and a train-the-trainer curriculum to teach other parents to teach the course. This product served several purposes: (1) it recruited more family members into the leadership, (2) it taught parents how to be advocates, and finally, (3), it taught parents how to navigate the service system appropriately. Because the leadership of SUCCESS participated in many of the meetings and training events associated with the grant, both locally and at the state level, the organization built a reputation for being not only an advocacy group, but also one that approached issues from a knowledge base that is equal to that of the professionals. The leadership also developed a reputation for fairness in relationships with the service system and professionals. This reputation prevented the development of the adversarial relationships that had characterized previous family groups that had made similar efforts to become an advocacy organization in the community.

SUCCESS also took the lead in the development of youth advocacy groups and youth training. The professionals attempted to bring youths who were receiving services together for one night a week to learn about System of Care so that they could become self-advocates. It was not until the parents and the youths themselves led the effort to develop a youth group that it succeeded. The youths formed a local group initially, but their work quickly escalated to the development of a statewide group, Powerful Youth Friends United. This group became nationally recognized for its development as a youth group and received funding to support their efforts from the State Division of Mental Health, Developmental Disabilities, and Substance Abuse Services in a very difficult funding year. Finally, the Powerful Youth Friends United coordinator was the daughter of a parent who was involved in the county community collaborative. Over time, through the involvement of the grant activities locally and at the state level, this group made state and national presentations at conferences, advocated at the state and national levels for funding for improved services for youths with mental illness, and served as advocates for other youths with serious emotional disturbances who need services.

The Collaborative (Grant Goals 3 and 4)

The community collaborative struggled for some time, but the members were committed to becoming a functional group that could lead others through change in implementing the values and principles of System of Care, work through problems, and identify and advocate for services. As a group, they held the power to bring about a better child-serving system for children with serious emotional disturbances. In acknowledging this important purpose, the members agreed on their mission as follows:

> *The mission of the Community Collaborative is to promote the sharing of resources and accountability across agencies and programs on behalf of families and children who have significant mental health needs and to build community capacity to provide effective, community-based, family and youth driven services that are delivered within a system of care philosophy.* The Community Collaborative will serve as the local management structure for the System of Care, as specified in the State Child Mental Health Plan and as designated by the County Mental Health Center. (GCCC, 2002)

After its successful first retreat, each subsequent year of the System of Care grant the community collaborative scheduled a 1-day retreat. This provided an opportunity to revisit goals, develop a strategic plan, and update the memorandum of agreement that specified the responsibilities of the participating agencies to the implementation of the values and principles of System of Care into their respective service systems. The retreat also served as an appropriate place to air differences and address issues as an entire group. The community collaborative members had to learn to share and work together.

Lesson learned: One person does not get all the credit, nor does one person ever take a fall.

As a group, the members learned to support each other and share successes. They also learned that "collaboration is a mutually beneficial and well-defined relationship entered into by two or more organizations to achieve results they are more likely to achieve together than alone" (Winer & Ray, 2002). In every collaborative group, one will find that not all members are invested at the same level. Also, not all members carry the same decision-making power, as defined by their role in their agency or in the community. Some members will have power within their agencies because of their role within the agency. Some members will be key leaders among the grassroots community, and some members will quietly move mountains behind the scenes. However, none of the members will be able to do anything alone as well as when working together as part of a group.

This community collaborative ended up as a high-functioning group. The members used data from the evaluation process to make informed decisions. The collaborative became a recognized advocacy group in the community for children's mental health. The members piloted new processes among agencies to attempt to reduce duplication of services, especially in the areas of case management and care coordination. They informed themselves and the community about mental health reform that was being implemented by the State Division of Mental Health Services, Developmental Disabilities, and Substance Abuse. They pooled money from each agency in order to continue paying stipends for parents' time served on committees after the grant funds ended. They created a case review process that would serve as a decision-making place for case managers and families to review "hard-to-fund" treatment plans for children whose needs could not be addressed through traditional services. This group also began to coordinate other grant application efforts to ensure that System of Care was included in other work of the agencies and that similar efforts to develop family-centered services were well coordinated. Finally, it had become a collaborative group and had used the grant to serve its community as a catalyst for change.

Data Collection (Grant Goal 5)

Data collection was a requirement of the grant goals and expectations. This was a process by which identified and enrolled children and their parents participated in lengthy interviews every six months to determine the improved functioning of the children and their families. In the second year of the grant, the first of two excellent data directors was hired. The first data director set up an evaluation committee to provide oversight of processes for gathering data, performing quality improvement activities, and creating presentations of that data to the community collaborative and other audiences.

Data collection through the longitudinal study of the grant period consisted of interviews of enrolled families every six months for three years. Unlike other sites implementing the grant in other places in the state, Guilford County had a commendable reputation for families remaining in the longitudinal study for the full three years. This was in part due to the persistence of the data collectors and also due to the relationships developed between data collectors and case managers. If a family moved, case managers knew where a family had relocated. Case managers collected some of the semiannual data and updated diagnosis and Child and Adolescent Functioning Scale (CAFUS) scores. The National Evaluation Team at ORC Macro International selected the 22 required data collection measures that were used for the study. Because the interviews often took two hours, stipends were provided to children and their parents for their time. Monthly outcomes reports were presented to the collaborative, and over time a process was developed to provide feedback to the individual families.

Lesson learned: Before presenting data to a group, be sure that the group knows how to read graphs and data reports.

Although this may seem basic, it is good practice. The reports became useful to the community collaborative members after they could read and understand them. Eventually, the community collaborative members asked for more specific reports on certain topics to inform them of areas of concern. Also, they requested data that were useful to determine and to fill service gaps in the community. The quarterly data reports were circulated to agency directors and community partners and were important in public relation campaign efforts about the changes in the service systems.

Another key aspect of the data collection was quality improvement activities. The group needed to know whether practice within the agencies was actually changing over time. This meant that it was important to read family treatment plans and to observe child and family team meetings to assure that the values and principles were being applied.

Lesson learned: This process may threaten case managers; thus, plan carefully to make it as strength-based as possible.

The process of observing team meetings and reviewing charts began early in the second year of the grant. In retrospect, the groundwork for these activities should have been laid with supervisors. The approach behind the quality-improvement activities was that the individual form completed after file review and team observations was copied and sent to case managers and their supervisors. An aggregate report was compiled every six months and copied for the training committee and the collaborative. Figure 3-1 illustrates the flow of information, which worked very well.

The case-level data portion of this flowchart was implemented with appropriate training on utilization of the tools to supervisors and case managers. The quality-improvement data reflected strengths of the individual case managers, as well as areas for improvement. Ideally, the supervisors could use the information gathered from the tools to

Mechanism for Utilization of Quality Improvement Data in the System of Care

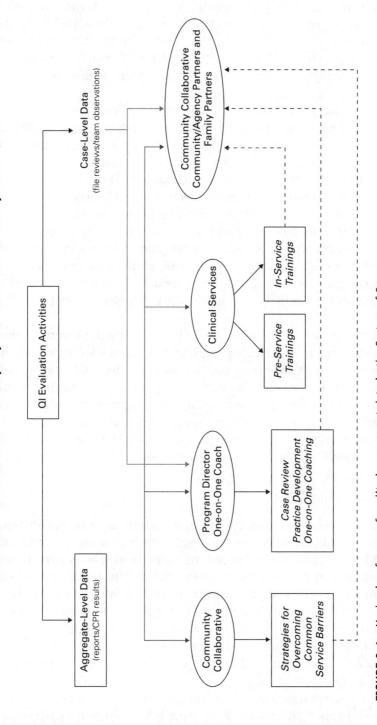

FIGURE 3-1 Mechanism for use of quality improvement data in the System of Care.

Source: Guilford County Collaborative Evaluation Committee (2000).

coach and mentor the case managers in building their skills. Professional practice will not change until new skills are built and old habits are broken. Some of the case managers and supervisors began to use the information to shape practice. The activities assessed through the quality-improvement process were as follows:

- Are the parent and child included in the meeting?
- Does the team consist of informal, nonpaid supports, such as a family friend or a minister, as well as the professionals representing service agencies?
- Do team members represent the culture of the family?
- Did the youth and parent participate in the team meeting?
- Did team members listen to the child and parent?
- Were child and family strengths reviewed in the meeting?
- Were strengths used when developing strategies for the plan?
- Was a crisis plan developed in case strategies do not work?
- Did the case manager facilitate input from everyone and redirect team members when nonproductive discussions took place?

Every agency or business should have quality-improvement procedures to ensure that quality work and outcomes are being reached. However, at the time, this process was new for case managers but proved to be most helpful in determining the case management unit's training needs. Before System of Care, case managers were "process oriented"—that is, focused on how things were done rather than outcome- or results-oriented. In the end, the success of the plan was measured by how well the child and family were doing.

Training (Grant Goal 6)

Training was an extremely important component of the System of Care transformation in the county. In the beginning, a collaborative training committee was formed. Its early focus was on two areas: (1) to assess training needs for agency staff, family members, and community partners, and (2) to infuse principles into the university curricula within numerous academic departments: nursing, social work, psychology, specialized education services, counseling, curriculum and instruction, exercise and sport science, parks and recreation, public health education, and human development and family studies, music education, and dance.

For in-service training, the community collaborative contracted for several years with a trainer from outside the community who had experience delivering training on System of Care topics. In-service training assessments showed that initially System of Care overview training was necessary for employees. The mental health center staff had first priority, and the agency mandated that every employee, regardless of professional role or age of consumer served, would participate in the System of Care overview training. In addition, there was intense training for the professionals in the child and family unit. Over time, the training efforts provided System of Care to professionals in the schools and in other public agencies. This training plan worked well for 4 years, with the site director and training committee working closely with the training consultant to tailor topics to the specific, requested needs.

Lesson learned: When contracting for your training delivery, plan early for how to sustain training once the grant is over.

The preservice training component was intense. The university engaged numerous departments to develop curricula for undergraduate and graduate level students to learn System of Care principles and practice. An interdisciplinary course in System of Care was developed and adopted by six academic departments. From the beginning of the development of the course and teaching the course, parents were involved with the faculty in presenting the course content, and over time, the parents became an integral part of the interdisciplinary teaching team. The collaboration between faculty and parents initially was not easy but was incredibly successful, resulting in a course that has been taught annually with parents as co-teachers for several years.

Another important partnership between university training and community agencies was intern placements. Initially, this was unsuccessful because the agencies had not incorporated System of Care into their practice. Therefore, students were not experiencing the System of Care values and principles during their internships. However, in time, as System of Care practice developed, more options for successful student placements became possible. Several interdisciplinary placements were developed, placing social work, nursing, psychology, and recreational therapy students in a single agency working collaboratively with families and children.

The university leadership for the training became especially critical as the end of the grant neared. The committee discussed ways to maintain the level of training offered by the training consultant as well as ways to develop new training topics as data in outcome reports identified needs. The committee contracted with a trainer to teach representatives of the collaborative in training and presentation skills. Many professionals in the community understood the content that was necessary for System of Care implementation into practice, but they were not comfortable in delivering training to others. The train-the-trainer course provided opportunity to learn how to train others in the System of Care.

The participants included four parents and representatives from the Department of Social Services, the Center at the University of North Carolina at Greensboro, the mental health center, and private provider agencies. The selection process for training was critical because it was necessary to have exposure to System of Care and be able to commit to conducting training workshops after the course was completed. The training team spent five days over the course of two months learning training skills and training development. In this process, training curriculum in core topics of System of Care practice was developed. The consultant taught the course, assisted the team in the development of the first training topics, including instructional guides for future trainers to use, and coached the new team in training delivery. The initial training group split into small training teams, and each practiced training existing topics with the contractor and eventually delivered the training alone, with the contractor observing and giving final feedback. This process produced a team of trainers in the community that continued to deliver the core training necessary to orient new employees and community partners.

The training has continued, and numerous topics have since been developed based on data collected. The array of topics included System of Care overview, keeping children in the community, developing crisis plans, engaging families, conducting strengths-based assessments, and using informal supports, all of which threaded cultural competency throughout.

Key Points to Sustaining Systems of Care in the Community

- Give the parent-involvement process enough time to truly build trust and relationships. Everyone learns better in a patient, accepting environment.
- Parents and youths provide excellent guidance to professionals on how systems can be redefined—when professionals are willing to listen.
- Monitor the practice change closely through quality improvement activities, even if employees are uncomfortable during

the process. Otherwise, you will not know that the employees have changed from traditional service delivery to family-centered services.

- Collect data based on useful outcomes, and use the information to make beneficial changes in the system. Often data are collected, but the outcomes gathered are not based on what was needed or helpful.
- Circulate data reports everywhere that they could possibly make an impact: judges, agency directors, family advocacy groups, state leaders, grassroots leaders, and so forth. Data reports serve no purpose if they get placed in a desk drawer.
- Agency directors and managers must understand System of Care comprehensively enough to know where changes in the agencies must be made to support the practice changes made by front line staff.
- Organized family groups are the best advocates for legislative influence. Support and partner closely with them.
- As agencies rewrite policy and procedures to support System of Care principles, they must financially support it. This can be done through advocacy of noncategorical funding through legislative budgeting or pooling of funds locally.
- Go into this work knowing that it will not be easy. If you really want to see the work done right, you will not be popular all of the time. Know that this work is slow.
- Acknowledge, celebrate, and advertise every success along the way, no matter how small.

Summary

The challenge for a group of community agencies, with their professionals accustomed to conducting business a certain way and for parents whose children have been "recipients of services," is to begin to establish a relationship that can lead to trust and mutual respect. Once this occurs, a community can begin to collaborate on issues. Then it will continue to find success when implementing System of Care. This county is far from finished, but it has processes in place to advocate, brainstorm, and create change to better serve the children and families in need of services in their community. Reflecting the System of Care core values and guiding principles in everything that is expected, acted on, and created is the key to success.

At the end of the 6-year funding of the System of Care grant, Guilford County invited community partners to a celebration. The Guilford County Community Collaborative members brainstormed about what they should do at the celebration. Should they tell everyone that the grant was over and show what they did? Should they give out the data reports compiled over the years? Should family members "tell their story about their family" to people at the party?

When the celebration plans were finalized, the invitations were entitled "Where We've Been and Where We're Going." The community collaborative members gave brief presentations on each goal of the grant and provided everyone in attendance with a copy of *The Kaleidoscope*.

The celebration ended with everyone acknowledging that this had been hard work worth doing. The community collaborative members, parents, community partners, and the child-serving agencies would continue to make the county a place where System of Care supports its children with serious emotional disturbances and their families. Each agency had realized its mission.

Lesson learned: Never give up.

This chapter tells the story of the implementation of System of Care into the public human service agencies and school system of Guilford County, North Carolina, as reflected by the site director, Elizabeth (Bibba) Dobyns, and the editor and Director of Training, Margaret Bourdeaux Arbuckle, who were both involved in the process throughout the grant period.

References

Guilford County Collaborative Evaluation Committee. (2000). *Quality improvement evaluation activities flowchart: Mechanism for utilization of quality improvement data in the system of care.* Unpublished report.

Guilford County Community Collaborative. (2002). *GCCC memorandum of agreement: GCCC mission statement.*

Medicaid Service Guidelines (rev. ed.). (1999, July). Division of Mental Health, Developmental Disabilities and Substance Abuse: Management Services Section.

Winer, M., & Ray, K. (2002, April). *Collaboration handbook: Creating, sustaining, and enjoying the journey.* Amherst H. Wilder Foundation.

Chapter 4

Parents' Voices

Kids Who Are Different

Here's to the kids who are different,
The kids who don't always get A's
The kids who have ears twice the size of their peers,
And noses that go on for days . . .
Here's to the kids who are different,
The kids they call crazy or dumb,
The kids who don't fit, with the guts and the grits,
Who dance to a different drum . . .
Here's to the kids who are different,
The kids with the mischievous streak,
For when they have grown, as history's shown,
It's their difference that makes them unique

> Written by group of children living in Guilford County
> who came together in a group for children with serious
> emotional disturbance. Unpublished poem.

Parent Reflections on Issues for Families Who Have Children with a Serious Emotional Disturbance

FREDERICK DOUGLAS

For many years, children and families with mental health challenges were seen as problems. The children were labeled as "bad" because of their behavior. Many times, the parents were blamed for not managing their children, or even worse, the concerns and issues of children and parents went unnoticed because the illness was not visible to others. Often parents are told that nothing is wrong with their child and that the child "will outgrow it." The parents know that something is wrong, but doctors perceive them as anxious parents. Thus, the parents feel inadequate because they do not understand the medical profession. Just as a physically handicapped child uses a wheelchair to tell others that he or she is physically different from some other children, the mentally ill child's behaviors tell others that he or she is emotionally different and needs special assistance.

Over time and with a great deal of work from mental health advocates, mental illness has been accepted as a disability. However, the focus has been on symptoms or behaviors that are manifested from the disability rather than the disability itself. For example, a child who is unable to walk and who is bound to a wheelchair is seen much differently than a child with an attention deficit disorder (ADD), depression, or manic depression (bipolar disorder).

Over time, programs were developed that were based on the philosophy of System of Care values and principles and that resulted in the ability of professionals to look at these children with a greater understanding about the child's disability. People began to acknowledge that children with mental illnesses and emotional disorders should no longer carry unwanted stigmas that are not associated with other disabilities. These children are finally beginning to receive the proper treatment that they so desperately need.

The System of Care process brings together professionals from many of the health care disciplines who are involved with these children and their families. They form partnerships with the family and use strategies to establish common goals for the family's success. The System of Care process can be very successful and can be used by any of the helping disciplines, such as teaching, social work, nursing, psychology, and psychiatry.

In this chapter, I give my perspective on System of Care core values and principles. Some of the barriers that I have seen that hinder the process from being effective are identified. "My story" reflects some of the many experiences that my family has endured throughout the years.

Core Values and Principles

Family-Focused Child-Centered Services

One of the most important ideas that System of Care promotes is the provision of services for children and families with mental health needs, keeping the focus on the entire family and centering services around the child.

The previous way of providing services had been professionally driven: all services were provided according to the opinions and suggestions of the professionals involved. The professionals chose the services for the child without consulting the family. Although professionals have been trained and obtained professional degrees, their perspectives are not the only ones that should be considered. As a matter of fact, the perspectives of the child and family should drive the process in selecting and obtaining services. Many might ask how the child and family's perspectives can be beneficial to the process. After all, parents are not formally trained and supposedly do not know what is best. Professionals have attended universities and have studied many years to obtain the knowledge that they possess in working with mental health issues.

However, the child and family also have studied long and hard. These families have something that no one else possesses: experiences. The saying that "experience is the best teacher" rings clearly in many cases. Although professionals in mental health agencies, the school system, the juvenile justice system, and other health care agencies are more familiar with the services that they offer, children and families know what they need. After all, families live in their child's world every day. They have managed their lives many times with little or no resources. Many times, families handle situations for years before professionals intervene. All may agree that appropriate choices are difficult to make when families face extreme circumstances; somehow, someway, they are able to survive and keep their families together.

The System of Care philosophy acknowledges that the families are the experts about their lives. Not only are the needs of the identified person who qualifies for services acknowledged, but also the needs of the entire family are addressed. The plan that is developed with System of Care values always remains flexible. The plan fits the child and family—not the agendas of the professionals or the agencies.

Focus on the Strengths

One of the greatest principles of System of Care is that services are identified and offered based on the strengths of the child and family. Usually when the traditional system comes into the lives of families with mental health issues, the focus is on what is going wrong. The question remains, "How can we fix the problem?" Decisions are often made without the valuable information that children and families can bring to the table. In the old way of service delivery, a mental health professional or other service provider interviews a family, discusses the case with other professionals from agencies involved with the family, and then returns to the office to write a plan of care. This care plan is expected to meet the child's needs and to be well received and carried out by the family. However, we know from the history of mental health services that the plan is often not appropriate for the child and family and that the child does not improve. In fact, many times, the family did not or could not adhere to the recommendations written in the care plan and thus were considered "noncompliant" by the professionals.

The System of Care approach examines the strengths that are already present within a family before planning and interventions begin. Because the traditional system does not recognize these strengths does not mean that they are not there. Sometimes the family is also surprised at its own strengths because its strengths have never been explored. Over time and during the many struggles that families experience while living with a child with a mental illness, something brings these families through great hardships. It is their strengths! The key is not just to identify the strengths of the children and families, but to use these strengths in order to solve problems when implementing the plan. Acknowledging the strengths of the child and family and the strengths of the system offers the team players more options in preparing a more successful plan.

A Child and Family Team

The ideal in the system of care planning is for all persons involved in a family's services, and the natural supports of that family, to come around the table together at one time and share. This prevents the child and family from attending so many meetings and from presenting the same information many times. This even helps professionals to understand each other better and to work smoothly together, acknowledging the strengths of the child and the family and the strengths of the system. This offers the collaborative team more options in preparing a successful plan. However, we must always remember to keep the child and family first!

Also, the System of Care philosophy understands that the families are the experts of their lives. Not only are the needs of the identified person who qualifies for services acknowledged, but also the needs of the entire family. The plan that is developed with System of Care values always remains flexible. The plan fits the child and family, not vice versa. The partners understand that at any given time the child and family can request that the team come back together if the plan is not working. In the traditional service delivery system of the past, plans were considered constant. The child and family had to adapt to the plan. Previously, services were selected from a narrow list in the continuum of care. Usually these lists only consisted of formal supports. Natural support systems were not included in the care plan.

A successful plan depends on the community offering a wide range of services that meet the needs of children and families. Services should be individualized and not confined to traditional treatment, thus encouraging the team to investigate many ways of meeting a family's needs. Creativity is used to develop a plan that is unique and individual. Often the plans are considered "out of the box." For example, the faith community is an extremely valuable resource when developing care plans, as this community resource can be a source for personal assistance and support, based on friendships. Plans can also include art, recreation, and music as strategies to build on the strengths of children with mental health challenges.

Working in Partnerships

Another exciting component in the System of Care process is recognizing the child and family as partners with the professionals and community resources. Families are no longer inside the circle being bombarded with services, but they have now joined the circle. Families are no longer treated as "cases" to be studied. They are not a problem to be fixed. The child and family emerge as valuable members of the team, offering insights that are crucial to their plan of care.

The System of Care process encourages cross-agency coordination because the professionals from several disciplines and agencies who are involved with the family are meeting together regularly. Consequently, professionals are better able to communicate and share information that is beneficial to the success of the child and family. Families believe that when everyone works together, barriers such as "turf" issues (agencies concerned about only their own specific needs) are broken down. This process allows agencies to put aside their own agendas in order to understand better how to meet the needs of the child and family and all concerned. It is usually the families that lead agencies to this threshold because it is through the families that the collaboration has occurred and all begin to work together. Although agencies still have guidelines and mandates that they must follow, professionals are able to consider the perspectives of others who are seated around the table in order to work toward a common goal, which is to improve the quality of life for the child and family.

Cultural Competence

Finally, cultural competence is the foundation on which System of Care rests. Most people feel that they are culturally competent if they have friends of another race or culture. Still others feel culturally competent if they know about people from other countries or even neighborhoods. However, culture means more than ethnicity, place of origin, or even language. Culture extends beyond the perimeters of geographic areas. Cultural competence cannot be achieved by reading books. It is a lifestyle. It is a way of interacting with others. Cultural competence is not something you learn. It is something that you experience.

Within a System of Care framework, in order to become culturally competent, the mind is opened to explore other ways of thinking that must be considered. Do we understand the culture of a family with a blind child or a single-parent household? Do we understand the culture of a family that has experienced a family member with a drug addiction? Have we considered that people who live in poverty have a culture of their own? What about a university or a service agency? Are there different cultures among different professions, different service agencies, and institutions?

Looking closely at cultural competence, we find that it is not merely about acknowledging people who are different from ourselves; it is also about changing and broadening our frames of reference to respect these differences. We can then use these differences to influence the decisions that are made in developing a plan for the delivery of services to children and families.

Cultural competence means that one person has only one voice. One person cannot speak for an entire race or for a group of people with similar interests. In addition, one parent who has a child with mental health challenges cannot speak for all families who have a child with a similar condition. Even if their situations are similar, many factors determine their different perspectives. Factors that influence different perspectives are how people were raised, their personal experiences, and their resources. These different factors all play a role in how families respond to circumstances and crises. When professionals isolate a family and stereotype and use them to determine the prognosis for similar families, then the system fails the family who is seeking help. Always remember that one parent only carries one voice and speaks from one perspective. Remember, too, that each family brings its own unique and refreshing perspective to the healing process.

Barriers to the System of Care Process

Barriers to establishing a System of Care process must be explored if this journey is to be completed. Any time different ways of conducting business or doing things are introduced to a community, opposition and resistance to change usually exist. Changing attitudes is not easy. The professionals, the agencies where they work, and even the families must release the past and embrace the future. They must give up what is familiar for something that they have never experienced. Sometimes it is easier to hold on to what you know, even if you know that it is not working. Thus, we are challenged with the old saying that "a bird in the hand is better than two in the bush." People feel safer with the familiar because they do not know what the future holds.

Establishing a trusting relationship between parents and professionals may be difficult because of the past experiences of both. Many times, staff members do not feel comfortable discussing a family's circumstances in front of the family. However, they do not have a problem sharing information about the family with other professionals. Often families do not trust providers because of many of their past experiences. They have not experienced providers who are willing to accept families as partners. Therefore, family/professional relationships may begin on a negative note because of mistrust. Often families themselves do not recognize all of the strengths that they can bring to the table. The relationship of trust is established only through time and by sharing experiences.

System of Care is not a short-term process that quickly fixes the mental health delivery system, and therefore, it can be difficult to implement. Professionals and family members must continue returning to the table, even when all looks hopeless. When there is little or no success, the question must always be, "What is the next strategy?" The answer should never be, "We've done all we can do." Rather, the team should consider how to change the plan because the previous plan is not working.

Realistically, sometimes the limit on time and resources makes success extremely difficult. However, System of Care presents the team with an ideal. System of Care promotes looking outside of traditional funding sources and community resources. For instance, if funds are not available to pay for an activity for a child, is it possible that it could be provided through a church or a recreation center for little or no cost?

One of the greatest ideals of System of Care is to address barriers creatively and nontraditionally. There are many barriers that continue to rank at the top of the list. Child care and transportation must always be considered when families are expected to be active members of the System of Care process. These two issues play a major role as to why family involvement continues to be one of the greatest struggles in implementing System of Care. Frequently, parents are unable to take time from work or their families to be involved in outside activities that take them away from their homes. Consequently, there are many levels of family involvement and participation. Families should be valued at whatever level they are able to participate.

Many other barriers should be examined. However, I believe that there are two that need special consideration and discussion. They are (1) the stigma of living with a mental health diagnosis, and (2) the understanding of the dynamics of a specific mental illness.

The world for a child who is mentally disabled is completely different from other disabilities. First, having a child with mental illness automatically labels the entire family as dysfunctional. This labeling usually does not happen to families whose children have physical disabilities. Attitudes from professionals and, yes, even other family members, begin to take a completely different direction once the diagnosis is known. Many families do not seek help because of the stigma that is associated with a mental illness.

For example, one situation occurred when my daughter was in the hospital. Each day I would meet with the social worker to discuss my daughter's progress. We always met in the worker's office for privacy. On one particular meeting, I happened to mention that I, too, was diagnosed as being manic depressive. The next day the social worker staged a completely dramatic scene in order to prop the door open to her office while we met. It was as if she was following a script. Suddenly she was afraid of me. The only thing that had changed was the additional information. That changed her perception of me as a person. Now I was diagnosed with a mental illness. How can a social worker do her job effectively if she is afraid of people and their circumstances? It may not be only the illness that she fears.

The community's perception of mental illness has evoked all kinds of negative images even before the Columbine tragedy. These preconceived images cause stigmas that follow families throughout their lives. Prejudices appear in many forms. They also create roadblocks that prevent families from having successful careers. Mental health illness challenges a person's success in many areas of his or her life.

Understanding the illness itself is one of the most difficult tasks for both professionals and family members. Professionals who have intensely studied mental illness still do not have a clear understanding of all of the manifestations of the illness, much less the causes. Just as a psychiatrist expects the patient to take medicines because they have been prescribed, so does a social worker expect parents to provide discipline and structure as a normal part of the family routine. Many psychiatrists cannot accept that just because a medicine has worked for one child, it does not mean it will work for all. It is important for psychiatrists to understand that it takes time for children to overcome their fears of taking medicine when there has previously been an allergic reaction to a medication. The same may be said for a social worker who says, "You're enabling that child. You let her manipulate you too much." That may be true. However, what parent does not give into their child on occasion? Why should my situation be any different just because you, the professional, came into my family and looked at it under a microscope? Many times parents of children with mental illness move past power struggles and choose their battles. It is not as important to exercise authority as it is to help a child complete a task. Discipline has to occur at the appropriate time when the child is able to receive and benefit from it. How do you use a system of rewards and consequences in a family when every day seems to be a consequence within itself? In many service delivery systems, families are lumped together, using the same strategy for each family, never listening to the family as a guide for what it needs. System of Care provides a collaborative team that encourages professionals and families to work together to overcome barriers and to become partners in successfully developing productive communities for children suffering from a severe emotional disturbance.

My Story

- This concept of family-professional partnership as told by the Family Story is used frequently by those involved in System of Care who seek to better understand children and families and their mental health challenges.
- This concept connects families who experience these challenges, but it is the beginning of their uniqueness.
- The story exposes the many similarities of stigma, hardships, preconceived generalities, and feelings of guilt, hurt, and shame.
- The list goes on and on. However, it is also in these stories that the richness of each family's individuality can be found.

My story could begin with my birth because I am diagnosed with bipolar disorder, or it could begin with my deceased husband, whose diagnosis was never made. He later self-medicated with street drugs. The story could begin with my oldest daughter, Miss C, whose needs were never really addressed and who eventually left traditional school at 16 years old. Her diagnosis to this day is still unclear, but for the sake of time, we begin the story with Miss M, my youngest daughter who was the catalyst for my family's connection with the System of Care process in my community.

A few months after my husband's death, M, 5 years old, began to experience extreme depression and suicidal tendencies. At the time, I was not sure why my child was acting this way. I felt that she had become someone whom I had never met. All I knew was that this "new" addition to our family was very unhappy. She was increasingly unable to follow the simplest request and made that very clear through abusive language and physical outbursts. Once M began school, the experience turned into a nightmare. By this time, she was suicidal and was beating her head against the wall everyday. Initially, I was told that the M I knew at home was completely different from the one at school.

The next phase was the "psychological testing" stage. The school decided that psychological testing would determine how to serve M. In other words, the school had no problems using a biased test to decide whether my child qualified for special services or supports that the school may be able to provide.

Because my husband had recently died, M's teacher told me that I was setting a bad example for my daughter by grieving too long. She went on to say that my daughter needed things to get back to normal and that once that happened she would be fine. Needless to say, the teacher's perspective of the grieving process did not help my family heal; things then got worse. Although M's experiences at school worsened, the school administration never informed me. Three months passed, as I waited to hear from the school about the testing and any support that they would be able to offer M.

Finally, I did hear from the school, but it was not from her teacher, the principal, or even the counselor. I heard from the janitor, whom I knew from church. One day, she pulled me aside and told me horror stories about my child's experiences at school. I could not believe what I heard. Apparently, on several occasions, M had been missing from the playground. She would run away, and they could not find her. The school would have to organize a search party to look for her. I was also told that she would have intensive crying episodes. She would literally be "dragged" down hallways kicking and screaming. She was always somewhere other than her classroom. I spoke with the principal, trying to understand why he withheld this information from me.

It was at this point that we entered the next stage, which was "blame the parent." I was told that M had a severe behavioral problem and that I needed to discipline her more at home. Meanwhile, at home, M did not want to attend school at all. The morning ritual consisted of me dragging her from bed. Next I would drag her into the bathroom. Finally, I would drag her to the bus and run quickly back into the house. I would watch from the window in tears. She would beat on the bus door and try to push the door open to get off.

The morning ritual eventually became so painful that I finally gave up. I decided that I needed to protect my daughter both physically and emotionally. At this point, trust was a real issue for me, particularly related to the school, and thus, I decided that until I found a solution, I would keep her at home with me.

After approximately 2 weeks, a social worker from the school called and asked how she could help. She came to my home, and I began to confide in her. I was desperate for help. We discussed the fact that my furnace was broken and that I was low on food. I explained that I had been going through financial troubles since my husband had died. My daughter's problem was causing even more problems because I was unable to work. I did not know that all of this information would soon be used against me. Within 1 week, I received papers stating that I was in violation of truancy and was not properly providing for my family. I was devastated.

The next place I turned to was mental health. My daughter was diagnosed rather quickly as ADHD (Attention Deficit Hyperactivity Disorder). She was then prescribed Ritalin. I told them that M was having side-effects from the medication and that we needed to do something different. I was told with great authority and confidence that M had not been on the medication long enough to make an evaluation. Just keep on it; they said that she would be fine. It was not until I showed up in their waiting room with M foaming at the mouth that they finally listened. They called 911, and we were off to seek medical assistance.

Medication was a stressful issue for M for many years. Nothing seemed to work. Psychiatrists continued to tell me, "Let's just wait and see." Each time I would explain that the medication was making things worse for my daughter. Finally, they just labeled me "noncompliant." Even after one medication caused M to practically loose her mind and she pulled my rear view mirror completely from my windshield, they still would not acknowledge that I was the expert about my child and her response to the medication.

The problematic journey has continued for many years. Obtaining M's education has been the most difficult task. Year after year she has been denied access to the proper strategy and skills that would support her success in school. She has not been taught the necessary skills that she needs to make a smooth transition into adulthood.

With the process of System of Care and its values and principles, which were being incorporated into our community service systems, we have made great strides in our community to begin to introduce a new way of providing mental health care to children and adolescents. Parents and professionals have sat around the table together. I have met with people who are directly involved with M, and we have developed great plans that seemed appropriate for her. Implementation has been our downfall.

I recognized that some of my child's needs are different from the services that the system provides. These differences make her a special needs child. I will never understand why that concept is so hard to grasp. I know that it takes time and money to institute the System of Care process properly. What better way is there to spend time and money than on someone so "special?"

M is now 16 and has recently left school to be enrolled in vocational rehabilitation. We finally realized that the traditional school could not meet her needs. We decided that it was best for her to obtain some skills that would help her to be able to function in the workplace and in her community.

Even though M went through so many difficult times in school, she never gave up. When the decision was made for her to leave school, she cried. When a school professional asked what the school could provide for her, she replied, "an education."

I could tell you many stories that qualify us (M and me) for the "I can't believe they didn't lose their mind" award. However, I will leave you with only one other experience.

J is my middle child who never presented any real problems until her 11th-grade year. She became very depressed and was diagnosed with major depression and anxiety. She was homeschooled for the latter part of that year. However, this plan did not work well for J. She was only able to earn two credits for the year. The homeschool plan involved a homeschool teacher who came to our home 3 hours a week. The teacher was new to J, and therefore, bonding, which takes time, was necessary. Also, the fact that J had no contact with her previous classroom teachers left her feeling disconnected and unable to understand much of her school work. She was homeschooled for only the last 8 weeks of the school year. She had earned a B+ in her honors US History class. However, she did not receive credits for this class because the homeschool teacher and the classroom teacher did not communicate well enough to ensure that J was prepared for her final exam in that class. In the final analysis, there was nothing we could do. She did not take her exam. Thus, J is now retaking this class. The summer between her junior and senior years was very difficult for J, causing her senior year to begin with a lot of stress and anxiety.

However, because of the training and support that I received in System of Care, I called a team meeting. The team met and developed a plan. Unfortunately, J was placed on a medication that was producing some significant side effects. She was too tired to get up in the morning for school. She began to miss too many days of school. I spoke with her psychiatrist on her next visit and asked about hospitalization to stabilize her medication. She met with J and agreed to that step. She did, however, say that she would place her in a short-term treatment facility while she looked for a long-term facility. I was very concerned and told her that I felt that my daughter did not need long-term treatment. We agreed to short-term treatment, and she was hospitalized for what I thought would be a short-term medication stabilization period.

Three days later, when talking to the attending psychiatrist, I was told that J had been involuntarily committed and that they were seeking a long-term treatment facility. I was told that the staff had met on three different occasions and decided that this was the best plan. I was also told that there was disturbing information in J's record from her last meeting with her psychiatrist. This information is why she was involuntarily committed. The attending psychiatrist looked me straight in the eye and said, "There is nothing you can do."

Immediately, I searched my mind to retrieve information from System of Care trainings, workshops, and its core values and principles. I remembered that you should never go to meetings alone. Also, it is imperative to read any and all paperwork thoroughly. Several years ago I would have condemned myself and become extremely stressed. However, this time I felt confident that this situation would be resolved.

First, I asked the psychiatrist how information could be in J's record that would support this kind of action without her legal guardian, in this case, her mother, being notified. Second, I asked whether my daughter participated in the meetings. I was told that that was not "the way they do things here." I told the psychiatrist that the plan could not be comprehensive if a child and family members were not present. Finally, I asked whether she had ever heard of System of Care and that if she had not I had some information that I could share.

After arriving home that afternoon, the only thing that I could think of was the look on my daughter's face as I left her at the hospital. She was terrified! I had failed her. However, I picked myself up and called another family member from a community support group for families of children with mental health challenges. I also called professionals who had supported me in the past. After I spoke with them, not only did I feel better, but also we had developed a plan of our own. Because of my supports, I was able to get my daughter discharged the very next day. A mentor was found to help her with her senior year tasks and class work. Through my involvement with training in System of Care and my work with the community in adopting System of Care as the way to provide services to families and children with complex needs, I had acquired some of the skills and knew some people who could help us.

The System of Care process undoubtedly came straight from heaven. It has supported my family through many difficult times. It has taught us many important strategies and skills that have not only helped us but that we will be able to use to help others.

At this point in time, amazingly, all three of my girls are coping with their situations and I am able to work part time. Even though M has not yet successfully completed high school, she is 16 years old and is involved in a statewide organization for behaviorally challenged youth. Each child has developed skills in making presentations and is willing to tell her story so that other families, youth, and professionals can better understand the horrific challenges that she has faced. The children have been invited to speak all over the country. They train professionals and families to support children and families better and to understand their needs. C is 22 years old and has used an alternative school to complete her high school education and is in college training to be a physician's assistant. J is an honor student in high school and plans to attend college and study psychology.

The breadth of my family's experience through the process of System of Care has made us an asset not only to other families who face mental health challenges but also to the effective delivery of services in my local community.

What Have I Gained?

It was one night after teaching the System of Care interdisciplinary course at the university that I was faced with this question: "Is it really worth it?" This was my third year of teaching the course with the team of faculty members, and over time, we had become a teaching "team." My daughter had been invited to share her experiences in the class so that the students who are in college can learn how to be effective "helpers" in education, social work, nursing, psychology, recreation, or counseling.

On our way home, my daughter turned to me and said, "Momma, there were students, who sighed and rolled their eyes every time you spoke. They didn't do that when the professionals spoke." She asked me why I continue to tell people about our personal life. She said, "They don't really believe what we tell them anyway. They think we make up all of this stuff. They think we're a joke."

As I held back the tears, I told her that if sharing our experiences connects with only one student and better equips that one student to work with families that face mental health challenges, it is worth it. I explained to her how hard it is to co-teach a class with professors at the university level. At each class, I use my pain as my degree and my experience as my philosophy and theory. Yes. Sometimes I am only seen as the lady with the "sob story." However, I know that the story is real and that the truth will never go out and come back void. Thus, I thank God for allowing my family to be involved in such a life-changing process. I am supported by other families and professionals who acknowledge my family's strengths. I have recognized the need for the family perspective to be heard at the local, state, and national levels. Families are now members of collaborative committees and participate at all levels of decision making in the state's mental health system. Family members are participating in teaching college courses and training other professionals.

System of Care offers opportunities for building effective communities. Some say we cannot afford to implement System of Care. Those of us who have benefited from this process say, "We cannot afford *not* to."

Another Parent's Perspective: Living with a Child with Serious Emotional Disturbance

LIBBY JONES

The only thing that I really feel needs to be said is our children, the children with serious emotional disturbance, truly are the forgotten children. Our children are dying. The schools, court counselors, and social workers try. They have the knowledge, but they have not lived what we have lived. They have not lived with a child who cries all night and does not know why. They have not lived with the school calling every day saying, "Come get your child." We truly feel that professionals only see our children as "behaviors"—our children are more than that. They are beautiful, loving children who are hurting inside where no one can see. Because of that, people tend to label them as bad and forget about them. As parents, we feel so often that schools and other agencies want our children to go away because they do not know how to deal with them. We feel that professionals think that our children "could control it or do better if they just tried." Then we as parents are treated as if it is our fault or as if we caused it. Mental illness eats away at your soul. These children and families need so much love, support, and caring. Too often, that is the last thing they get. Instead they get blamed.

If you had held a 10-year-old boy in your arms as he cried all night because he just wanted to die and he said that no one liked him and all you can do is cry with him, you, too, would be angry at the "system." If you attend a meeting and your advocate asks the teacher to "tell me some strengths of this child" and the teacher looks you in the eyes and says (with the child sitting right there) that "this child has no strengths," you, too, would be angry.

If you sat in a meeting with the principal of your child's high school and begged him with tears streaming down your face to please find him a buddy or mentor or just another student to show him around and support him and the principal said, "If I do it for one, I have to do it for all," you, too, would be angry. (My response to him was that not all children need mentoring, just this one, and he still refused.) When I found out several months later, in the school newspaper, that there was a "buddy" program in which they matched kids with kids who were having difficulty and my child was denied this opportunity, I was mad and you, too, would be mad.

When your child is kicked out of school and blamed for something horrendous that he did not do and you know that the suspension could have been avoided if only school officials had taken the time to get to know him, you, too, would be angry.

When your son comes home every day and tells you that students pushed his chair out from under him as he goes to sit down, making him fall to the floor, while everyone laughs and the teacher says, "You need to toughen up," you, too, would be angry.

It seemed that no one really saw this young man who came to school every day. He had no friends and no one to eat lunch with or talk with at break. He was picked on and harassed, and was told that because his hands shook (a side effect of the medicine) and because he had no friends and was a loner, he might cause the next Columbine. How horrible for someone to give a young boy a label and send that message!

Still he went to school everyday. No one saw the child's strengths. He went to school each day to face such adversity—there is strength in that!

The greatest joy that I have had or the greatest satisfaction came when I was able to go to that principal (who had moved to another school) and I sat down to talk with him. I told him it was my time to talk. It was the summer, and my son had not been at his school for two years, as he had transferred to an alternative school, the middle college high school program. I told him that I felt like he had let my child down and that I felt sorry for him as a school leader because he did not take the time to get to know my son who is such a wonderful person. I told him how angry I had been when he had my son in a class in the 10th grade designed for kids who had not passed the 8th-grade competency test, although my son had passed in the 8th grade. When my son did not want to do the work in that class, the teacher and principal were angry. When my son said, "I already know this," they responded, "Then do it." They told us at a meeting that he did not know the math. They said that they did not feel that my son would make it and really needed to look at other options, such as a GED (graduate equivalency degree). I cannot tell you the pleasure I had when I showed this man my son's report card from the middle college program. It was wonderful! (Remember, my son was now in a different school and had the support of a team—the System of Care team.) I sat there and watched this grown man cry—not just tears in his eyes, but literally cry, with big crocodile tears! It felt great! All the anger over the years melted away. I felt sorry for this man—sorry that he had missed an opportunity to get to know such a beautiful person and sorry for him that he thought my son could not do this and then to realize not only could he, but he did. Most importantly, he did it without the help of this man because, you see, this man was afraid of the term "emotional" or mental illness. He was afraid of the diagnosis of bipolar disorder. You see, my son graduated with honors in all honors classes!! They said it could not be done, but he did it!

It is easy to forget what you do not like or do not understand. Most people do not like our kids. They do not understand them. Our families need so much support, and they need to know that they are not alone. The children need to know that someone cares for them and understands what they are going through. There are no magical answers, but knowing that someone cares makes a difference.

I used to be an angry parent (that is not to say I do not still get angry!), but now I believe in working collaboratively with professionals, instead of just getting mad at them. We all have to work together to make changes happen, instead of trying to do it alone. We have to acknowledge that we all have strengths and that we all have areas of weakness. That is the beauty of the team. No one has all of the answers, and no one should take all of the blame.

For so long, parents had to speak for their children. Now children are beginning to speak for themselves. We have had the youth come to speak at our class at the university. It began with the siblings of a brother or sister who suffered from an emotional disturbance; they came to a class called Interdisciplinary Practice: Systems of Care to talk about what it is like to live with a brother or sister who struggles so much. Then the youth who have mental health challenges came to talk about what they go through, having to deal with being different from their classmates. How powerful! It was wonderful that they were so open and honest!

My son came to a university class to talk. He was told that he could talk about whatever he wanted. He did not have to share if he did not want to—it was his choice. Of all the wonderful things that he said, the most touching was when one of the students asked him what helped him the most when he was struggling so hard with school or what made the biggest difference to him. Without blinking or pausing, he said, "My mom; she always believed in me. Even when no one else did, my mom was there to support me and believe in me."

The Collaborative

Professionals do not realize how hard it is for parents to come and be a part of this process. When we attend the meetings, we share our stories, and then we become vulnerable. We are naked and exposed. No one else is. The other team members, who are professionals, do not share their personal stories. It is hard! It is incredibly difficult to say, "My child was arrested for. . . ." Even if it happens in their lives, we do not hear about it. It is almost as if we, the families of children with emotional challenges, are on display, naked for all to see, which is painful. However, we have to do it for the sake of our children and for the other families. We cannot sit back and watch our children become the forgotten children.

Since System of Care came to our county, things are better now, but we have a long way to go. Families cannot do it alone. We—families, professionals, and politicians—need to work together to make change happen. As the saying goes on the posters for System of Care, "In a child's life, everyone is accountable." It can no longer be just the parent or just the teacher or just the therapist or just the social worker or just the doctor who work to make changes occur. We have to do it together!

Today, two of my children are grown (the third is just 18 years old, so to me he is not grown yet!) and have entered the adult world. My daughter is the youth coordinator for the statewide youth group Powerful Youth Friends United, which is part of the parent organization NC Families United. My son is now working and just bought a car so that he can go to college and not have to borrow our car to do it! I still cry when I remember what my children faced. I cry when I see all of the other youths hurting so much. However, I feel that there is hope—hope for a better system and a better future for children and their families. I see doors opening, but we have a long road ahead.

I pray the day will come when our children are no longer the forgotten children. I look forward to the day when people can understand that these children are hurting inside and do not know how to express what they are feeling.

I pray for a system that will embrace our children and will want to hold them when they cry and not try to force them to do things in a certain way, but to understand that we all are different and we all do things in different ways. Different is good. In System of Care, differences are respected and valued.

I pray for the families—not just the parents, but the siblings, too. Mental illness does not hurt only the child going through it; it hurts the parents and the siblings as well. All family members are affected by it. All families and children need support and love. Too many times the family, especially the siblings, of a child suffering from a mental illness is overlooked.

I pray for a time when our children—all children—are able to stay at home (no more residential treatment centers) with supports in place that provide services that are wrapped around them like a quilt on a snowy day so that they are comforted and supported and can be successful. Our children deserve to be at home or in school, safe and happy.

Children need to know that it is okay to have this challenge. However, we all need to strive for mental health and wellness for our children, our families, and ourselves!

Ms. Frederick Douglas and Ms. Libby Jones are parents of children with serious emotional disturbances. Both of them have participated in the implementation of System of Care values and principles through involvement with their own children, participating as parents on the community collaborative and its committees, leadership in training activities both in the community and in the university System of Care course, and in the development of a family support system for families with children with serious emotional disturbance.

II

Building a System of Care from the Professionals' Perspectives: An Approach to Caring for Clients and Families with Complex Needs

Chapter 5

The Implications of System of Care for Psychologists

Terri Lisabeth Shelton

Objectives

■ Discuss the many roles of the psychologist.
■ Describe how to design research that is consistent with System of Care values and principles.
■ Identify the benefits of strength-based approaches.
■ Discuss the challenges, barriers, and consequences of conducting strength-based assessments.
■ Explain why it is important to provide to youth and families information about the results of the research.
■ Identify models of helping.
■ Compare and contrast relational and participatory practices.

The philosophy of service delivery, variously called System of Care or family-centered care or sometimes wraparound, has been applied in a number of fields, including nursing, social work, education, and psychology as well as with a number of consumer groups (e.g., children with chronic illness or disabilities, children with learning disabilities, adult chronic illness such as cancer, children with serious emotional disturbance). This approach has implications for professionals of all disciplines, but there are particular implications for psychologists. These implications are as varied as the roles that psychologists may play. The purpose of this chapter is to review briefly how System of Care principles might be operationalized in various roles of psychologists, the empirical support for this approach in those contexts, as well as a discussion of the specific barriers that might make implementation difficult and ways in which these barriers might be addressed.

The Role of the Psychologist in Research

One of the roles that many psychologists have is as a researcher. Whether employed full time in a research position or as part of their job in a university or even in examining the efficacy of their work in direct private practice, many psychologists are engaged in the process of setting forth questions and hypotheses and testing these. How might the System of Care principles and tenets play out in research?

One obvious role is in the examination of the efficacy of System of Care approaches. As the field grapples with operationalizing the principles of System of Care, there is an ongoing need to examine the following: what is the impact of this type of service delivery? What are the key active ingredients of the approach that leads to improved outcomes? What is the cost-effectiveness of such an approach? Perhaps more importantly than the active investigation of System of Care efficacy is the import of this philosophy to the way in which research is conducted.

Conducting research consistent with System of Care fundamentally reflects basic good research practice, such as being open to what the data are truly telling you. However, doing this is not as easy as it may appear. A wonderful example of this relates to the perception of families reflected in two research articles published many years ago examining the impact of having a child with a disability on the family. In the first article, Wikler, Wasow, and Hatfield (1981) conducted a study examining the "chronic sorrow" that parents of children with mental retardation experience. Although most parents reported feelings of sadness, they also indicated that they had become much stronger individuals because of their experiences. The authors chose not to report these more positive findings because the result so contradicted their prior assumptions. They attributed these unanticipated findings to methodological problems. However, in an unprecedented move, the authors published another article two years later in which they re-analyzed the data. They reported that they "consider this initial dismissal to be another example of a pervasive stance adopted among professionals, in which problems instead of strengths and instances of coping are concentrated on" (Wikler, Wasow, & Hatfield, 1983, p. 313). The authors illustrated how important our assumptions are in everything psychologists do, including research. Because there is the perception that data that are published are "truth," having an open, strength-based, and more objective approach to what data may tell us is vitally important.

To their credit, these researchers asked a range of questions that resulted in a rich set of data even if they did not recognize the findings initially. Sometimes, however, these assumptions can even constrain the outcomes that are possible. As the saying goes, "Garbage in, garbage out." If a broad range of questions or measures or interviews that even tap strengths are omitted from a research study, then the results are partially determined before the first analysis begins.

Thus, how do we guard against these potential downfalls in research? System of Care principles provide an excellent map. First, whenever possible, research, particularly that about families and child outcomes, is greatly improved when families and youth participate in the design and interpretation of the data. Because of their unique perspective, families and youth add richness to the hypotheses that are generated, to the inclusion of strength-based measures, and in the actual interpretation of the results that is not possible when research is designed and psychologists alone analyze the data. Similarly, research that is conducted with other professional disciplines may be more likely to lead to a fuller understanding of any question.

As mentioned earlier, it is especially important to include measures or mechanisms in which strengths can be identified. As discussed later here, a growing number of measures tap strengths and a broader perspective. With regard to measuring family-centered care or System of Care approaches specifically, several assessment approaches are available, including the tools developed by Dunst and colleagues (e.g., Family Resource Scale, Support Functions Scale, Family Needs Scale, Family Support Scale, Inventory of Social Support, Family Functioning Style [Dunst, Trivette, & Deal, 1988b]; Helpgiving Practices Scale [Dunst, Trivette, & Hamby, 1996]; Family-Oriented Early Intervention Program Practices Scale [Dunst & Trivette, 1998]; A Measure of Processes of Care [King, Rosenbaum, & King, 1995]; and Enabling Practices Scale [Dempsey, 1995; Dempsey & Dunst, 2004]).

Another approach is to partner with families in the collection of data. Particularly with sensitive data, or when families who are receiving services receive them from the same providers that are conducting the research, families and youth may feel more comfortable in being open in their responses when the questions are asked by other families. This is particularly important when psychologists are involved in evaluating the program or services where the families or youth are being served. Again, this is just good practice, but particularly with families and youth who are consumers of services from the same professionals who are conducting the research, great care must be taken to ensure that families and youth are truly comfortable in choosing whether to participate. For example, it is important to separate service delivery from research requests as much as possible or to at least consider the dual messages that might be communicated (e.g., recruiting during an office visit or having the direct service provider be the one to ask for participation). Having family members review recruitment procedures and research protocols and written communication for length and potentially offensive language can go a long way to ensure that research is conducted in as family-centered a way as possible.

Another important practice applies after the research is completed. Are there mechanisms for youth and families to provide feedback about the research experience, and is this information incorporated into the remainder of the research? Although it seems elementary, it is important to share the results of the research with the youth and families who participate. Too often, many of the families and their children who participate in research never receive any information about the results. The checklist for conducting research (Table 5-1) demonstrates how the somewhat abstract principles of System of Care can be operationalized within this role of psychologist as researcher.

The Role of the Psychologist in Assessment

Another frequent role for psychologists is that of assessment, which may involve determining a diagnosis, establishing eligibility for services such as social security income (SSI) or educational placement and support, or evaluating progress on a treatment plan. This may be one of the most challenging roles to ensure that System of Care principles are truly being followed, particularly with regard to the use of strength-based approaches and partnering with families in gathering and interpreting the information.

One potential barrier to using strength-based approaches has to do with the very purpose of the assessment, which is usually the identi-

Table 5-1	Checklist for Research

- What are the ways in which families and youth collaborate with professionals in the design of the research?
- How do the research design and data analysis allow for a balanced approach, focusing on family and child strengths as well as needs?
- What steps are taken to ensure that families feel that they will not jeopardize the quality of services they receive if they do not wish to participate?
- What are the mechanisms for ensuring that consent forms are easy to understand and are translated into other languages or media as needed?
- If a number of research studies are being conducted in one agency or clinic, what are the mechanisms for ensuring that families are not overwhelmed with multiple requests?
- What are the mechanisms for ensuring that the results of the research are communicated and explained to the families and youth who participated?
- How do families provide feedback to the researchers on their perceptions as participants?

Adapted from Shelton and Stepanek (1994).

fication and description of a problem. Moreover, authorization and payment for mental health services, whether Medicaid or third-party payers, are frequently dependent on the severity of a child's needs. In fact, identifying a child's strengths can make it more difficult to access services in some situations.

Another potential barrier is the traditional deficit-based approach taken in many professional training programs. Although some practices are changing, many psychologists trained in assessment follow what Tallent (1958) referred to as the "prosecuting attorney brief" (p. 243). Clearly, services are not provided when there is an absence of a problem. In addition, clear documentation of the problem is necessary and certainly helpful when this information links with research on prognosis, course, and empirically supportive treatments. However, at times, the picture becomes imbalanced. Focusing solely on the presenting problem is not only inaccurate but can become a self-fulfilling prophecy and often undermines the hope and motivation that is key to turning that assessment's findings into a successful intervention for the child, his or her family, and providers (Kashdan et al., 2002).

Another challenge has to do with the availability of methodologically sound strength-based measures. Although increasing numbers of options are available—for example, subscales that tap positive behaviors on rating scales, such as the Behavior Assessment System for Children (BASC-2) (Reynolds & Kamphaus, 2004); measures directly devoted to strengths, such as the Behavioral and Emotional Rating Scale (Epstein, 1999); and the Child and Adolescent Strengths Assessment (Lyons, Uziel-Miller, Reyes, & Sokol, 2000)—professionals still have fewer options and historically less training on techniques to identify child and family strengths.

Even when methods are available, another potential barrier to conducting assessment in a System of Care way has to do with the degree to which psychologists believe in the veracity of the family's report. Interviewing parents about their perceptions or having them complete rating scales automatically leads to the question of whether or how to include parental report. In much the same way as the research study cited previously, some psychologists assume that parents cannot be reliable reporters. Interestingly, you will hear as many statements about families being in denial and underestimating a problem as those citing families for maximizing and shopping for a diagnosis. However, when studies have been conducted on the validity of parent report, these assumptions are challenged. For example, in examining the predictive validity of parent versus professional assessment of a child's developmental levels, a study conducted almost four decades ago (Honzik, Hutchings, & Burnip, 1965) found that families' reports had greater predictive validity of a child's future level of developmental functioning than that of professionals. The interpretation is that families recognize emerging skills, which form the foundation for future development. Because most best practices on assessment recommend multi-method, multi-informant approaches (e.g., Anastopoulos & Shelton, 2001), many psychologists will find themselves in the position of soliciting and interpreting feedback from families. Questioning the veracity of their report and denigrating the results when they are different from that of professionals does not honor the unique perspective of families makes getting a comprehensive picture more difficult and in many instances will make it more difficult to develop the type of collaborative partnership between the family and professional that will be needed to effect real change.

There are many advantages, however, to trying to overcome these barriers. With regard to strength-based assessment, including strengths will provide a more balanced and accurate picture than focusing on deficits alone. Second, it is definitely more motivating and provides a glimpse for all involved as to what is possible as an outcome. Third, and perhaps most important, it provides important clues for intervention. Assessment should not be an end in and of itself. It is supposed to lead to a greater understanding of the presenting issues and access to services. However, particularly with regard to children and youth with serious emotional disturbances, identifying strengths and ascertaining when and under what circumstances they occur despite the serious emotional challenges provide important information on direction for intervention. Finally, there is accumulating evidence that strength-based approaches are not only more effective than traditional pathology-driven interventions (Burns, Goldman, Faw, & Burchard, 1999; Dunst, Trivette, & Deal, 1994), but that they are more acceptable to children, families, and teachers (e.g., Jones, Eyberg, Adams, & Boggs, 1998; Miller & Kelley, 1992; Power, Hess, & Bennett, 1995; Tarnowski, Simonian, Park, & Bekeny, 1992). It is a key part of recognizing and acknowledging the client's competencies. As is outlined later with regard to treatment, assuming client competencies, particularly with regard to their ability to use these assets in addressing the problem, is vitally important.

How can a psychologist reflect the philosophy of System of Care in assessment? One way to do this is through functional behavioral assessment. Most psychologists are familiar with functional behavioral assessment, an approach required under certain conditions of the Individuals with Disabilities Education Act (IDEA). Although this approach is applied primarily to problem or target behaviors (e.g., ABCs: antecedents, behavior, consequences), it can be easily applied to identifying the important circumstances that elicit and support strengths in the child and/or the family (discussed later). Imagine how much more successful an intervention would be if the intervention were based not only on knowledge of the antecedents and consequences of the problem behavior but also on the antecedents and consequences of strengths (Table 5-2).

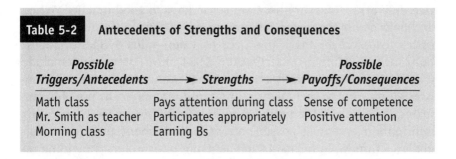

Table 5-2	Antecedents of Strengths and Consequences	
Possible Triggers/Antecedents ⟶	*Strengths* ⟶	*Possible Payoffs/Consequences*
Math class	Pays attention during class	Sense of competence
Mr. Smith as teacher	Participates appropriately	Positive attention
Morning class	Earning Bs	

The Center for Effective Collaboration and Practice has a mini web-site focusing on functional behavioral assessment (e.g., http://www.air.org/cecp/fba/default.htm), and many of the helpful appendices can be applied with strengths as well as problems (e.g., Behavior Pathway Charts).

Another way to employ System of Care principles is in the choice of techniques used in assessment. As mentioned, a growing number of methodologically sound instruments permit an assessment of strengths—some that simultaneously permit identification of concerns (e.g., BASC-2: Reynolds & Kamphaus, 2004). However, it is important for psychologists to be skilled in other strength-based techniques, such as interviews or strength-based discoveries. Sometimes, it is very difficult for families and children to identify their strengths. They have typically had little experience in identifying strengths in the therapeutic process and may have lost touch with those strengths as a function of struggling with the problem that brought them into contact with professionals. This is not sufficient justification to abandon strength-based approaches, but rather, the psychologist may have to elicit strength-based observations from others (e.g., friends, teacher, extended family) or offer their own observations. However, the psychologist must consistently move this question back to the family and child and not rely only on the observations of others for the empowering aspects of strength-based assessment to occur.

As mentioned earlier, assessment is not an end in and of itself. An assessment process is only as good as the way that assessment is used and a big part of that is how results are communicated. The feedback session becomes the link between the assessment process and the beginning of a collaborative treatment planning and implementation—if not with you the psychologist, then with another professional. How this feedback is provided is crucial. This is especially evident when one reviews the research on parental satisfaction with feedback. It is surprising to see how dissatisfied most families are with this part of service delivery. However, there are some keys to good practice. When one looks across the research literature, several practices are associated with successful feedback practices (Anastopoulos & Shelton, 2001; Cunningham, Morgan, & McGucken, 1984). Key components include scheduling adequate time, ensuring that families' questions are answered, offering to include as many family members as possible, ensuring that the child is provided with information as well, providing information as soon as possible after the assessment, providing information in multiple formats such as using interpreters, providing information on audio, and using outlines to accompany the report.

Brenner (2003) elaborated on English's (2000) recommendations to (1) eliminate jargon, (2) focus on referral questions, (3) individualize assessment reports, (4) emphasize client strengths, and (5) write concrete recommendations. The assessment process can also provide an opportunity to build relationships with consumers by formulating referral questions, and through the manner, feedback is provided. According to Brenner (2003), collaborative approaches to providing feedback enhance relationships and increase the utility of assessments by increasing consumers' ability to understand and use assessment findings. Another suggestion is to gather feedback about the quality of the assessment or how the diagnosis was delivered. This enables psychologists to improve the quality and accuracy of assessments continually (Lanyon, 1972), which is consistent with most approaches to quality management, as well as with the Boulder model of clinical psychology (i.e., scientist–practitioner role in psychology), which encourages psychologists to use research to guide clinical practice. However, psychologists cannot assume that consumers will comment on the quality without some prompting. Brenner (2003) suggested using some of the same methods used to assess consumer satisfaction in health care service delivery such as personal interviews, focus groups, and surveys (Savitz, 1999). Building this collaborative relationship during assessment and diagnosis is critical to the child and family's willingness to enter into a collaborative partnership during treatment. However, System of Care principles must also be present in treatment and care coordination if the benefits are to continue throughout the therapeutic process.

The Role of the Psychologist in Treatment and Care Coordination

In this role, the System of Care principle of collaboration and partnership with youth and families is paramount. Across multiple fields, including developmental disabilities, early intervention, and pediatrics, research supports that best practice and effective mental health services require successful partnerships among youth, families, and their service providers. Defined as working together or joining in the pursuit of a common goal (DeChillo, 1993), these collaborative partnerships reflect a shift from viewing the family as the source of the problem to making the family the focus of therapy or another "service provider," to viewing the family as a fully participating partner in the design delivery and evaluation of care (DeChillo, Koren, & Schultze, 1994; Dunst, Johanson, Trivette, & Hamby, 1991; Shelton & Stepanek, 1994). Families who are respected members of their child's treatment team report increased satisfaction with services. Moreover, collaborative treatment planning is related to both improved service coordination and to addressing children's needs successfully (Koren et al., 1997; Rosenblatt, 1996). It is paramount to providing culturally responsive treatment, another key principle of System of Care (Dunst, Trivette, Davis, & Cornwell, 1988a; Hernandez, Isaacs, Nesman, & Burns, 1998; Hodges, Nesman, & Hernandez, 1999). Finally, it is the primary vehicle for developing interventions that truly reflect the family's priorities, values, and hopes for their child and "satisfies an ethical obligation to parents and families in our society" (Heflinger, 1995, p. 6).

As with the other roles discussed, there are barriers to ensuring that System of Care principles are reflected in how the psychologist operates in therapy or intervention. One powerful barrier is the assumption that help-giving is always helpful. In an extensive series of systematic studies, Dunst et al. (1988a, 1991, 2002) and Dunst and Trivette (1996, 1998) have identified the ways in which certain behaviors on the part of help-givers can actually lead to harmful consequences. Most of these nonhelpful behaviors relate to the quality of the relationship between client and professional and the assumptions that the professional makes about the client's fault for the "problem" and his or her capability for participating in the solution. Help-giving is likely to have harmful consequences such as undermining efficacy and encouraging dependency when professionals take relative or absolute control over the process, if they convey that the client is inferior or incompetent, such as not being capable of participating in developing treatment priorities, when they prevent or interfere with the acquisition of new competencies such as advocating directly for their child among others (Dunst et al., 1988b, 1994).

This view of the client is somewhat understandable. As Merton, Merton, and Barber (1983) noted, "(Because) the professional consulted when the client needs help, may never (have) seen the client in a state of general well-being, therefore (he or she) can have only an indirect sense of the client's capabilities and strengths. This limited perspective reinforces the already ingrained tendency for the professional to exercise paternalistic authority" (p. 21). Nevertheless, as with assessment, it is not an accurate view and perhaps more importantly does not lead to the type of outcomes that both consumers and professionals desire. As outlined in the discussion of assessment, strength-based approaches are key.

Another barrier is the perception that this type of relationship is only possible with "certain kinds of clients." Too often psychologists report that System of Care is fine with some families but not with the ones that they see. When questioned, they usually report what they see as characteristics that preclude families and children from participating as true partners. One example is when families are overwhelmed, such as in the middle of a crisis or at the time of diagnosis. At these times, families will sometimes ask professionals to take charge or to advise them on the course of action. Whatever the reason, psychologists cannot use one situation to lessen what should be a commitment to building the capacity of the clients they serve.

Thus, how can treatment or intervention be delivered in a way that is consistent with System of Care philosophy? First and foremost is valuing and supporting a true collaboration in all aspects of the treatment process. Taking the previous example of a family or client in crisis, there are ways in which family preferences can be elicited as part of crisis planning. Crisis intervention preferences can be discussed when the crisis is not occurring. Several states even have legislation that permits this to be on record, and it is the responsibility of the psychologists and other professionals to inquire as to whether these preferences have been declared.

Another is to meet the family where it is at any given step. Even if balance between professionally driven and family-driven processes might momentarily shift toward professionals, System of Care practice expects that the psychologist continues to offer opportunities to share decision making at whatever level is comfortable for the family and to revisit this once the crisis has past.

System of Care and family-centered care does not mean that there is no role for the psychologist. It is in the *partnership* that the best outcomes are realized, but how these priorities are established can either strengthen or weaken the partnership and can actually determine whether a treatment is implemented. Youth and families that have a key decision-making role in treatment decisions are more likely to be satisfied with services, and this satisfaction is related to a number of outcomes. More specifically, parental satisfaction with treatment has been shown to be related to changes in child compliance and to improved child outcomes according to parent behavior ratings (Brestan, Jacobs, Rayfield, & Eyberg, 1999). Adolescent satisfaction has also been associated with a change in parent-reported behavior problems, parental satisfaction, parental ratings of treatment progress, and therapist ratings of progress (Shapiro, Welker, & Jacobson, 1997). Parents' views of treatment and their view that the treatment being offered is compatible with their conceptualization of the problem are important predictors of treatment adherence and dropout (Hoza et al., 2000; Nock & Kazdin, 2001).

However, a growing body of research points to specific practices and assumptions that are more or less likely to lead to the type of collaborative partnerships consistent with System of Care. In one of the earliest investigations, Solomon (1976) found that the degree to which individuals see themselves as responsible for change and the degree to which true partnerships are developed were central components leading to empowerment. An extension of that line of thinking is found in the research on helping models by Brickman et al. (1982, 1983); Karuza, Zevon, Rabinowitz, and Brickman (1982); and Rabinowitz, Karuza, and Zevon (1984). They found that the degree to which the consumer is held responsible or blamed for causing problems, as well as the degree to which the consumer is viewed as being capable of participating in the solution, determines to whom the consumer attributes any change. These attributions, in turn, have differing behavioral outcomes and result in differing helping models.

Helping Models ⟶ *Self-Efficacy* ⟶ *Behavior Outcomes*

More specifically, as outlined in Table 5-3, when professionals adopt a blaming approach and see the consumer as responsible for the problem or need that they are bringing to the professional for assistance *and* they see the client as being totally responsible for remedying the situation (i.e., no partnership in solution), the result is understandably one of isolation, loneliness, or physical exhaustion. In the *moral model,* if the outcome of the consumer's efforts is good, the consumer is likely to attribute efficacy to himself or herself. However, if the outcome is not good, the consumer is also likely to attribute the failure to himself or herself.

In the traditional *medical model,* the assumption is that consumers are not responsible for the problem or need, but neither are they responsible or capable of participating in the solution. As a result, the professional or "expert" is in charge, and thus, any change is attributed to the professionals' efforts. The outcome then is one of dependency on the expert and loss of competencies. The type of despair and learned helplessness families of children with serious emotional challenges often report may be due not only to the magnitude of the stress surrounding their child's difficulties but also to the manner in which therapy or supports have been provided. A real danger in this model

Table 5-3	Models of Helping		
Consumer's Responsibility for the Problem	**Consumer's Responsibility for the Solution**	**Consumer's Attributions About Self-Efficacy**	**Outcomes**
High	High	High	Isolation, exhaustion, loneliness
Low	Low	Low	Dependency, learned helplessness
High	Low	Low	Low self-esteem, guilt, low maintenance of gains
Low	High	High	Empowerment, maintenance of gains, increased competence

Adapted from Dunst et al. (1988 a & b).

is that the more that the consumer experiences it with each succeeding interaction with the professional community, the less likely he or she will be to participate as a full partner even when the opportunity is there.

In what has been termed the "enlightenment" model, consumers are seen as responsible for their problem but not in the solution. This is perhaps the most debilitating of the models because this model results in consumers having an increasingly negative image of themselves and in order to change that image they must be dependent on professionals who prescribed the solutions as they see them. As with the medical model, any change is likely to be ascribed to external factors, with the consumer outcomes being guilt, a sense of incompetence, and depression.

In the final model, which Dunst and Trivette have adapted somewhat from Brickman's original concept and called the *enabling or empowering model* (Dunst et al., 1988a), the assumption is that the consumer is not blamed for the problem or the need for which they are seeking assistance, but most importantly, they are assumed to be competent or capable of being competent. The model focuses on the promotion of growth-producing competencies and on promoting and strengthening functioning. They are expected to be active partners in the process and as a result are more likely to attribute accurately the improvements to themselves and their competencies. The outcome of this approach, which is philosophically similar to the tenets of Systemof Care, is one of enhanced well-being and an increased sense of empowerment (Table 5-3).

In an extension of this line of research, Dempsey and Dunst (2004); Dunst (2002); Dunst et al. (2002); and Dunst and Trivette (1996) have investigated the actual behaviors or practices that are associated with this effective help-giving. This research provides one way of operationalizing System of Care as well as highlighting the importance of providing services in this manner and the dangers when these practices are not followed. More specifically, to be maximally effective, psychologists must have three components: technical quality, certain help-giver traits/attributions, and participatory involvement practices.

Technical quality relates to the knowledge, skills, and competencies of the professional. This is a basic requirement and one that has been part and parcel of the various iterations of the American Psychological Association's (APA) *Code of Ethics* (2002). First and foremost, psychologists must not practice outside their level of competence. If training and supervising other psychologists, they are also responsible for ensuring that the supervisee is competent to provide treatment.

Help-giver attributions refer to those outlined previously—that is, the degree to which the professional attributes intent or blame or responsibility to the consumer for the problem and the degree to which they assume that the youth or family is capable of participating in the solution and in exercising or acquiring new competencies. Help-giver traits relate to relational skills, such as warmth, caring, active or reflective listening, compassion, and empathy. Participatory practices are just that—the degree to which the professional provides opportunities for consumers to participate in the process, whether it is in sharing information, in setting priorities for treatment or in evaluating outcomes. It is reflected in shared decision making and collaboration (Dunst & Trivette, 1996).

Research has demonstrated the added value when all three characteristics are evident within services such as therapy or case management or care coordination. For example, in services that have a high technical quality (e.g., empirically supported treatments) but are devoid of empathy or participatory caregiving (e.g., high tech/low touch), the child may show some improvement, but family anger and resentment are likely to increase. Without family input and participation in the decision making, it is unlikely that the child gains are as great as they could be (Whitcher-Alagna, 1983). As already outlined, positive help-giver traits along with attributions that increase self-efficacy are more likely to be associated with some of the best outcomes (e.g., Levinson, 1994).

Seemingly more difficult to achieve are the participatory behaviors, and these are key to practicing in a way that is consistent with System of Care philosophy. For example, in an article summarizing quantitative and qualitative research on family-centered practices, Dunst (2002) highlighted that attitudes and behaviors among elementary school professionals reflect knowledge and practice of relational behaviors (e.g., frequent communication, positive comments), but there was less evidence of participatory behaviors such as parent input about school policy and practices. This pattern of a lack of participatory practices was even more evident in high school. Although relational skills are important and contribute to psychological health, participatory behaviors are the ones that are most associated with the consumer's feelings of self-efficacy and empowerment. Perhaps most importantly, when families receive services in a way that is participatory, there is a synergistic effect. Professionals who truly believe in the competencies of the families with whom they work are more likely to work in a collaborative way. Families are more likely to increase their self-esteem and their self-efficacy, and as a result, they become more competent and seek other participatory experiences. The increased competence will then reinforce others' perceptions of them as capable partners. Thus, empowerment is a "regenerative process, in which outcomes produced at one stage in the process in turn contributes energy to further participation in the process" (Cochran, 1992, p. 9; in Dunst & Trivette, 1996). Furthermore, there is increasing evidence that it is this increase in empowerment or self-efficacy that may be the active ingredient in successful therapeutic interventions (Dunst & Trivette, 1998). For example, in a recent study of 79 families receiving services within a System of Care philosophy, results indicated that the degree to which families reported feeling empowered mediated the link between fidelity to System of Care in service delivery and improvement in child outcomes at one year (Rogers & Shelton, 2004).

The child and family team is an ideal place to practice participatory behaviors. Whether as a team member or as the facilitator, psychologists should ensure that family members have sufficient information to be informed partners, that the child and family have the formal and informal supports present, that their opinions are heard, and that their priorities for treatment are respected. Thus, to practice in a way that is consistent with System of Care philosophy, psychologists need to have technical expertise (e.g., knowledge of empirically supported treatments, knowledge of assessment techniques), but they also have to have the ability to truly listen, to be empathic and compassionate, and to truly believe in the capacity of the children and families they are serving to participate as partners (Table 5-4).

As outlined in the following case study, psychologists have a great opportunity to practice in a way that is consistent with System of Care philosophy. As Dunst et al. (1988a) noted, "It is not just an issue of whether needs are met but rather that manner in which mobilization of resources and support occurs that is a major determinant of enabling and empowering families" (p. 44).

Table 5-4	Psychologists Characteristics for System of Care Practice
Help-Giving Component	*Help-Giving Practices*
Relational traits/attributions	• Tries to understand client's concerns • Listens to concerns • Views client as capable • Believes in client's role in achieving outcomes • Is warm and caring • Is honest, sincere, and supportive • Focuses on strengths
Participatory involvement	• Regularly provides information to client necessary to make informed choices • Elicits and respects priorities • Encourages client decision making • Encourages use of existing client capabilities • Encourages client to acquire new skills • Builds on strengths

Adapted from Dunst (2002); Dunst et al. (2002); and Dunst and Trivette (1996).

Case Study

Angie Freeman is a 21-year-old single mother of two boys: Jordan, who is 4.5 years old, and Sam, who is 3 years old. She is currently living with her mother, Mary, and her younger brother James, who is 15 years old. Angie is working on her GED (Graduate Equivalent Degree), having dropped out of school when she was pregnant with Jordan. She also works part time at a fast-food restaurant for minimum wage. Mary also works. The three-bedroom home is crowded, with Angie and her two sons sharing one room. Both Jordan and Sam are enrolled in the local Head Start program. Jordan was referred for evaluation and treatment because of concerns about his behavior in the classroom. His teacher reports that he is very active, inattentive, and refuses to follow the classroom rules, and when frustrated, he may hit other children. Angie is reluctant to pursue the referral. Before enrolling the children in Head Start, Jordan and Sam were in another daycare where they also had behavior problems. The daycare director referred them to a psychologist in town for assessment because of concerns that the children might have attention deficit/hyperactivity disorder. Angie met with the psychologist who interviewed the children and based on his interview and the report from the daycare provider diagnosed the children with attention deficit/ hyperactivity disorder (AD/HD) and recommended medication. He did not gather much information from Angie, and when she asked whether there was some other option beside medication, such as working with the daycare staff, the psychologist indicated that Medicaid did not reimburse classroom consultation. When Angie refused to put the children on medication, the daycare asked her to remove her children because they were disruptive, and she was, according to the daycare director, "resistant" to the recommendations after she went to the trouble to set up the evaluation. Thus, when the Head Start teacher suggested that Angie take Jordan to a psychologist, she was quite reluctant and not optimistic about the outcome.

Dr. Johnson, the psychologist working with the Head Start program, who had received training in System of Care, called Ms. Freeman to see what might be the most convenient time and place to meet. After discussing several options, they both decided to meet at the Head Start Center after Dr. Johnson's observation of Jordan and on a day when Ms. Freeman would not be in school or at work in the afternoon. Ms. Freeman thought to herself that this was already different from her previous contact with the other psychologist, but she still was quite wary. This became obvious to Dr. Johnson who found Ms. Freeman a bit cool when they met. Her initial responses were short and curt, and she went out of her way to point out to

Dr. Johnson that she did not have any trouble with Jordan at home. She also said that if Dr. Johnson was going to suggest medication then the interview would be over. Dr. Johnson was a bit taken back but realized from these comments that Ms. Freeman must have heard this before. She turned to Ms. Freeman and asked whether someone had suggested that before, because Dr. Johnson recognized that Ms. Freeman's responses did not have anything to do with her, as they had just met. Dr. Johnson did not respond in anger or assume, as so many professionals might, that Ms. Freeman was resistant. However, it was clear that previous contact with a professional had not been positive or collaborative and that Ms. Freeman was feeling blamed for Jordan's problems. From her training regarding the work of Dunst and colleagues on the different help-giving models, Dr. Johnson realized how important it was to use both relational as well as participatory practices and to communicate to Ms. Freeman her belief that she was not to blame for Jordan's current challenge but that she needed Ms. Freeman as a partner in order to help Jordan be successful. She decided that it was important to ask Ms. Freeman about what had previously transpired.

After that discussion, Dr. Johnson asked Ms. Freeman whether she and Jordan's teacher could complete some rating scales on Jordan. Dr. Johnson chose the BASC-2 because it tapped both problem behaviors and strengths and had a reading level that was within Ms. Freeman's capabilities. She also asked whether Ms. Freeman and Jordan's teacher could meet to discuss their respective observations. Dr. Johnson completed her classroom observation using a functional behavioral analysis to begin to set some expectations about when Jordan was likely to have the most difficulty as well as to identify his strengths and when and under what conditions those were evident. After collecting and analyzing the data, Dr. Johnson suggested that Jordan's teacher, Ms. Freeman, and any other family members or friends meet to discuss the various results and to begin to develop a plan toward addressing the current concerns. Ms. Freeman indicated that she would like her mother to come as well as a neighbor who often babysits. They planned to meet the following week to accommodate all of the schedules.

In preparation for the meeting, Dr. Johnson provided Ms. Freeman with a copy of her written feedback on the results thus far. She also gave her a tentative agenda of what Dr. Johnson planned to cover and elicited her feedback about the process. All is planned, but the morning of the meeting Ms. Freeman calls to indicate that she cannot make the meeting because she was called to work. Jordan's teacher is upset because Jordan's behavior is becoming increasingly more disruptive. She suggests that Dr. Johnson and she meet anyway because she has arranged for a substitute in the classroom. Dr. Johnson considers this request because she has some ideas for classroom interventions and Ms. Freeman has already said that she does not have concerns about Jordan's behavior at home. It also would help to address the stress that Jordan's teacher is experiencing in the classroom. However, Dr. Johnson is worried that meeting without Ms. Freeman, particularly at this stage, would seriously hinder her ability to develop a collaborative partnership and might reinforce Jordan's teacher's perspective that Ms. Freeman is not that interested in doing anything about the behavior. Dr. Johnson decides not to meet without Ms. Freeman, and they are able to reschedule the meeting the day after.

Dr. Johnson opens the meeting by asking Jordan's mother and teacher to talk about the strengths that they have noticed in Jordan. Ms. Freeman is pleasantly surprised when she hears Jordan's teacher talk about how smart he is and his interest in being the teacher's helper. In turn, Jordan's teacher is surprised when Ms. Freeman compliments her and says how much better Jordan is doing in this setting than in his previous daycare. With that as a background, Dr. Johnson offers her analyses from the rating scales and her observations. She takes care to double check with both Ms. Freeman and Jordan's teacher as to whether the summary is consistent with their view of Jordan. Dr. Johnson recognizes that there needs to be consensus on the veracity of the findings in order for there to be "buy in" on any interventions. Both women as well as Jordan's grandmother and neighbor agree that Jordan has many strengths but does have a tendency to become aggressive when frustrated or when he does not get his way.

Dr. Johnson then starts to move into a discussion about possible intervention strategies. She observes, however, that as the discussion continues that most of the comments are being made by Jordan's grandmother and Jordan's teacher and that Ms. Freeman is becoming very quiet. She has pushed her chair back from the table. Dr. Johnson redirects that discussion by asking Ms. Freeman if she would mind sharing what goes on at home. Although Jordan's teacher indicated that she thought the reason that Jordan had no difficulty at home was because he probably got his way, Dr. Johnson knows that it is important to use Jordan's strengths (not being aggressive at home) to elucidate strategies for the classroom. Ms. Freeman talks about how she gives Jordan choices, and this seems to help. She also admits that Jordan does better when it is just the two of them and that problems seem to arise when he has to share adult attention. Jordan's teacher says that she has seen the same thing, and this information then becomes the basis for designing a series of interventions in the classroom. A number of behaviors are identified, including his overactivity, his aggression toward other children when frustrated, and his crying and withdrawal when he is reprimanded for inappropriate behavior. Dr. Johnson asks Ms. Freeman which ones she would like to prioritize. She also solicits the same information from Jordan's teacher. Through discussion, Dr. Johnson provides her own suggestions based on the research on early childhood behavior and her opinion. Collaboratively, the group decides on the first behavior to target. They agree to try the intervention for the next two weeks and then all meet together to review how things are going.

After the meeting, Ms. Freeman acknowledges to Dr. Johnson that she is somewhat concerned about Jordan's behavior at home but was reluctant to say anything because of her previous experience and her worry that medication would be recommended. She said that because she did not feel that she was being blamed for being a single mother and not finishing high school, she felt more comfortable in sharing this with Dr. Johnson. They decide on a time for a home visit where Dr. Johnson says that they can use the same strength-based process to design a series of interventions to address any concerns at home.

Summary

What are the implications of System of Care to the work of psychologists? The key System of Care principles outlined in the earlier chapters provide guidance as to the ways in which psychologists should conduct research, assessments, as well as treatment and care coordination. Psychologists are likely to be most effective if they envision what is quality care. The principles of System of Care become a road map to reach that vision. As illustrated in the case study, System of Care becomes a way to link the research on effective help-giving with what is a growing body of literature on empirically based treatments. Knowledge of a research-based treatment or assessment technique is not sufficient to bring about change without a true and respectful collaborative partnership between psychologists and the children and families they serve. Almost as important is the quality of the collaborative partnership with colleagues from other disciplines. What is also clear is that for this type of practice to occur, we need to examine current approaches to training, both preservice and inservice. As Dunst et al. have outlined, we need competence in the techniques and treatments of our field, grounding in the help-giving practices but, perhaps most importantly, expertise in how to truly build respectful partnerships with our colleagues, the children we serve, and finally, their families.

Activities to Extend Your Learning

- What are some examples of conducting research that are consistent with a System of Care philosophy?
- Identify three benefits of strength-based approaches.
- Describe when help-giving can have negative consequences.
- What are the three components of effective help-giving?
- What are some examples of relational practices?
- What are some examples of participatory practices?
- Identify three examples of how Dr. Johnson reflected System of Care principles in her work.

References

American Psychological Association. (2002). *APA code of ethics*. Washington, DC: Author.

Anastopoulos, A.D., & Shelton, T.L. (2001). *Assessing attention-deficit/hyperactivity disorder*. New York: Kluwer.

Brenner, E. (2003). Consumer-focused psychological assessment. *Professional Psychology: Research and Practice, 34*(3), 240–247.

Brestan, E.V., Jacobs, J.R., Rayfield, A.D., & Eyberg, S.M. (1999). A consumer satisfaction measure for parent-child treatments and its relation to measures of child behavior changes. *Behavior Therapy, 30*, 17–30.

Brickman, P., Rabinowitz, V.C., Karuza, J., Jr., Coates, D., Cohn, E., & Kidder, L.H. (1982). Models of helping and coping. *American Psychologist, 37*, 368–384.

Brickman, P., Kidder, L.H., Coates, D., Rabinowitz, V.C., Cohn, E., & Karuza, J., Jr. (1983). The dilemmas of helping: Making aid far and effective. In J.D. Fisher, A. Nadler, & B.M. DePaulo (Eds.), *New directions in helping: Vol. 1: Recipient reactions to aid* (pp. 18–51). New York: Academic Press.

Burns, B.J., Goldman, S.K., Faw, L., & Burchard, J. (1999). The wraparound evidence base. In B.J. Burns & S.K. Goldman (Eds.), *Promising practices in wraparound for children with serious emotional disturbance and their families: Systems of care: Promising practices in children's mental health* (1998 Series, Vol. IV, pp. 77–100). Washington, DC: Center for Effective Collaboration and Practice, American Institutes for Research.

Cochran, M. (1992). Parent empowerment: Developing a conceptual framework. *Family Science Review, 5*, 3–21.

Cunningham, C., Morgan, P., & McGucken, R. (1984). Down's syndrome: Is dissatisfaction with disclosure of diagnosis inevitable? *Developmental Medicine and Child Neurology, 26*, 33–39.

DeChillo, N. (1993, February). Collaboration between social workers and families of patients with mental illness. *Families in Society: The Journal of Contemporary Human Services*, 104–115.

DeChillo, N., Koren, P.E., & Schultze, K.H. (1994). From paternalism to partnership: Family and professional collaboration in children's mental health. *American Journal of Orthopsychiatry, 64,* 564–576.

Dempsey, I. (1995). The enabling practices scale: The development of an assessment instrument for disability services. *Australia and New Zealand Journal of Developmental Disabilities, 20,* 67–73.

Dempsey, I., & Dunst, C.J. (2004). Helpgiving styles and parent empowerment in families with a young child with a disability. *Journal of Intellectual and Developmental Disability, 29,* 40–51.

Dunst, C.J. (2002). Family-centered practices: Birth through high school. *Journal of Special Education, 36,* 139–147.

Dunst, C.J., & Trivette, C.M. (1996). Empowerment, effective helpgiving practices, and family-centered care. *Family Matters, 22,* 334–337, 343.

Dunst, C.J., & Trivette, C.M. (1998). *Family-oriented early intervention program practices scale.* Unpublished scale available from the authors through the Orelena Hawks Puckett Institute, 18A Regents Park Boulevard, Asheville, NC 28806. E-mail: dunst@puckett.org.

Dunst, C.J., Trivette, C.M., Davis, M., & Cornwell, J. (1988a). Enabling and empowering families of children with health impairments. *Children's Health Care, 17,* 71–81.

Dunst, C.J., Trivette, C.M., & Deal, A.G. (1988b). *Enabling and empowering families: Principles and guidelines for practice.* Cambridge, MA: Brookline Books.

Dunst, C.J., Johanson, C., Trivette, C.M., & Hamby, D.W. (1991). Family-oriented early intervention policies and practices: Family-centered or not? *Exceptional Children, 3,* 115–126.

Dunst, C.J., Trivette, C.M., & Deal, A.G. (1994). *Supporting and strengthening families: Methods, strategies and practices.* Cambridge, MA: Brookline Books.

Dunst, C.J., Trivette, C.M., & Hamby, D.W. (1996). Measuring the helpgiving practices of human services program practitioners. *Human Relations, 49,* 815–835.

Dunst, C.J., Boyd, K., Trivette, C.M., & Hamby, D.W. (2002). Family-oriented program models and professional helpgiving practices. *Family Relations, 51,* 221–229.

English, J. (2000). The four "Ps" of marketing are dead. *Marketing Health Services, 20,* 21–23.

Epstein, M.H. (1999). The development and validation of a scale to assess the emotional and behavioral strengths of children and adolescents. *Remedial and Special Education, 20*(5), 258–262.

Heflinger, C.A. (1995). Studying family empowerment and parental involvement in their child's mental health treatment. *Focal Point, 9*(1), 6–8.

Hernandez, M., Isaacs, M.R., Nesman, T., & Burns, D. (1998). Perspectives on culturally competent systems of care. In M. Hernandez & M.R. Isaacs (Eds.), *Promoting cultural competence in children's mental health services* (pp. 1–25). Baltimore: Brookes.

Hodges, S., Nesman, T., & Hernandez, M. (1999). Promising practices: Building collaboration in systems of care. *Systems of care: Promising practices in children's mental health* (1998 Series, Vol. IV, pp. xi–18).

Honzik, M.P., Hutchings, J.J., & Burnip, S.R. (1965). Birth record assessment and test performance at eight months. *American Journal of Diseases of Children, 109,* 416–426.

Hoza, B., Owens, J., Pelham, W.E., Swanson, J.M., Conners, C.K., Hinshaw, S.P., Arnold, L.E., & Kraemer, H.C. (2000). Parent cognitions as predictors of child treatment response in attention-deficit/hyperactivity disorder. *Journal of Abnormal Child Psychology, 28*(6), 569–583.

Jones, M.L., Eyberg, S.M., Adams, C.D., & Boggs, S.R. (1998). Treatment acceptability of behavioral interventions for children: An assessment by mothers of children with disruptive behavior disorders. *Child and Family Behavior Therapy, 20,* 15–26.

Karuza, J., Jr., Zevon, M.A., Rabinowitz, V.C., & Brickman, P. (1982). Attribution of responsibility by helpers and recipients. In T.A. Wills (Ed.), *Basic processes in helping relationships* (pp. 107–129). New York: Academic Press.

Kashdan, T.B., Pelham, W.E., Lang, A.R., Hoza, B., Jacob, R.G., Jennings, J.R., Blumenthal, J.D., & Gnagy, E.M. (2002). Hope and optimism as human strengths in parents of children with externalizing disorders: Stress is in the eye of the beholder. *Journal of Social and Clinical Psychology, 21*(4), 441–468.

King, S., Rosenbaum, P., & King, G. (1995). The measure of processes of care (MPOC): Means to assess family-centered behaviours of health care providers. Unpublished manual. Hamilton, Ontario, Canada: McMaster University, Neurodevelopmental Clinical Research Unit. E-mail: ncru@fhs.mcmaster.ca.

Koren, P.E., Paulson, R.I., Kinney, R.F., Yatchmenoff, D.K., Gordon, L.J., & DeChillo, N. (1997). Service coordination in children's mental health: An empirical study from the caregiver's perspective. *Journal of Emotional and Behavioral Disorders, 5,* 162–172.

Lanyon, R.I. (1972). Technological approach to the improvement of decision making in mental health services. *Journal of Consulting and Clinical Psychology, 39,* 43–48.

Levinson, W. (1994). Physician-patient communication: A key to malpractice prevention. *Journal of the American Medical Association, 272,* 1619–1620.

Lyons, J.S., Uziel-Miller, N.D., Reyes, F., & Sokol, P.T. (2000). Strengths of children and adolescents in residential settings: Prevalence and associations with psychopathology and discharge placement. *Journal of the American Academy of Child and Adolescent Psychiatry, 39*(2), 176–181.

Merton, V., Merton, R.K., & Barber, E. (1983). Client ambivalence in professional relationships: The problem of seeking help from strangers. In B. De Paulo, A. Nadler, & J. Fisher (Eds.), *New directions in helping: Vol. 2: Help-seeking* (pp. 13–44). New York: Academic Press.

Miller, D.L., & Kelley, M.L. (1992). Treatment acceptability: The effects of parent gender, marital adjustment, and child behavior. *Child and Family Behavior Therapy, 14,* 11–23.

Nock, M.K., & Kazdin, A.E. (2001). Parent expectancies for child therapy: Assessment and relation to participation in treatment. *Journal of Child and Family Studies, 10,* 155–180.

Power, T.J., Hess, L.E., & Bennett, D.S. (1995). The acceptability of interventions for attention-deficit hyperactivity disorder among elementary and middle school teachers. *Journal of Developmental and Behavioral Pediatrics, 16,* 238–243.

Rabinowitz, V.C., Karuza, J., Jr., & Zevon, M.A. (1984). Fairness and effectiveness in premeditated helping. In R. Foger (Ed.), *The sense of injustice* (pp. 63–92). New York: Plenum.

Reynolds, C.R., & Kamphaus, R.W. (2004). *BASC-2: Behavior assessment system of children* (2nd ed.). Circle Pines, MN: American Guidance Service.

Rogers, K.N., & Shelton, T.L. (2004). Family empowerment as a mediator between system of care and changes in child functioning: Identifying an important mechanism of change. Unpublished manuscript.

Rosenblatt, A. (1996). Bows and ribbons, tape, and twine: Wrapping the wraparound process of children with multi-system needs. *Journal of Child and Family Studies, 5,* 101–116.

Savitz, L. (1999). Measuring consumer satisfaction. In C.P. McLaughlin & A.D. Kaluzny (Eds.), *Continuous quality improvement in health care* (pp. 129–146). Gaithersburg, MD: Aspen.

Shapiro, J.P., Welker, C.J., & Jacobson, B.J. (1997). The youth client satisfaction questionnaire: Development, construct validation, and factor structure. *Journal of Clinical Child Psychology, 26,* 87–98.

Shelton, T.L., & Stepanek, J.S. (1994). *Family-centered care for children needing specialized health and developmental services.* Bethesda, MD: Association for the Care of Children's Health.

Solomon, B.B. (1976). *Black empowerment: Social work in oppressed communities.* New York: Columbia University Press.

Tallent, N. (1958). On individualizing the psychologist's clinical evaluation. *Journal of Clinical Psychology, 14,* 243–244.

Tarnowski, K.J., Simonian, S.J., Park, A., & Bekeny, P. (1992). Acceptability of treatments for child behavioral disturbance: Race, socioeconomic status, and multicomponent treatment effects. *Child and Family Behavior Therapy, 14,* 25–37.

Whitcher-Alagna, S. (1983). Receiving medical help: A psychological perspective on patient reactions. In A. Nadler, J. Fisher, & B. DePaulo (Eds.), *New directions in helping: Vol. 3: Applied perspectives* (pp. 131–161). New York: Academic Press.

Wikler, L., Wasow, M., & Hatfield, E. (1981). Chronic sorrow revisited: Parent vs. professional depiction of the adjustment of parents of mentally retarded children. *American Journal of Orthopsychiatry, 51,* 63–70.

Wikler, L., Wasow, M., & Hatfield, E. (1983). See strengths in families of developmentally disabled children. *Social Work, 28*(4), 313–315.

Chapter 6

System of Care in Nursing: Across the Life Span and Across Practice Settings

CHARLOTTE A. HERRICK, T. ROBIN BARTLETT,
GERALDINE S. PEARSON, CAROLYN SCHMIDT, AND JOY CHERRY

Objectives

■ Examine the history of a System of Care approach in nursing.
■ Define System of Care values, principles, and concepts within a nursing paradigm.
■ Explain the role of the professional nurse as a generalist and as an advanced practice nurse in delivering nursing care based on System of Care values and principles.
■ Describe a model for nursing case management in a community-based, interdisciplinary, wraparound program for foster children.
■ Discuss how the integration of System of Care principles and values into nursing can help in the development of evidenced-based practice.

System of Care values and principles fit "hand in glove" with nursing values, such as providing holistic care, being an articulate communicator, and conveying a caring spirit. Traditionally, nurses have focused their care on underprivileged groups, including the emotionally disturbed, the financially disadvantaged, the homeless, and fragile older adults— all of whom are at risk for health problems and can benefit from a System of Care approach. As a framework for education and practice, however, the System of Care philosophy applies to all nursing care and can be viewed as "best practice"—whether the nurse is a generalist, a nurse case manager or a specialist in advanced practice. Although System of Care was developed for the care of children and their families, in this chapter, the focus is across the lifespan and health–illness continuum. The purpose of this chapter is to integrate System of Care principles and values (e.g., family-centered and community-based care, cultural competence, interdisciplinary practice) into a framework for nursing practice.

Nursing and System of Care Values

Even though core System of Care values and beliefs have not been specifically identified in the nursing literature in the same way that they are listed in System of Care texts, these principles have always guided nursing care. Family-centered and community-based care that strives for cultural competence found in the nursing literature can be equated with System of Care values described by other disciplines. Thus, this chapter begins with a description of family-centered and community-based care from a historical perspective.

Family-Centered Care

Historically, hospitals isolated children from their parents because of the threat of infection. Now it is understood that isolating children from their parents has devastating psychological effects (Francis, 1993), and hospitals have developed rooming-in policies so that parents can stay with their children, provide opportunities for pre-hospitalization visits, and have sibling visitation policies (Ahmann, 1994; Hanson & Boyd, 1996).

Knitzer's (1982) exposé (see Chapter 1 *System of Care Principles and Practice*) sheds light on the overuse of inpatient residential settings for emotionally disturbed children. These settings were often located far from where families resided and served to isolate these children from their families. The publication *Unclaimed Children* set the stage for the advent of the System of Care movement in children's mental health (Stroul, 2003). It has now become clear that nurses need to invite family members to collaborate in the care of their loved ones so that families, nurses, and other health care professionals work together to deliver quality, safe, age-appropriate, culturally sensitive care in all agencies across the health care continuum. A goal of System of Care collaboration is to provide care in the least restrictive setting, preferably the home (Stroul, 1996).

One of the essential functions of the family is to provide for the health of its members. In a family-centered paradigm, families partner with professionals to plan, implement, and evaluate the child's care and are the "experts" because they know their child's health and behavior before the onset of illness. The nurse provides accurate information about the disease process so that the parents can participate in decision-making. According to Washington (2001), families need information and hope for the future. The nurse assists the family in exploring potential resources, including both health care and natural support systems to meet their needs. An illness of any kind, whether emotional or physical, demands changes in the function and structure of the family (Meleski, 2002). Family-centered health care enables family members to take on the additional role of care provider so that they can participate in their loved one's care whether in the hospital or at home. Participating in caregiving enhances parents' and families' sense of their own abilities to care for their loved one (Ahmann, 1994; Hanson & Boyd, 1996). Table 6-1 addresses the principles of family-centered nursing care.

The principles of family-centered nursing care (Table 6-1) can guide the nurse in providing family-centered care that promotes the well-being of both the child or other-aged client and his or her family. However, barriers remain that must be overcome when providing family-centered care. Those are listed in Table 6-2.

Community-Based Care

The generalist nurse provides care in community settings. Nurses provide community-based care through public health departments, visiting nurse services, home health services, schools, occupational health services in businesses or corporations, rural health services, community mental health centers, and other community-based programs. The recent congregational nursing movement has placed nurses in churches as parish nurses (Brown & Magilvy, 2001). Opportunities for

Table 6-1   Principles of Family-Centered Nursing Care

- A family is the constant stabilizing force in a client's life.
- Establishing a caring atmosphere fosters collaboration.
- Communication is bidirectional—open and honest.
- Trust and mutual respect are conveyed from family to professional and vice versa.
- The family's cultural, ethnic, and socioeconomic values and beliefs are honored.
- The diverse needs of family members, including siblings, are considered when planning care.
- The family's strengths and individuality are respected. By focusing on assets rather than problems, families feel empowered.
- Unbiased information is provided, including all available options for treatment, risks, and potential outcomes.
- All decisions must rest with the family or those legally responsible when the care receiver is a child. Nurses and other health professionals respect the family's decisions, setting aside personal biases.
- Nurses and nurse case managers provide emotional support to families so that they can nurture each other, flourish, and survive in periods of crises. Family-to-family networking is encouraged. Normal family functioning is supported as much as possible.
- Family perceptions and opinions are solicited.
- The nurse or nurse case manager ensures that the client's and family's goals are identified and addressed.
- The nurse or the nurse case manager assists families to care for themselves.
- Holistic care is provided for children, clients, and families.
- Policies are flexible to meet individual needs for emotional, physical, and financial support.

Adapted from Ahmann (1994); Francis (1993, 1995); Hanson and Boyd (1996); Powers, Goldstein, Plank, Thomas, and Conkright (2000); and Stroul (1996, 2003).

nurses to work in community settings continue to grow as admissions to hospitals and hospital stays decline.

Community health nurses work with populations, aggregates or groups, families, individuals, and other professionals. The goals of community health nursing are health promotion, health maintenance and disease prevention, health education, and assistance to people in achieving their highest level of wellness. Care is holistic and continuing, not episodic, and may or may not be disease-based. Holistic health care addresses a broad range of interacting needs that affect health, and

Table 6-2	Barriers to Family-Centered Nursing Care

- The traditional structure for providing health care, which is individually focused, professionally centered, in-patient oriented, and paternalistic.
- Resistance to a paradigm shift from the traditional provider-recipient conceptual framework to a collaborative partnership between nurse and family.
- A lack of research and evidence-based outcomes to support family-centered care.
- Parental anger, which is often directed at the nurse or the care coordinator because he or she is often the health professional who is most available.
- A lack of resources to address children's health and mental health needs.

Adapted from Foster (1993); Francis (1993, 1995); and Green (2003).

the focus varies from setting to setting. Nurses working in the community take a global approach that fosters both the health of the community and the health of individuals and groups of people residing in the community.

Public health nursing differs from community health nursing. Public health nursing synthesizes knowledge from public health science and professional nursing theories to improve the health of the entire community. Public health nurses have as their goals the prevention of illness and injury and health promotion (American Nurses Association [ANA], 2004; cited in Klainberg, Holzemer, Leonard, & Arnold, 1998). Community health nurses provide care and promote wellness for individuals, groups, and families within the context of the larger community's needs (Klainberg et al.). The focus of public health nursing is on the community or population as a whole to maintain the health of the community and prevent the spread of disease, whereas the focus of community health nursing is on individuals, families, and groups to teach health promotion and prevention, identify those at risk for illness, and meet the health care needs of individuals who reside in communities. What the two approaches have in common is that both are community based.

System of Care strategies must be incorporated into community health programs to provide for the health care needs of the mentally ill residing in the community. Community health nurses focus on maintaining or improving the health of the mentally ill, whereas public health nurses address the epidemiology of mental illness and the mental health of communities.

Future trends for community health nursing include a continuing focus on keeping people healthy in the community in order to contain health care costs. There will continue to be an emphasis on primary care in the community, nursing case management, long-term care, and home health care because of an increase in the number of older people with chronic illnesses or mental health problems (Kuhlman & Wilson, 2004). Community-based care addresses these and other health concerns with the following: (1) health and mental health promotion and illness prevention for individuals, families, and communities through education, counseling, immunizations, and periodic screenings; (2) care for the sick in community settings, including early diagnosis and prompt treatment; (3) fostering of healthy lifestyles; and (4) care for the chronically ill and the severely and persistently mentally ill in the community with the goal of limiting their disabilities (Klainberg, 1998).

It is interesting that 8 of the 10 leading health indicators in the *Healthy People 2010* report have to do with mental health issues or lifestyle (Office of Disease Prevention and Health Promotion, US Department of Health and Human Services, 2000). The indicators include obesity, tobacco use, substance abuse, irresponsible sexual behavior, mental health, access to care, injury, and violence. One of the goals of this report is to rebuild health care systems to maintain healthy communities (Clark, 2003; Spector, 2004). Progress toward addressing this and other *Healthy People 2010* initiatives can be improved by including a System of Care perspective in community-based programs planned to address them.

Psychiatric Nursing: Hospital to Community

Although all areas of nursing can benefit from a System of Care approach, psychiatric nursing seems to fit particularly well with this paradigm. A view of the recent evolution of psychiatric nursing in the United States illustrates this point.

Historically, psychiatric nurses not only worked but also were educated in psychiatric asylums. In these settings, nursing care was custodial and focused primarily on assisting patients in activities of daily living (Herrick, 1985). The 1950s brought fundamental changes to the care of the mentally ill. Congress passed the Community Mental

Health Centers Act (88-164), which initiated the community mental health movement known as deinstitutionalization (Kneisl & Wilson, 2004; Lourie, 2003). Psychiatric care moved to local communities. The role of the case manager developed to facilitate the transition of the mentally ill from state hospitals to their communities (Kersbergen, 1996). During the 1960s, the federal government funded stipends for psychiatric nursing masters degree education and also provided matching funds to states to establish community mental health centers (Herrick, 1985; Kneisl, 2004). The intent was to provide comprehensive community-based care to the mentally ill. Movement of care for the mentally ill to local communities continued throughout the 1970s (Herrick).

Specific to child mental health care, before the System of Care movement, there were few local services, except for a few private psychiatric centers or child guidance clinics, that were available for children (Lourie, 2003; Pothier, 1974). Residential treatment programs were rarely local and were mostly staffed by social workers, psychologists, and psychiatrists—not nurses (Stroul, 1996). Then, during the 1970s, nurses began working in psychiatric programs that were established for children. During this same time, more nurses received master's degrees. Advanced practice nurses began working in a number of roles with a variety of populations in diverse settings, including community-based settings.

In the next era, psychiatric–mental health nurses are expected to work in new and nontraditional settings (Kneisl & Wilson, 2004). Opportunities will be available for nurses to provide mental health care in primary care settings and other community-based programs. Nurse practitioners, clinical nurse specialists, psychotherapists, case managers, and generalist nurses will be needed to provide care for high-risk populations. Providing a caring system for the mentally ill remains a goal today (Herrick, 1985).

Culturally Competent Care

Nurses have addressed the cultural dimensions of nursing care since Florence Nightingale went to the Crimea. Through the Visiting Nurse Association of New York City, nurses cared for immigrant populations from Europe beginning in the late 1800s (Herrick, 1985; Swanson, 1993). In the 20th century, the simultaneous arrival of the civil rights and the community mental health movements raised the awareness of the need for culturally competent care (Tripp-Reimer & Lively, 1993).

During the 1960s Madeline Leininger, a nurse anthropologist, established the Transcultural Nursing Society and published the first nursing journal that addressed cultural issues in nursing, *The Journal of Transcultural Nursing*. Leininger developed a theory titled "Culture Care Diversity and Universality" (Andrews, 1999, p. 7; Leininger, 1991). She challenged nurses to gain knowledge of a person's cultural values, beliefs, and practices and to integrate that knowledge into nursing care based on an understanding of the humanity of every individual.

Cultural competence has been defined as "a complex combination of knowledge, attitudes and skills" (Spector, 2004, p. 31). A number of models provide guidelines to promote culturally competent nursing care (Andrews, 1999; Boyd, 1998; Campinha-Bacote, 1997; Giger & Davidhizar, 2004; Leininger, 1991; Spector). Campinha-Bacote's model includes the following components: cultural awareness, cultural knowledge, cultural skill, cultural encounters, and cultural desire (Boyd, 1998; Campinha-Bacote, 1997). Developing cultural competence is a process that includes learning about other cultures by listening intently to the client's and family's concerns, reading about other cultures, and participating with clients from diverse backgrounds as they strive for the best level of health that they can achieve within their own frame of reference.

The System of Care Principles That Guide Nursing Practice

A goal of this chapter is to illustrate the utility of a System of Care approach in providing nursing care across the lifespan. Sometimes the best way to demonstrate this usefulness is in nursing care of children. Here are some details about how a System of Care can be implemented effectively in the care of the child and his or her family, and with adults with various health concerns.

System of Care principles are the same across all disciplines, but they are implemented in different ways in different disciplines. In a System of Care framework, professional services are comprehensive, occur in the least restrictive setting, are both individualized and normalized, and are delivered using an interdisciplinary approach. Services are seamless, wrapped around the child and family, so that transitions can be made smoothly. A case manager, often referred to as the care coordinator among System of Care experts, is assigned to the child and family to coordinate care, acts as a liaison between agencies and families, and provides an empowering environment for self-care. According to Stroul and Friedman (1986), "The case management function is critical for the effective operation of the System of Care" (p. 12). The case manager may be a nurse or a professional from another discipline, such as social work.

Comprehensive Services

The principle of comprehensiveness mandates that services be all-inclusive across the continuum of care. A continuum of care includes the variety of health care services that may be found across inpatient and outpatient settings that may be needed by an individual at any point in his or her illness (Finkelman, 2001). At one end of this health care continuum are the least restrictive settings, including schools, churches, recreational, and other community settings, where the focus is on prevention. School and parish nurses, health educators, and community health and mental health nurses teach people healthy living. Further along the continuum are community-based systems of care, such as child health services, social services, public health clinics, outpatient clinics, community mental health centers, special education programs, hospital outpatient clinics, and day care programs for severely emotionally disturbed or physically disabled children, the older, and chronically mentally ill adults. Two goals of these programs are to keep people at their maximum level of functioning and out of inpatient settings. Proceeding further along the continuum are more restrictive acute care and chronic care settings, including inpatient hospital units for the acutely ill, residential treatment centers for children and adults who are severely and persistently mentally ill, and nursing homes for the cognitively impaired or physically fragile older persons (Finkelman).

Clients and families must have access to an array of services that address their physical, emotional, and social needs. In addition, educational services for children and vocational and rehabilitation services for disabled or mentally ill adults must be an integral part of care, with linkages between agencies and programs in order to plan, develop, and coordinate services to meet individual and family needs. The goal is to provide *continuity of care* across the health care continuum, using a variety of agencies and service providers while preventing the duplication of services and reducing fragmentation (Powell, 1996; Stroul, 1996, 2003). Nurses work with other professionals in many settings across the health care continuum.

Individualized Care

At the bedside and in the community, nurses individualize care to meet the needs of the client and family, treating each person as a unique person. The goal is for the client who is ill to regain health, guided by an individualized care plan. Services and interventions are coordinated around the *strengths* and needs of the client and family (Stroul, 2003). Clients' and their families' values and beliefs are respected (Powers et al., 2000), and clients are treated as individuals. The nurse is nonjudgmental and empathizes with clients, conveying a caring attitude (Kneisl & Wilson, 2004).

The Setting: The Least Restrictive
Alternative, Most Normal, and the Most Therapeutic

The care coordinator (case manager) selects a health care setting that meets the client's needs based on the acuity of symptoms. The goal is to treat the client in a setting that least restricts his or her rights (Kneisl, 2004) and that is safe and therapeutic. The client and family make decisions collaboratively with the care coordinator or health care provider. Information on the various options is discussed, and an appropriate setting is selected. Psychiatric nurses, nurse case managers, clinical nurse specialists, and nurse practitioners work with teachers, school nurses, and public health nurses to select services for children with complex physical and mental health needs that can be obtained in the most appropriate educational setting.

Whenever possible, the clients should be cared for in their homes with the assistance of nurses and other health care providers. The nurse/care coordinator facilitates the use of available community resources so that a child or adult can remain at home. System of Care philosophy stresses the importance of using natural and nontraditional support services in the community, along with the traditional services (Pumariega & Winters, 2003).

Interdisciplinary Care

Interdisciplinary health care teams provide care that is organized as a seamless system across the health care continuum. Nurses are one part of this seamless system and often serve as advocates for the client/family and/or as leaders of the team. There is a strong tradition among mental health professionals to work collaboratively (Cheven & Brady, 2003). The representative from each discipline contributes his or her expertise to develop the plan of care, and the role of each team member is identified in the plan. Family members and significant others are equal partners and members of the team. Families are also participants in the delivery of care, as much as possible, and there is growing evidence that collaborative models are the most effective in delivering health care (Koenig, 2001).

Seamless Care

An integrated health case system, such as System of Care, provides clients and families access to all components of the health care system through collaborative relationships among professionals and agencies (McLuhan, 1995). A coordinated System of Care wraps services around the client and family so that they do not get lost going from one provider or agency to another. System of Care programs for children with complex emotional needs are often referred to as wraparound programs (see Chapter 2 *Building Collaborative Relationships*).

A seamless health care delivery system also provides *continuity of care* during transitions. These may include going from childhood to adulthood, using different Systems of Care, or transferring from one system, for example the mental health system, to another system like social services or from an outpatient community mental health setting to an inpatient setting. A wraparound program is individualized and provides comprehensive services across the health care continuum (Handron, Dosser, McCammon, & Powell, 1998).

Care Coordinated by a Case Manager (or Care Coordinator)

Case management is the "linchpin for an effective interagency system" (Winters & Terrell, 2003, p. 171). Case management models have evolved to serve diverse populations who are considered at high risk for physical and mental health problems. A variety of models have been developed, including "within the walls" (acute care) (Cohen & Cesta, 2001), "beyond the walls" (chronic, community-based care) (Michaels & Lamb, 2001), "the broker model" (linking clients to services), "the collaborative model" (interdisciplinary), and "the disease management model" (focused on a target population across the health care continuum) (Huber, 2002). The case manager's role depends on the model under which the nurse is operating, the organizational goals, the target population, and the setting (Herrick & Bartlett, 2004).

The case manager may play a variety of roles either at once or over time, including case finder, planner and broker, change agent, monitor and overseer, liaison and coordinator, care provider, collaborator, consultant, advocate, resource manager, financial advisor, evaluator, researcher, and educator (Conti, 1996; Herrick & Bartlett, 2004; Mullahy, 2004; Ritter-Teitel, 1996). The case manager is a source of support and stability for the client and the health care system (Thurkettle & Noji, 2003).

In a System of Care, the model is collaborative. The nurse may be a team leader or a member of a collaborative partnership. The family and all team members are collaborative partners.

Psychiatric case management —developed during the 1950s when veterans returning from World War II were in need of psychiatric services—is designed to provide continuity of care for the chronically mentally ill. The Veterans Administration designed a model for psychiatric case management, which addressed veterans' needs for health, mental health, and social services (Herrick & Bartlett, 2004; Kersbergen, 1996). During the community mental health movement of the 1960s, case management services were developed in community mental health centers as support systems for the deinstitutionalized mentally ill. According to Tahan (1998), the concept of a continuum of care emerged during deinstitutionalization, with emphasis on client-centered, coordinated, and comprehensive care. Psychiatric case management is critical to the integration of health, mental health, educational, and social services for the mentally ill. The goal of psychiatric case management is to keep the client out of the hospital and in his or her own community (Platter, Vaughn, & Young, 2001). Unfortunately, such services were unavailable to children until the 1980s, when System of Care programs were developed to address the needs of children, adolescents, and families with complex mental health concerns (Stroul, 1996, 2003).

The purpose of case management is to deliver a coordinated System of Care that is therapeutic and cost-effective. The case manager in a psychiatric setting matches the client's needs to the appropriate resources, which may be health or mental health care, housing, or financial aid (Powell, 1996). The psychiatric case manager assists clients in accessing services and enables them to move smoothly through the health care system in accordance with their changing needs (Stroul & Friedman, 1986; 1996).

The case manager ensures a "seamless transition to the right services and right providers at the right time" (Michaels & Cohen, 2001, p. 31). The psychiatric case manager coordinates and integrates care across agencies and disciplines, facilitates interdisciplinary care, conducts strength-based assessments, plans interventions and supervises their implementation, monitors and evaluates progress, and assesses outcomes in terms of effectiveness (Herrick & Bartlett, 2004; Platter et al., 2001). Psychiatric case management has become an essential component of inpatient psychiatric treatment since the advent of managed care, in order to move the patient from hospital to community care as quickly as possible (Herrick & Bartlett).

Early case finding and early interventions are areas in which public health nursing and nursing case management overlap. As public health nurses focus more on aggregate populations and health systems become more complex, the case manager becomes more important as a liaison between the client and family and the various components of the health care system. The need for case management is expected to continue to grow in response to changing demographics, an aging population, more clients who are chronically ill, continued emphasis on cost containment, and reduction in the length of stays in hospitals. Case management is viewed as "best practice" in part because it provides quality care that is also cost-effective (Herrick & Bartlett, 2004).

System of Care as a Framework for Nursing Practice

The Professional Nurse

The professional nurse is prepared with a minimum of a baccalaureate degree in nursing and may have a master's degree in nursing or a doctoral degree (American Association of Colleges of Nursing [AACN], 1998; American Nurses Association [ANA], 2004). System of Care values are consistent with the foundational values of nursing and, therefore, fit naturally within a nursing framework to guide practice. The nurse who integrates all of the elements of System of Care into practice provides holistic and compassionate nursing care.

The Advanced Practice Nurse

The advanced practice nurse has, at minimum, a master's degree; some advanced practice nurses have doctoral degrees. The advanced practice nurse can be an nurse practitioner, a certified nurse midwife, a clinical nurse specialist, or a certified registered nurse anesthetist. In psychiatric mental health nursing, the advanced practice nurse is generally a nurse practitioner or a clinical nurse specialist. The psychiatric nurse practitioner and the clinical nurse specialist are frequently involved in community-based care. The focus of the nurse practitioner's practice is the physical health of someone who is mentally ill. The clinical nurse specialist is educated to provide psychotherapeutic interventions for adults, children, adolescents, families, and older persons, provided to individuals and/or groups. Both of the advanced practice nurses are knowledgeable about psychopharmacology. Advanced practice nurses are innovators, carving out new roles in delivering timely, cost-effective, quality health care to the poor, including children, the older population, people living in rural areas, or those residing in urban slums (ANA, 2004). Advanced practice nurses in community-based clinics are in a position to integrate System of Care principles within a framework for holistic nursing practice.

Why is the advanced practice nurse particularly suited to integrate System of Care principles into nursing practice? Puskar and Bernardo (2002) noted that vulnerable populations such as racial and ethnic minorities, individuals with chronic mental illness, and those living in rural or inner city areas may be ignored and receive neither high-quality health care nor coordinated care, the latter a hallmark of System of Care service delivery. Advanced practice nurses partner with consumer groups, advocating for the unmet health needs of high-risk populations. Advanced practice nurses have the skills and training to provide coordinated care, integrating System of Care concepts with models from psychiatric and primary care, focused on the "whole" person—the mind, body, and spirit. Because advanced practice nurses are familiar with both inpatient and outpatient settings, they can easily assist clients and families to make the transition from one setting to another.

In many states, the advanced practice nurse has prescriptive authority and is able to integrate medication management into his or her practice. Consequently, advanced practice nurses are able to provide clients and their families health and medication education and to monitor the client's response to medication while also addressing psychosocial needs. Advanced practice nurses incorporate leadership skills along with their therapeutic skills, which allow them to set the tone for health care teams and to coordinate care for their clients. They may also use their leadership skills as advocates for the underserved.

Integration of System of Care Principles with Competencies for Professional and Advanced Practice Nurses

The American Association of Colleges of Nursing (1998) has identified three important components of nursing practice: (1) care of the sick in diverse settings, (2) health promotion, and (3) population-based care. Nurses strive toward competence as advocates, educators, and communicators, and as care providers who are culturally sensitive and client and family-centered.

Advocacy is the hallmark of professional nursing (AACN, 1998). As advocates, nurses provide emotional support to the most vulnerable in society. They advocate on behalf of those who cannot advocate for themselves, speaking publicly as needed. Because advanced practice nurses have acquired leadership skills, including public speaking and writing skills, they are uniquely positioned to be advocates. Johnson (1995) noted that as child advocates, nurses must advocate for both the child and the parents. Nurses also advocate for the profession through lobbying activities and professional organizations, such as the American Nurses Association or the International Society of Psychiatric Nurses.

Nurses and nurse case managers are educators and communicators as well as care providers (AACN, 1998). Nurses manage information to increase their own expertise and to educate clients, assisting them to understand, evaluate, and apply information to make decisions about their own care and to improve their state of health. Nurses teach health promotion and disease prevention to promote healthy lifestyles across the lifespan and to decrease health disparities frequently found among minorities. They inform the client and family about the illness and the available resources. Nurses establish therapeutic relationships with clients and families that empower them for self-determination and self-care. Nurses provide care *with* the client and family, rather than *for* them (Cohen & Cesta, 2001). Self-care has a long tradition in nursing, dating back to the early days of the visiting nurses on Henry Street in New York City, where the goal was "helping people help themselves" (Swanson, 1993, p. 32). That goal continues today.

Nurses convey health information verbally and in writing to clients, families, groups, and other professionals. Nurses develop active listening skills in order to understand the perceptions of others. Advanced practice nurses have been educated to provide psychotherapy to individuals and groups who are mentally ill. Throughout the course of a nurse's education, communication skills and the therapeutic use of self are stressed so that all nurses can be effective as care providers, educators, and communicators (McMahon, 1997).

The professional and advanced practice nurse delivers holistic care, integrating biopsychosocial and spiritual concepts with concepts related to physical care of the sick (AACN, 1998). As a care provider who is client- and family-centered, the nurse provides clients and families with opportunities that lead to empowerment by encouraging them to identify their strengths, before defining the problem so that assets rather than deficits are the foundation of the care plan. The care plan, which guides nursing interventions, is developed in collaboration with the client and family so that it is customized to meet individual and family needs (Brun & Rapp, 2001; Stroul, 1996).

Nurses work with a variety of populations from various cultures to deliver culturally sensitive care that respects the client's and family's beliefs. Nurses combine their knowledge of human development, cultural competence, and their medical and nursing knowledge about disease states with the use of the latest biotechnology to enhance their ability to deliver expert care. As expert clinicians, nurses apply technical skills as they deliver health care in diverse settings, based on scientific principles. The acquisition of new skills continues throughout the nurse's career, as new technologies are developed (AACN, 1998). These skills are continually integrated into the overall practice of professional nursing.

Nurses develop, monitor, manipulate, and manage environments to promote health (AACN, 1998) in order to meet individual needs and collective needs of the community related to health and safety. Nurses strive to design an environment that is comfortable and supportive (as normal as possible) that promotes health and healing, one that protects the client's safety, as well as one that protects the client's rights. Discharge planning starts with the initial nursing assessment. Nurses work with other professionals to facilitate a smooth transition from one health care environment to another, to ensure continuity of care. Nurses work independently and also interdependently with professionals from other disciplines as members of interdisciplinary teams. The goals are to design, manage, and coordinate a quality health care system (AACN, 1998). As collaborative partners, nurses work with clients, families, and other professionals to assist the client and/or family to reach the highest possible state of health (AACN).

Nurses apply standards of practice and a professional code of ethics, take actions to prevent or limit unsafe or unethical practices, and enable individuals and families to make choices based on their own values. Nurses evaluate patient care outcomes and are accountable for them. It is nurses' professional responsibility to participate in lifelong learning and to use research findings to determine "best practice" (AACN, 1998). All of these roles and responsibilities are consonant with a System of Care approach.

The following are some exemplars of nurses working within a System of Care framework.

Case Study 1: Undergraduate Nursing Students Participate on an Interdisciplinary Team—A Unique Clinical Experience

---

Although interdisciplinary teams are taught in schools of nursing, actually having a clinical practicum with a team of students from other disciplines is rare. Undergraduate nursing students, social work master's students, early childhood education students, and recreational therapy students, with their assigned faculty, worked alongside the staff of the Second Chance House as an interdisciplinary team to care for women recovering from substance abuse and their children. The Second Chance House was the only home for homeless women in the community. The group integrated System of Care principles into the holistic care of these women and children in a community-based living and treatment setting.

This unique educational experience was designed to emulate a well-functioning interdisciplinary team. Faculty, students, and staff held regular collaborative meetings to plan interventions. The students worked at the house with the residents and the staff, and the faculty served as consultants. All students participating in the interdisciplinary practicum at the Second Chance House took a System of Care course at the university before enrolling in the practicum. Each student brought to the student team his or her unique expertise, and students had the opportunity to apply what they had learned in the classroom to a "real-life" setting. The faculty was experienced in teaching System of Care strategies and worked together to serve as role models for the students, across the disciplines.

In the true spirit of System of Care, regardless of their discipline or level of study, all students worked together to meet the needs of staff and clients at the Second Chance House. Undergraduate student nurses focused on meeting the health care and psychosocial needs of clients but also helped out with projects initiated by students from the other disciplines. Nursing student activities at the house included providing education on the care of the newborn for new mothers, helping residents access health care and navigate the challenging waters of public health care assistance programs, helping to care for residents' children when the residents were engaged in learning activities with students from other disciplines, planning and implementing leisure activities for the residents with the other students, and providing educational activities for staff on the medications being taken by the residents and their children.

The experience at the Second Chance House exemplifies the tenets of System of Care, including collaborative, interdisciplinary practice, community-based care, and building on individual strengths. Although different student groups entered the experience with different goals, the students reported that they had gained expertise in providing care, based on the System of Care values and principles, and that they had benefited from working with students and faculty from other disciplines.

Case Study 2: A Wraparound Program for Foster Children at the Department of Social Services— The Development of a Nurse Case Management Model

Another example of System of Care principles in nursing practice is a wraparound program to address the health, mental health, and psychosocial needs of foster children. A nurse case manager from the health department was assigned as a liaison to the Department of Social Services (DSS) to coordinate the care of foster children, with a focus on health promotion and early case finding. The goal was to coordinate psychosocial and health care by wrapping services around the foster and biological families in order to provide holistic care to both families so that the children could grow and develop in a healthy environment. The nurse care manager coordinated services, including physical, psychosocial, developmental, educational, and family services, working side by side with social workers for the welfare of the children they served.

According to Marx, Benoit, and Kamradt (2003), children in foster care need more health and mental health services than their peers; however, the available services are frequently "inadequate, fragmented and poorly coordinated" (p. 338). Children who enter foster care are often the victims of abuse and neglect and have never experienced a nurturing or stable environment. The children have rarely had consistent primary and preventive health care and, consequently, are at high risk for physical, developmental, and behavioral health problems (Marx, Benoit, & Kamradt). Two of the authors of this chapter, Schmidt and Cherry, developed the Wraparound Triangle of Care Model to illustrate how a nurse case manager coordinates services to meet the multiple needs of children and their families, both the biological and foster parents (see Figure 6-1). Furthermore, the model illustrates how a nurse case manager operates in a collaborative role between the Public Health and Social Services Departments in addressing the needs of children in foster care.

Wraparound Triangle of Care Model to Assist the Child, Family, and Community

Objectives

Child—Nursing case management services are family-centered, culturally competent, strength-based, and outcomes-driven.

Family—Provide family with resources and knowledge to facilitate empowerment toward self-care.

Community—Partner with community organizations who have similar goals for children and families.

Implementation

Child—Collaborate, manage, implement, monitor, and evaluate health care needs.

Family—Identify family stressors that prevent adequate parental care of the child.

Community—Educate the public, public officials, and health care providers to barriers of care for high-risk child populations.

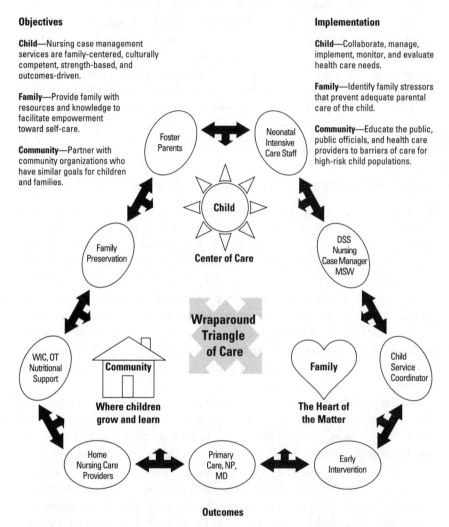

Outcomes

Health needs will be coordinated and implemented in a timely, cost-effective manner. Services provided will be culturally sensitive, meaningful to the family, and valued by the community.

Data will be collected and studied for demographic information, outcomes, and trends to better serve the community in the future.

(Read clockwise, beginning with the Neonatal Intensive Care Staff)

The diagram illustrates the Wraparound Model, based on System of Care, as a framework for the care of foster children and their families and how it guided the care of baby Anne.

FIGURE 6-1 Schmidt, C. & Cherry, J. The Wraparound Triangle of Care Model to Assist The Child, the Family, and the Community, 2004.

The Wraparound Triangle of Care Model was designed to address the health care needs of young children with a focus on prevention, to educate the community about the needs of foster families whose children are "at risk," and to teach them about potential health and developmental problems in these children. The model is a collaborative interdisciplinary health care model based on System of Care values. The model provides guidelines for nursing interventions that are family-centered, culturally sensitive, and coordinated within the community to improve the care of foster children and their families. The Wraparound Triangle of Care Model provided guidelines for working with baby Anne.

Working with a Foster Child Exemplifies the Wraparound Triangle of Care

Baby Anne was the second daughter of a 37-year-old mother who was not only a single parent but was also an insulin-dependent diabetic. Prenatal care was started late in the pregnancy. The first child had died of sudden infant death syndrome 2 years before the birth of this baby. Baby Anne was born at 31-weeks gestation by caesarean section, weighing 4.7 pounds. She was large for her gestational age, had hypokalemia, hypoglycemia, respiratory distress syndrome, and anemia. She remained in the hospital for 11 weeks. Baby Anne was discharged on a sudden infant death syndrome monitor, Neosure, a 22-calorie formula, and a gastrostomy tube (feeding tube) because she experienced significant feeding problems.

Social services became involved with this family after referral from the neonatal intensive care unit. Despite the mother's regular hospital visits, there were questions about her ability to adequately care for the baby and take care of her own medical problems. The Department of Social Services assigned a nurse case manager and a social worker to baby Anne. The social worker was from the Multiple Response System, a strength-based, family-centered, wraparound program that promotes the development of collaborative partnerships with parents and other service providers. Other services for baby Anne and her mother included a child service coordinator, early intervention services, a primary care provider, home nursing care, food from the Women, Infant, and Children Program, occupational therapy, and Family Preservation Services. Members of the wraparound team conducted regular home visits. Eventually, hospitalization was recommended to assess for failure to thrive because of the baby's poor weight gain. During several visits to the hospital, the mother's diabetes was observed to be out of control. Several hypoglycemic episodes required emergency care in the emergency department of the local hospital.

Before discharge, a team decision-making meeting was conducted at the hospital, attended by the Department of Social Services nurse case manager, the Department of Social Services social worker, staff from the neonatal intensive care unit, involved community agencies, and the parents. A safety plan that was agreed on at the decision-making meeting failed, and subsequently, baby Anne was placed in foster care. It was found during the meeting that the mother had not been under a doctor's care for her diabetes since the birth of baby Anne, which resulted in uncontrolled diabetes. As a consequence of this meeting, the Department of Social Services nurse case manager arranged and accompanied the mother to a doctor's appointment to gain an understanding of how to help the mother stabilize the diabetes. A new self-care regime was developed, and the nurse case manager regularly monitored the mother's progress. The mother gained control of her diabetes. Hypoglycemic episodes ceased, and the team began to work toward reunification of the mother and baby.

Both the foster parent and the biological mother attended all of the baby's medical appointments, each contributing to decisions about the baby's care. At the first permanency-planning meeting, the foster mother reported that baby Anne had severe reflux. A few weeks later, during a brief hospitalization for flu, dehydration, and pneumonia, the reflux problem was deemed serious enough to warrant a surgical procedure. A follow-up swallowing study several weeks later confirmed normal swallowing. Five months after the Department of Social Services assumed custody of baby Anne, custody was returned to the biological mother. Mother had been adherent to her medical regime, and her diabetes was under control. Baby Anne's medical problems had been resolved. She was gaining weight, feeding orally, and reaching developmental milestones. The Department of Social Services nurse case manager and social worker continued to facilitate the wraparound services. Department of Social Services' services were eventually discontinued when the mother demonstrated the necessary skills to care for herself and the baby. Tables 6-3 and 6-4 define the terms for the case study discussed above.

System of Care as Evidence-Based Nursing Practice

Evidenced-based practice is the integration of research findings and clinical expertise to provide optimal care (Stuart, 2001). According to Goode

Table 6-3   Definitions of Medical Terms for the Case Study About Baby Anne

- Anemia: A condition in which the blood is deficient in red blood cells, hemoglobin, or in total volume.
- Hypoglycemia: An abnormal decrease of blood sugar.
- Hypokalemia: A decrease of potassium in the circulating blood. Respiratory distress syndrome: An acute lung disease. Difficulty breathing occurs because of a malfunction of the lungs, which frequently occurs in premature infants. The lungs do not expand properly, which causes rapid shallow breathing. The condition can be fatal. It has also been called hyaline membrane disease.
- Sudden infant death syndrome: The unexpected death of an apparently healthy baby, during sleep, before the age of 1 year from an unknown cause.

These definitions were adapted from Merriam-Webster (2002).

Table 6-4   Other Terms Related to the Case of Baby Anne

- Child service coordination: A child service coordinator at the local Department of Public Health is assigned to a child who is at risk for developmental delays. A nurse or a social worker facilitates the coordination of all of the community services that are required to meet the needs of the child and the family.
- Permanency planning: It is the continuous practice of interdisciplinary planning, monitoring, and decision making in order to insure that the best interests of the child, including health and safety and other vital interests are addressed. The permanency planning meeting involves all of the people important to the child, including the parents, who contribute their expertise to developing the plan. The permanency planning interdisciplinary team continuously conducts reviews to update the plan.

Adapted from Guildford County Social Services at http://www.co.guilford.nc.us/government/socservices/#childpro; Legal authority; US Public Law 96-272; the Social Security Act; and North Carolina General Statutes. Retrieved August 10, 2004.

(2001), outcomes from current research provide the evidence for making the best decision about nursing care. Practice guidelines are developed after defining the clinical question, finding the evidence, analyzing, and evaluating it. The replication of findings increases confidence that certain therapeutic strategies have validity (Wilson, 2004). Outcome studies regarding System of Care programs are being conducted across the country. Friesen and Winters (2003) reported that most programs clearly demonstrate a reduction in costs and quality of care improvement. Today, nurses, especially nurse case managers and administrators, are involved in collecting and analyzing data, developing outcome management strategies, and examining the effectiveness of nursing interventions to determine best practice (Brodie, 2001; Goode, 2001).

Summary

Implementing System of Care principles and values into the care of all persons constitutes the "best practice" in nursing. Not only do these principles fit with traditional nursing practice and values such as family-centered and community-based care, but they also promote practices that provide for cost-efficiency and improved client and provider relationships. They also offer great promise in helping address the *Healthy People 2010* goals for America (Clark, 2003; Spector, 2004). Most importantly, System of Care principles and values promote the belief that all persons are worthy of dignity, respect, and self-determination, values instilled into the nursing profession by its original designers such as Florence Nightingale.

Activities to Extend Your Learning

- Select a nursing agency that provides services for children and spend some time observing the nursing care. Discuss with the personnel the program, mission statement, and philosophy of care. Compare it with the System of Care philosophy. Discuss System of Care values and principles with the agency personnel.
- Interview nurses working in pediatric settings or children's health or community mental health settings.
  - How do they incorporate families in the care of the child?
  - How do they address cultural issues?
  - Does the inpatient setting interface with the community-based setting to coordinate a smooth transition from one treatment setting to another?
- If you have the opportunity, talk with a family of a sick, disabled, or emotionally disturbed child.

- What does the family know or believe about the child's health and illness?
- Were the family's ideas solicited when the plan of care was formulated?
- Did the family participate in the decision making?
- Was the family satisfied with the nursing care?

The authors give special thanks to Elizabeth Tornquist and Kimberly Shealy for their editorial assistance.

Suggested Reading

Case Manager

Bodgett, B.P. (1993). Case management in mental health: The pendulum still swings. *Journal of Case Management, 2*(3), 95–100.

Malone, S.B., Reed, M.R., Norbeck, J., Hindsman, R.L., & Knowles, F.E. III. (2004). Development of a training module on therapeutic boundaries for mental health clinicians and case managers. *Lippincott's Case Management, 9*(4), 197–202.

Child Abuse and Foster Care

Pelzer, D. (1995). *A child called "It": One child's courage to survive.* Deerfield Beach, FL: Health Communications, Inc.

Pelzer, D. (1997). *The lost boy. A foster child's search for the love of a family.* Deerfield Beach, FL: Health Communications, Inc.

Pelzer, D. (2004). *The privilege of youth: A teenager's story of longing for acceptance and friendship.* New York: Dutton, Penguin Group, Inc.

Children with a Severe Emotional Disorder

Flach, F. (1990). *Rickie.* New York: Publishers Weekly, Ballantine Books.

Freeman, S. (1997). *The cuckoo's child.* New York: Paperbacks for Children.

Schnurr, R.G. (2000). *Asberger's, Hugh: A child's perspective.* Canada: Anisor Publishing.

Culturally Competent Care

Campinha-Bacote, J. (1998). *The process of cultural competence in the delivery of health care services: A culturally competent model of care* (3rd ed.). Cincinnati, OH: Transcultural C.A.R.E. Associates.

Campinha-Bacote, J. (2000). *Readings and resources in transcultural health and mental health* (12th ed.). Cincinnati, OH: Transcultural C.A.R.E. Associates.

SAMHSA. (1998). *Developing culturally competent systems of care for state mental health services.* Washington, DC: Western Interstate Commission for Higher Education.

Family-Centered Care

Koplewicz, H.S. (1996). *It's nobody's fault: New hope and help for difficult children and their parents.* New York: Random House.
Kozol, J. (1988). *Rachel and her children: Homeless families in America.* New York: Crown Publishers.

Systems of Care

Focal Point: The National Bulletin on Family Support and Children's Mental Health. Research and Training Center on Family Support and Children's Mental Health. Available from: www.rtc.pdx.edu.

References

Ahmann, E. (1994). Family-centered care: Shifting orientation. *Pediatric Nursing, 20*(2), 113–117.
American Association of Colleges of Nursing (AACN). (1998). *Essentials of baccalaureate education.* Washington, DC: Author.
American Nurses Association (ANA). (2004). *Nursing facts: Advanced practice nursing: A new age in health care.* Retrieved September 19, 2004 from: http://www.nursingworld.org/readroom/fsadvprc.htm.
Andrews, M.M. (1999). Theoretical foundations of transcultural nursing. In M.M. Andrews & J.S. Boyle (Eds.), *Transcultural concepts in nursing care* (3rd ed., pp. 3–22). Philadelphia: Lippincott.
Boyd, M.A. (1998). Cultural issues related to mental health care. In M.A. Boyd & M.A. Nihart (Eds.), *Psychiatric nursing: Contemporary practice.* Philadelphia: Lippincott.
Brodie, B. (2001). Developing outcome management strategies. In E.L.Cohen & T.G. Cesta (Eds.), *Nursing case management* (3rd ed., pp 563–572). St. Louis: Mosby.
Brown, N.J., & Magilvy, J.K. (2001). Parish nursing as community-focused case management. In E.L. Cohen & T.G. Cesta (Eds.), *Nursing case management* (3rd ed., pp. 155–163). St. Louis: Mosby.
Brun, C., & Rapp, R.C. (2001). Strengths-based case management: Individual's perspectives on strengths and the case manager relationship. *Social Work, 46*(3), 278–289.
Campinha-Bacote, J. (1997). Understanding the influence of culture. In J. Haber, B. Kranovich-Miller, A.L. McMahon, & P. Price Hoskins (Eds.), *Comprehensive psychiatric nursing* (5th ed., pp. 76–90). St. Louis: Mosby.
Cheven, M., & Brady, B. (2003). Collaboration across disciplines and among agencies within systems of care. In A.J. Pumariega & N.C. Winters (Eds.),

The handbook of child and adolescent systems of care: The new community psychiatry (pp. 66–81). San Francisco: Jossey-Bass.

Clark, M.J. (2003). The context for community health nursing. In M.J. Clark (Ed.), *Community health nursing: Caring for populations* (4th ed., pp. 4–14). Upper Saddle River, NJ: Prentice Hall.

Cohen, E.L., & Cesta, T.G. (2001). Contemporary models of case management: Within the walls case management: An acute care based nursing case management model. In E.L. Cohen & T.G. Cesta (Eds.), *Nursing case management* (3rd ed., pp. 51–71). St. Louis: Mosby.

Conti, R.M. (1996). Nurse case manager roles: Implications for practice and education. *Nursing Administration Quarterly, 21*(1), 67–81.

Finkelman, A.W. (2001). *Managed care: A nursing perspective.* Upper Saddle River, NJ: Prentice Hall.

Foster, S. (1993). Partnering with children and families for evidence-based practice. *Journal of Pediatric Nursing, 9*(1), 3–4.

Francis, S. (1993). The child at risk: Illness, disability and hospitalization. In B.S. Johnson (Ed.), *Adaptation and growth: Psychiatric-mental health nursing* (3rd ed., pp. 799–815). Philadelphia: J.B. Lippincott.

Francis, S. (1995). Disability and chronic illness. In B.S. Johnson (Ed.), *Child, adolescent, and family psychiatric-mental health nursing* (pp. 146–173). Philadelphia: J.B. Lippincott.

Friesen, J.J., & Winters, N.C. (2003). The role of outcomes in systems of care: Quality improvement and program evaluation. In A.J. Pumariega & N.C. Winters (Eds.), *The handbook of child and adolescent System of Care: The new community psychiatry* (pp. 459–486). San Francisco: Jossey-Bass.

Giger, J.N., & Davidhizar, R.E. (2004). *Transcultural nursing.* St. Louis: Mosby.

Goode, C.J. (2001). Outcomes effectiveness and evidence-based practice. In E.R. Cohen & T.G. Cesta (Ed.), *Nursing case management* (3rd ed., pp. 573–580). St. Louis: Mosby.

Green, T. (2003). Facing challenges to family-centered care II: Anger in the clinical setting. *Pediatric Nursing, 29*(3), 212.

Guilford County Social Services. Title IV A. Legal authority: US Public Law 96-272, The Social Security Act and North Carolina General Statutes. Retrieved August 10, 2004 from: http://co.guilford.nc.us/government/socservices/#childpro.

Handron, D.S., Dosser, J.R., McCammon, S.L., & Powell, J.Y. (1998). "Wraparound" the wave of the future: Theoretical and professional practice implications. *Journal of Family Nursing, 4*(1), 65–86.

Hanson, S.H., & Boyd, S.T. (1996). *Family health care nursing: Theory, practice, and research.* Philadelphia: F.A. Davis Co.

Herrick, C.A. (1985). *The role of the Illinois community mental health nurse.* Unpublished doctoral dissertation. Carbondale, IL: Southern Illinois University at Carbondale.

Herrick, C.A., & Bartlett, T.R. (2004). Psychiatric nursing case management: Past, present and future. *Issues in Mental Health Nursing, 25*(6), 589–602.

Huber, D.L. (2002). The diversity of case management models. *Lippincott's Case Management, 7*(4), 212–220.

Johnson, B.S. (1995). Mental health of children, adolescents and families. In B.S. Johnson (Ed.), *Child, adolescent and family psychiatric nursing* (pp. 3–14). Philadelphia: J.B. Lippincott.

Kersbergen, A.L. (1996, August). Case management: A rich history of co-ordinating care to control costs. *Nursing Outlook, 44,* 169–172.

Klainberg, M. (1998). The nature of community health. In M. Klainberg, S. Holzemer, M. Leonard, & J. Arnold (Eds.), *Community health nursing: An alliance for health* (pp. 1–22). McGraw-Hill Nursing Core Series. New York: McGraw-Hill.

Klainberg, M., Holzemer, S., Leonard, M., & Arnold, J. (1998). *Community health nursing: An alliance for health.* McGraw-Hill Nursing Core Series. New York: McGraw-Hill.

Kneisl, C.R. (2004). Client's rights, ethics and advocacy. Creating a thera-peutic environment. In C.R. Kneisl, H.S. Wilson, & E. Trigoboff (Eds.), *Contemporary psychiatric-mental health nursing* (pp. 177–205, 207–231). Upper Saddle River, NJ: Prentice Hall.

Kneisl, C.R., & Wilson, H.S. (2004). The psychiatric–mental health nurse's personal integration and professional role. In C.R. Kneisl, H.S. Wilson, & E. Trigoboff (Eds.), *Contemporary psychiatric-mental health nursing* (pp. 4–22). Upper Saddle River, NJ: Prentice Hall.

Knitzer, J. (1982). *Unclaimed children: The failures of public responsibility to children and adolescents in need of mental health services.* Washington, DC: The Children's Defense Fund.

Koenig, E. (2001). Collaborative models of case management. In E.L. Cohen & T.G. Cesta (Eds.), *Nursing case management: From essentials to advance practice applications* (3rd ed., pp. 73–80). St. Louis: Mosby.

Kuhlman, G., & Wilson, H.S. (2004). Elders. In C.R. Kneisl, H.S. Wilson, & E. Trigoboff (Eds.), *Contemporary psychiatric mental health nursing* (pp. 639–657). Upper Saddle River, NJ: Prentice Hall.

Leininger, M.M. (1991). *Culture care diversity and universality: A theory of nursing.* New York: The National League of Nursing.

Lourie, I.S. (2003). History of community child mental health. In A.J. Pumariega & N.C. Winters (Eds.), *The handbook of child and adolescent systems of care: The new community psychiatry* (pp. 1–16). San Francisco: Jossey-Bass.

Marx, L., Benoit, M., & Kamradt, B. (2003). Foster children in the child wel-fare system. In A.J. Pumariega & N.C. Winters (Eds.), *The handbook of child and adolescent System of Care: The new community psychiatry* (pp. 332–350). San Francisco: Jossey-Bass.

McLuhan, M. (1995). Structuring for partnership: Defining the new organ-ization. In T. Porter-O'Grady & C.K. Wilson (Eds.), *The leadership revolu-tion in health care: Altering systems, changing behaviors* (pp. 70–105). Gaithersburg, MD: Aspen.

McMahon, A.L. (1997). The nurse-client relationship. In J. Haber, B. Karinovich-Miller, A.L. McMahon, & P. Price-Hoskins (Eds.), *Compre-hensive psychiatric nursing* (5th ed., pp. 143–159). St. Louis: Mosby.

Meleski, D.D. (2002). Families with chronically ill children: A literature re-view examines approaches to help them cope. *American Journal of Nursing, 102*(5), 47–54.

Merriam-Webster. (2002). *Langenscheidt's pocket medical dictionary.* New York: Langenscheidt Publishing Group.

Michaels, C., & Cohen, E.L. (2001). Two strategies for managing care: Care management and case management. In E.L. Cohen & T.G. Cesta (Eds.), *Nursing case management* (3rd ed., pp. 31–35). St. Louis: Mosby.

Michaels, C., & Lamb, G. (2001). Beyond the walls case management. In E.L. Cohen & T.G. Cesta (Eds.), *Nursing case management* (3rd ed., pp. 123–126). St. Louis: Mosby.

Mullahy, C.M. (2004). *The case manager's handbook* (3rd ed.). Boston: Jones & Bartlett.

Office of Disease Prevention and Health Promotion, US Department of Health and Human Services. (2000). *Healthy People 2010.* Retrieved September 24, 2004, from: http://www.healthypeople.gov.

Platter, B.K., Vaughn, K., & Young, B.C. (2001). The Colorado psychiatric health case management model: An innovative approach to client-centered care. In E.L. Cohen & T.G. Cesta (Eds.), *Nursing case management* (3rd ed., pp. 91–120). St. Louis: Mosby.

Pothier, P.C. (1974). Developmental reactions in infancy and childhood. In M.L. Kaukman & A.J. Davis (Eds.), *New dimensions in mental health-psychiatric nursing* (pp. 58–95). New York: McGraw-Hill Book.

Powell, S.K. (1996). *Nursing case management: A practical guide to success in managed care.* Philadelphia: Lippincott-Raven.

Powers, P.H., Goldstein, C., Plank, G., Thomas, I., & Conkright, L. (2000). The value of patient family-centered care: One hospital's innovative strategy for involving patients and families in care decisions. *American Journal of Nursing, 100*(5), 84–88.

Pumariega, A.J., & Winters, N.C. (Eds.). (2003). *The handbook of child and adolescent systems of care: The new community psychiatry.* San Francisco: Jossey-Bass.

Puskar, K.R., & Bernardo, L. (2002). Clinical practice: Trends in mental health: Implications for advanced practice nurses. *Journal of the American Academy of Nurse Practitioners, 14,* 214–218.

Ritter-Teitel, J. (1996). New challenges and opportunities in integrated health care system. In D.L. Flarey & S.S. Blancett (Eds.), *Handbook of nurse case management* (pp. 46–67). Gaithersburg, MD: Aspen.

Spector, R.E. (2004). *Cultural diversity in health and illness* (6th ed.). Upper Saddle River, NJ: Prentice Hall.

Stroul, B.A. (1996). *Children's mental health: Creating systems of care in a changing society.* Baltimore, MD: Paul H. Brookes Publishing.

Stroul, B.A. (2003). Systems of care: A framework for children's mental health care. In A.J. Pumariega & N.C. Winters (Eds.), *The handbook of child and adolescent systems of care: The new community psychiatry* (pp. 17–35). San Francisco: Jossey-Bass.

Stroul, B.A., & Friedman, R.M. (1996). The System of Care: Concept and philosophy. In B.A. Stroul (Ed.), *Children's mental health: Creating systems of care in a changing society* (pp. 3–21). Baltimore: Paul H. Brookes Publishing.

Stroul, B.A., & Friedman, R.M. (1986). *A System of Care of children and youth with severe emotional disturbances* (rev. ed.). Washington, DC: Georgetown University Child Development Center, National Technical Assistance Center for Child Mental Health.

Stuart, G.W. (2001). Evidence based psychiatric nursing practice. In G.W. Stuart & M.T. Laraia (Eds.), *Principles and practice of psychiatric nursing* (7th ed., pp. 76–87). St. Louis: Mosby.

Swanson, J.M. (1993). Historical factors: Community health nursing in context. In J.M. Swanson & M. Albrecht (Eds.), *Community health nursing: Promoting the health of aggregates* (pp. 13–40). Philadelphia: Saunders Co.

Tahan, H.A. (1998) Case management: A heritage more than a century old. *Lippincott's Nursing Case Management, 4*(6), 55–62.

Thurkettle, M.A., & Noji, A. (2003). Case management. A source of support and stability for the client and the health care system. *Lippincott's Case Management, 8*(2), 88–94.

Tripp-Reimer, T., & Lively, S.H. (1993). Cultural considerations in mental health-psychiatric nursing. In R.P. Rawlins, S.K. Williams, & C.K. Beck (Eds.), *Mental health psychiatric nursing: A holistic life cycle approach* (3rd ed., pp. 166–179). St. Louis: Mosby.

Washington, G.T. (2001). Families in crisis: Nurses say advocates help them meet families' needs without shortchanging patient care. *Nursing Management, 32*(5), 29–32.

Wilson, H.S. (2004). Evidence-based practice in psychiatric mental health nursing. In C.R. Kneisl, H.S. Wilson, & E. Trigoboff (Eds.), *Contemporary psychiatric mental health nursing* (pp. 42–56). Upper Saddle River, NJ: Prentice Hall.

Winters, N.C., & Terrell, E. (2003). Case management: The linchpin of community based System of Care. In A.J. Pumariega & N.C. Winters (Eds.), *The handbook of child and adolescent systems of care: The new community psychiatry* (pp. 171–202). San Francisco: Jossey-Bass.

The Development and Application of the System of Care Approach from the Perspective of Child and Adolescent Psychiatry

JACQUELINE ETEMAD AND SUSAN TACCHERI

Objectives

- Understand the System of Care as best practice and the application of System of Care principles beyond the seriously emotionally disturbed to a broader range of clinical interventions.
- Describe the development of System of Care principles through the course of child and adolescent psychiatry's history.
- Discuss
  - the addition of psychological, social, and cultural dimensions to the biological model of psychiatry;
  - the work of child and adolescent psychiatry with other disciplines, including psychology, social work, and nursing;
  - the development of work with families in child and adolescent psychiatry;

- ▣ the influence of the community mental health movement on the development of child and adolescent psychiatry;
- ▣ the alternative services movement's contributions to the System of Care approach.
- ▣ Explain the importance of experience with the System of Care method as a part of clinical training for all disciplines.
- ▣ Describe the contributions that a child and adolescent psychiatrist can make in specific System of Care clinical interventions.
- ▣ Discuss what the child and adolescent psychiatrist brings to the development and maintenance of System of Care community-based programs.
- ▣ Identify the barriers to child and adolescent psychiatrist participation in System of Care.
- ▣ Discuss the role of the specialty society in supplementing the training of child and adolescent psychiatrists for participation in System of Care.

The System of Care method has become the standard of care or best practice to address complex clinical situations among children with serious emotional disturbances and their families. System of Care emphasizes collaboration among caregivers of many disciplines, empowerment of families, and a commitment to do what it takes to achieve a positive result. It is an approach that identifies and capitalizes on strengths rather than focusing on pathology. System of Care is flexible and creative, tailoring an intervention to the needs of the specific clinical situation. System of Care is sensitive to specific factors, broadly identified as cultural, that may influence which interventions are more likely to achieve a positive response.

The history of System of Care is one of progressive discovery and improvement of practice over the past century. The development of System of Care has not been linear, as principles learned have at times been ignored or forgotten, only to be rediscovered at a later time. The child guidance movement, the community mental health movement, and the alternative services movement have each added dimensions that have become part of System of Care as we know it today.

Child and adolescent psychiatry is the medical specialty that addresses the psychiatric needs of developing individuals. The profession of child and adolescent psychiatry traces its roots back to the late 19th century. Many interconnections can be identified between events in the history of child and adolescent psychiatry and the development of the System of Care approach, such as work with other disciplines, consultation to schools and agencies, and the inclusion of families in the treatment of their children. A review of the history of child and adolescent psychiatry sheds light on how the various elements of the System of Care method have been discovered and integrated into a coherent approach.

The particular combination of medical, psychodynamic, and developmental expertise of the child and adolescent psychiatrist is well suited to contributing to the creation and implementation of the System of Care approach. Recent trends in child and adolescent psychiatry have moved the profession away from its roots in interdisciplinary practice in favor of a medical model. Nonetheless, child and adolescent psychiatrists have the potential to make effective contributions to the System of Care approach at specific levels, including clinical interventions, program development and implementation, and advocacy.

At the clinical level, the child and adolescent psychiatrists can role model and teach the System of Care concepts and encourage appropriate application of System of Care principles to provide better standards of care. As consultants to programs, the child and adolescent psychiatrists can contribute to effective implementation, and through participation in specialty societies and in their own communities, child and adolescent psychiatrists will find opportunities to advocate for children and adolescents by promoting the development of comprehensive mental health services that apply System of Care principles.

The Child and Adolescent Psychiatrist's Perspective

Historical Development of System of Care

Roots of Child Psychiatry in Psychology and Medicine

Musto (2002) traced the history of child psychiatry to its roots in both psychology and medicine. The contribution from psychology focused on the study of normal development, as reflected in the work of G. Stanley Hall (1904). At the end of the 19th century and later, the focus was on the normative work of his student Arnold Gesell (1952), who in 1911 established the precursor to the Yale Child Study Center in New Haven, Connecticut. In contrast, the medical/psychiatric contribution to child and adolescent psychiatry approached the understanding of children through the study of mental disorders. Both of these paths have been active in the development of training, research, and clinical practice in child and adolescent psychiatry, and both have relevance for active participation in community-based System of Care.

Biological and Psychodynamic Approaches

In the history of psychiatry, psychopathology has been viewed in two ways. The first is often termed the biological approach and tends to view psychiatric disorders as based in the structure of the brain and nervous system. The second is generally referred to as the psychodynamic approach and places emphasis on the impact of experience or life events as a factor in the development of psychopathology.

During the 19th century, American psychiatrists, known as alienists, leaned strongly toward a view of biological determinism for mental disorder. Then in the early 20th century, the teachings of Sigmund Freud reached America and rapidly came to dominate the field of psychiatry. Although Freud had begun his career with an emphasis on biological determinism, later, through the development of psychoanalysis, he focused attention on the impact of life experiences on the development of psychopathology. His psychodynamic view held that appropriate psychological intervention could be effective in reducing mental disorder (Andreasen & Black, 1991; Freud, 1925; Freud, 1955–1972).

Although child psychiatry has its roots in the biomedical sciences, the behavioral and biosocial sciences are equally important. According to Adams and Fras (1988), "Without a firm knowledge [of both biomedical and biosocial sciences], the child psychiatrist may be hampered" (p. 569). The interplay between the biological and psychodynamic approaches embodied in Freud's work (1955–1972) is a persistent thread throughout the development of psychiatry. At times, the field of psychiatry has favored one over the other. The psychodynamic approach held sway through the first half of the 20th century, until the discovery of medications that were effective in the treatment of psychosis, which marked the beginning of a swing back toward biology. Although psychiatry as a whole has leaned toward one or the other extreme, many have been drawn to the idea of a combined psychobiologic approach. George Engel's (1980) description of the psychobiological model addressed the individual, the family, and the community. An increased understanding of all of the elements that impinge on any given clinical situation, with the addition of social and cultural dimensions, is an appropriate extension of this perspective.

Developments in the understanding of brain structure and function, coupled with advances in psychopharmacology, have led to increasing emphasis on the benefits of pharmacologic interventions over the past 50 years. Recently, considerations have been given to the possibility that pharmacologic interventions may influence the structure as well as the function of the brain, particularly in the developing individual (Andreasen & Black, 1991). Integrating both the biological and psychological approaches, plus the addition of social and cultural dimensions, is necessary to provide the comprehensive treatment that is the goal of System of Care.

Interdisciplinary Tradition in Child Psychiatry

Jones (1999) traced the history of the child guidance movement. Social forces in the late 19th and early 20th century had a role in determining that mental health services for children and adolescents, which moved beyond the treatment of a few individuals to the development of community services for children and families. Industrialization, immigration, and urbanization gave rise to large populations of city children with significant mental health needs. Out of this need, the child guidance movement was born.

William Healy established the Chicago Psychopathic Institute in 1909 to serve the Juvenile Court (Adams & Fras, 1988, p. 589). This clinic was a prototype for the many clinics established in the 1920s that provided an interdisciplinary (psychiatry, psychology, social work) treatment model to address children's mental health needs. The development of services for children in the criminal justice system also harks back to Healy's later work with the Judge Baker Foundation in Boston. In both the child guidance and juvenile justice system, an interdisciplinary model was paramount. In these early years, child psychiatrists were individual physicians who chose to work with children. They came to child psychiatry from both pediatrics and from psychiatry. Many were trained in psychoanalysis, but it was also common for them to get some or all of their child psychiatry training in child guidance clinics where they worked together with psychologists and social workers (Adams & Fras, 1988). Meanwhile, in inpatient facilities, nurses became a part of the interdisciplinary team (see Chapter 6, *System of Care in Nursing*).

Working with the Family

Although the primary focus of Freud's (1955–1972) work was adult psychopathology, child psychoanalysis can be traced back to his case study of "Little Hans" in 1909, a child he treated indirectly through work with the patient's father (Adams & Fras, 1988, p. 589). Freud's daughter Anna went on to develop child psychoanalysis as a treatment modality for children. Anna did not work with the parents but focused primarily on children, seeing the child as frequently as possible, as many as four times per week. She stated that the outlook for the child's recovery was more hopeful if the parents had been or were concurrently in psychoanalysis when the child was seeing a child therapist (Szurek, 1967).

Child psychoanalysis was primarily an intervention with the individual child patient. Later, work emphasized seeing children in the context of their family. In the 1940s, Stanislaus Szurek and Adelaide Johnson pioneered the idea of understanding psychopathology in children as an expression of conflict within and between their parents (Szurek & Johnson, 1952). By that time, it was not unusual for mothers to be involved in the treatment of their children. Szurek (1952) went one step farther by emphasizing the importance of involving fathers, as well as mothers, in treatment. Szurek suggested that therapies that failed to include the significant adults in the life of a child were less likely to be successful than those that did. It is a small step to consider that when treatment focuses only on the individual or family and fails to include the other agencies, institutions, and caretakers involved in the life of the child, the result will be less successful than when a comprehensive System of Care approach is implemented. Thus, a System of Care approach can be seen as a natural evolution from working with children and families.

Several approaches to working with families were developed through the 1950s and 1960s. A treatment model called conjoint therapy described work with all members of a family as a group (Satir, 1967). Szurek (1952) championed the technique, sometimes called collaborative family therapy. A single therapist worked individually with both the child patient and the parents and then periodically saw the entire family. In some cases, different therapists saw family members individually and then met together in family sessions. Often these therapists came from different disciplines, creating a powerful vehicle for learning an interdisciplinary approach. Child and adolescent psychiatry trainees who worked together with others in the treatment of a family developed collaborative and consultative skills that are important to the System of Care approach. During the 1970s, the field of family therapy evolved further toward the System of Care through the work of Salvador Minuchin (1974) and his systemic family therapy. Minuchin's school was the first to include representatives from relevant agencies in the family therapy process.

Family-centered care has slowly gained wide acceptance in child and adolescent psychiatry and is now central to the System of Care approach (Huffine & Anderson, 2003). There was a time when the focus on the family as part of a child's treatment was interpreted as blaming the parents. Even today, caregivers who lack appropriate training and clinical experience may at times overidentify with clients, split families, and assign blame.

Child and adolescent psychiatrists are just beginning to come to terms with the notion of empowering families and identifying them as equal partners in the treatment of the child. As physicians, they may be influenced by a tradition of paternalistic medicine that assumes the doctor knows best. Along with other physicians, they are learning that families are a center around which treatment must be built and whose benefit to the child can only be enhanced by encouraging their participation as equal members of the treatment team.

Community Psychiatry and Child and Adolescent Psychiatry

Lourie (2003) traced the history of community child mental health that eventually led to the development of System of Care. During the 1950s, with the advent of phenothiazine medication and its applications to large populations of the mentally ill, many chronically ill patients were released from mental institutions and returned to their communities. This population shift stimulated a major change in mental health policy in the United States. Beginning in 1963, federal funding was provided for the development of approximately 1,200 community mental health centers. However, the inclusion of services for children was delayed until the mid 1970s, by which time a drop of enthusiasm and funding for community psychiatry had supervened. Despite the foresight of the Joint Commission on Mental Health of Children (1965–1970), the promise of comprehensive child mental health services was not realized. Yet many innovative programs were created, and much was learned about how services could be delivered most effectively. Concepts used in the community mental health movement were built on the tradition of child guidance, but implementation was lacking because of the low priority of services for children.

Even though community mental health services for children tended to lag behind those for adults, during the 1950s and 1960s, training in child psychiatry was influenced by the community mental health movement. Funds for training that emphasized community psychiatry were available, and experience in community consultation was an integral part of most training programs. Also during the 1950s and 1960s, in the heyday of federal training grants, residents in child psychiatry had many opportunities to acquire skills in individual and family psychotherapy and to do interdisciplinary work in consultation with schools, agencies, and hospitals. Consultation skills learned in the community mental health setting have become important in the implementation of programs of mental health care. Today, psychiatric consultation to school programs is prevalent, as mental health professionals assist teachers to deal with children who have learning and behavioral disorders (Porter, Pearson, Keenan, & Duval-Harvey, 2003).

The community mental health movement marked the shift of populations of children with serious emotional disturbances out of large institutions and back into communities. It was necessary to develop services to meet the needs of these children, and the pressure to meet these needs ultimately contributed to the development of better and more comprehensive models of service (Lourie, 2003).

Alternative Services for Youth Movement

Lourie (2003) described the history of the alternative services for youth movement, which began in the 1970s during the time that funding for community mental health services was waning and alternative sources of care were being developed for a growing population of alienated youth. In the absence of appropriate government-supported services, drop-in clinics or runaway shelters sprang up in areas where disaffected youth congregated. These ad hoc programs often started with general health care and only later moved to consideration of meeting mental health needs. Programs emphasized flexibility and meeting the expressed needs of clients rather than applying traditional models of care. The alternative services movement fostered many of the approaches later evident in the wraparound approach so characteristic of the System of Care model.

As was true with the other traditional disciplines, child and adolescent psychiatry's participation in this movement was initially limited to a few individuals who participated in local community programs on a volunteer basis. However, as the alternative services movement took hold, community service opportunities were increasingly seen as a worthwhile adjunct to the training or practice for some. Those with a special interest in such groups as ethnic minorities, inner city children, runaway or throwaway children, or gay and lesbian youth sought opportunities for training and service in local programs that were increasingly organized and better funded. Gradually, these activities became part of some child and adolescent psychiatry training programs that were enriched by these experiences with new and diverse populations. Trainees were able to increase their level of cultural competence as well as to learn the "new" techniques (many actually an extension of earlier child guidance principles) that were the underpinnings of what later became known as the System of Care approach (Lourie, 2003).

Increasing Fragmentation of Community Mental Health Services

Lourie (2003) discussed the increasing fragmentation of community mental health services during the 1970s and 1980s. Despite renewed interest and a series of legislative efforts, the goal of comprehensive mental health services for children remained elusive, and in 1981, direct federal funding was abandoned in favor of block grants to the states. State programs tended to emphasize existing services and often failed to reach congressional goals for inclusion of services for children.

Meanwhile, existing services were increasingly fragmented. The remains of the community mental health centers were poorly funded and offered few services to children. Child guidance centers and other clinics that operated on a similar model received little funding and tended to serve mainly middle-class and only moderately disturbed children. Many disturbed older children and adolescents with severe behavior problems entered a juvenile justice system that, apart from a few exceptional programs, placed increasing emphasis on punishment to the detriment of mental health care. In 1974, under pressure from civil rights advocates for the disabled, schools had been mandated to provide special education services for all disabled children, including those with serious emotional disturbances. However, the rise of special education also tended to break down traditional consultative relationships between mental health professionals and schools, as educational rather than mental health models were emphasized.

The majority of the most disturbed children gravitated toward a child welfare system that provided mental health services for abused, neglected, and abandoned children no longer cared for by families. As third-party payers reduced coverage for long-term residential care, such treatment became increasingly limited to the child welfare system. Unfortunately, in order to access services for their children, parents frequently had to give up "custody of their child with emotional disturbance to the welfare agency" (Lourie, 2003, p. 11).

Federal Action to Support System of Care Philosophy

The many problems and failures of mental health services for children were powerfully described in *Unclaimed Children,* a report by Jane

Knitzer (1982), who complied the findings of a 4-year study, supported by the Children's Defense Fund, regarding the national services for emotionally disturbed children and adolescents (Stroul, 1996). Inspired in part by findings from this study, renewed energy for child advocacy led to funding in 1984 of the Child and Adolescent Service System Program. This federal program represented a new level of integration of what had been learned from the child guidance movement and the Joint Commission on the Mental Health of Children as well as the alternative services movement. Child and Adolescent Service System Program principles, as described by Stroul and Friedman (1986), included support for interagency systems of care, improved mental health resources within Systems of Care, enhancing the role for the family, and assuring that services were culturally relevant. The ideal intervention began with a long-term commitment to a child with serious emotional disturbances and the family and worked outward to develop an integrated System of Care that could follow the child as long as help was needed. This wraparound approach became the hallmark of the first major implementation of Child and Adolescent Service System Program principles through the Mental Health Services Program for Youth of the Robert Wood Johnson Foundation. In 1992 Congress passed the Comprehensive Community Mental Health Services for Children and Their Families Program that continues to support local development of System of Care-based programs (Lourie, 2003; Stroul, 1996, 2003).

Given the more flexible approach to developing and maintaining a System of Care approach for individual patients including flexibility as regards role and funding, child and adolescent psychiatrists began to participate in some of the early Child and Adolescent Service System Program implementations. Individual case experiences led to increasing appreciation of the diverse skills of the child and adolescent psychiatrist and their potential contribution to a System of Care approach.

Implementation

The Child and Adolescent Psychiatrist's Contributions to Systems of Care

The Child and Adolescent Psychiatrist's Contributions to Clinical Interventions, Based on System of Care Values and Principles

By now, the System of Care method has been refined to a point in which it can be reproduced as a clinical intervention. A specific set of skills can be identified that are required for effective implementation of System of Care on a clinical level. These skills can be taught, and with a satisfactory combination of mandate, funding, and expertise, complex cases that seemed hopeless with more standard approaches can be treated with considerable success. As teams and their members become more experienced in the System of Care approach, the effort required to develop effective working relationships decreases. Problems may arise with personnel changes and the need to bring new people up to speed, but as long as the overarching System of Care program is adequately supported and working well, problems that arise in individual teams are manageable.

Although in some instances the child and adolescent psychiatrist operates primarily as the member of the wraparound team who provides the psychiatric services, in most cases, this role tends to expand to one of consultant and facilitator. Table 7-1 lists many of the skills that the child and adolescent psychiatrist may bring to specific System of Care clinical interventions.

Table 7-1   **What the Child and Adolescent Psychiatrist Can Bring to System of Care Clinical Interventions**

1. Understanding of severe disorders addressing both biological and psychodynamic components. Ability to perform and/or coordinate comprehensive evaluations and develop appropriate treatment plans.
2. Understanding psychodynamic approaches to mental disorders, including individual, group, and family and systems approaches. Ability to perform, to teach, and to supervise psychotherapies.
3. Understanding the biology of mental disorder. The ability to direct psychopharmacologic aspects of treatment. The ability to teach the role of medication to other System of Care participants and to help address issues of compliance.
4. Developmental perspective. Understanding of different expectations at different ages and stages of development.
5. Medical training that includes experience with severe disorder and life and death situations. Ability to maintain a cool head in a crisis. Modeling and teaching patience and perseverance.
6. Skills as a consultant or facilitator in a group process.

Case Study 1

The Child and Adolescent Psychiatrist as a Member of the Wraparound (System of Care) Team

This case illustrates the level of complexity for which the System of Care method is useful. It also shows the many ways in which the child and adolescent psychiatrist can advance the System of Care process by providing a combination of direct treatment, collaboration, and consultation. A wide range of experience and a high degree of flexibility are important to effective functioning of the child and adolescent psychiatrist in the System of Care setting.

RG is an 11-year-old boy with diagnoses of posttraumatic stress disorder, attention deficit hyperactivity disorder, generalized anxiety disorder, and bipolar disorder. He presented with disruptive behaviors in multiple settings. RG has a history of sexual abuse victimization by the father of his younger two siblings, who have also been sexually abused by their father. His mother abused drugs (benzodiazepines and methamphetamine) and was unemployed for years. His maternal grandmother, who was also involved in caretaking RG and his siblings, was also abusing methamphetamines and alcohol and would use drugs with RG's mother.

After several reports from child protective service, the children were removed from the home and put in foster care. RG's two siblings were placed in a regular foster care home, whereas RG required a therapeutic foster care home placement (a higher level of care home with just one foster child and specially trained foster parents) because of his disruptive behaviors.

Because of the complexity of this case, RG and his family were referred to the county wraparound services program. A case facilitator was assigned who developed a plan to include all treating providers, all involved agencies, the school, and the family in a multisystem (System of Care) approach to treatment.

With the leverage of child welfare, the mother was able to leave the abusing father and take out a restraining order on him when he stalked her. The child and adolescent psychiatrist worked with the rest of the team in strongly recommending addiction treatment for RG's mother. She entered addiction treatment in an intensive outpatient program that monitored her urine for substance use and required her to attend community recovery support groups—in her case, Narcotics Anonymous—in addition to attending the addiction treatment program three times a week for 3 months. Early on in treatment, when the mother relapsed, relevant providers were informed promptly, and the mother was made aware that she would be held accountable.

All child and adolescent psychiatrists are fully trained in general psychiatry before they begin the process of specializing in child and adolescent psychiatry. Thus, it is possible, where appropriate, for the child and adolescent psychiatrist to provide and support psychiatric services for adult family members as well as for children. The child and adolescent psychiatrist evaluated the mother and followed her for her co-occurring substance use and psychiatric disorders (depressive disorder and generalized anxiety disorder). When the initial problems were somewhat stabilized, the child and adolescent psychiatrist was also able to address ongoing treatment needs for the mother, such as the continued close monitoring of substance use (including regular urine drug screens) and ongoing individual therapy. The mother got a job at a local Dairy Queen and was able to maintain independent living in a rented apartment. After the mother completed 1 year of steady employment and continued abstinence, RG's three sibling were returned to her care with continued child welfare monitoring.

The child and adolescent psychiatrist evaluated RG and treated him with psychoactive medication. In addition, the child and adolescent psychiatrist collaborated with the teacher about RG's behavior in the classroom. Attempts were made by the child and adolescent psychiatrist to get RG transferred to another educational setting that could tolerate his disruptive behaviors on a full-day schedule, but these were unsuccessful. RG's aggressive and disruptive classroom behaviors persisted, and the school decreased his educational programming to half days. The therapeutic foster care mother then had to use afternoons to homeschool RG instead of getting much needed time for herself. Because he continued to be agitated and aggressive in the therapeutic foster home as well, both the therapeutic foster care parents and the agency that contracted with the parents felt that they could no longer provide foster care for RG. The child and adolescent psychiatrist attended multisystem provider meetings, discussed level-of-care needs for RG, and was able to facilitate admission for RG to a residential treatment program through clinical discussions with the relevant program staff.

During the course of work with RG and his family, the child and adolescent psychiatrist also collaborated with the family therapist about her work with the family, about the mother's clinical status, and about the need to address the grandmother's ongoing addiction if she was to resume her caretaking role with the children. After RG's admission to residential care, the child and adolescent psychiatrist discussed the case periodically with the residential treatment staff to facilitate their work with the family and with staff from the other agencies working with the family.

RG has been in residential treatment for 6 months. After 2.5 years of wraparound care, the family has stabilized, with mother and grandmother providing adequate care for RG's siblings and with their overall functioning much improved. Ongoing efforts are directed toward moving RG to a less restrictive level of care as soon as possible.

Case Study 2

The Child and Adolescent Psychiatrist's Contributions to Program Development in Communities Implementing a System of Care Approach

Although the System of Care method has developed to the point where it can be reproduced with relative assurance that a useful intervention can be achieved, the implementation of System of Care at the program level is another matter. The success of a System of Care program depends on the right combination of funding and political will coupled with strong leadership and the participation of capable professionals of all disciplines.

The child and adolescent psychiatrist can make important contributions at the level of System of Care program development and maintenance. Table 7-2 lists many of the contributions child and adolescent psychiatrists can make at the System of Care program level. At times, as in case study 2, the child and adolescent psychiatrist is given a specific role as facilitator. In other situations, as in case study 3, the child and adolescent psychiatrist may have to fashion his or her own role. The child and adolescent psychiatrists can also participate in advocating for better health care systems that incorporate the best practice principles of System of Care.

Table 7-2   What the Child and Adolescent Psychiatrist Can Bring to Programs That Are Implementing a System of Care Approach

1. A knowledge base that includes getting and managing funds, awareness of how to get things done, and details of administering a complex system. The child and adolescent psychiatrist does not necessarily have to do everything, but must have understanding of what needs to be done in order to facilitate a System of Care approach.

2. Consultative skills. The ability to assist others to move beyond turf battles to working cooperatively and the ability to reduce anxiety levels of patient, family, and professionals so that each can function more effectively.
3. Cultural competence. An awareness of characteristics of different cultures and implications for effective program development.
4. Leadership. The ability to be firm, decisive, authoritative. The leadership role often goes to the one with the highest level of training. However, also required is the recognition that traditional hierarchies may be less relevant than pragmatism with regard to who can do what best. The ability to follow as well as to lead.
5. Political savvy. The ability to assess complex systems, determine the political climate, and respond appropriately to that climate. The ability to develop networks that will be effective in achieving specific goals and to find a way into systems that are closed and/or dysfunctional.
6. Flexibility. Willingness to try new approaches, accept new roles, and learn from experience what works best in different settings. The ability to model flexibility for others.
7. Idealism. Dedication. Caring. Perseverance. Patience. Willingness to commit for the long haul and to continue working in the face of limited progress or reward.

Case Study 3

The Child and Adolescent Psychiatrist as an Agency Leader and Program Facilitator

This case demonstrates that the child and adolescent psychiatrist has unique skills to offer a community attempting to build a System of Care, especially as regards facilitating collaboration. It also illustrates a situation in which the child and adolescent psychiatrist is given the flexibility needed to operate effectively at all levels of the System of Care program.

In 1996, a $5 million demonstration grant in a suburban southeastern county supported development of a System of Care approach to work with children with serious emotional disturbances and their families. The availability of funds was contingent on collaboration among agencies. This mandate, coupled with a changing of the guard in the child welfare system, enabled agencies that had operated largely in isolation to develop collaborative relationships that broke down traditional barriers.

The county mental health center hired and later promoted to medical director an early career child and adolescent psychiatrist. Her job was to facilitate development of a System of Care approach. The psychiatrist was given flexibility to develop her role and had no specific demands to produce clinical work.

When the psychiatrist arrived, she found that children were being seen for play and individual therapy without a family component to treatment. At an early meeting of community stakeholders, a facilitator asked each person what they thought was most important to help the families in the county. The child and adolescent psychiatrist said, "My goal is to empower families." Some weeks later she encountered a child welfare supervisor who said, "I remember you; you're the empowering families person." Saying the words was just the beginning. The child and adolescent psychiatrist was able to model for and to teach the community to appreciate the importance of bringing families into the treatment process.

The child and adolescent psychiatrist also taught the art of "reframing," that is, looking at a situation in a new way. She encouraged "strength based" rather than "deficit" assessments, modeling this through her own evaluations.

When appropriate, the child and adolescent psychiatrist met with agency supervisors to collaborate on specific case plans or on overall System of Care issues. She also joined a community collaborative team with a staff from all the child service agencies. The process of collaboration helped to dispel negative expectations among personnel of different agencies and encouraged a cooperative approach focused on providing the care that was needed rather than struggling over who would pay for a given service. Building relationships took time; however, gradually, beachheads of credibility were established, and the ability to work together was strengthened. As various agencies learned to work together, the process with new children and families could be streamlined.

For the period that the grant was available, many children and families benefited from the higher level of commitment and continuity of care provided through the System of Care model. Outcome measures supported that under this system patients did better, and overall costs of care were reduced. Whether as team participant or community consultant, the child and adolescent psychiatrist was able to have a role in the evolution of various aspects of System of Care development. The flexibility of her role modeled the flexibility required of others who were increasingly being asked to go outside traditional roles, both in the collaboration process and in planning specific interventions.

When the grant funding terminated, the System of Care program was unable to continue operating at the same level. However, much of what had been learned was retained, and many principles of the System of Care method continue to be operative in the community.

Funding for mental health programs for children and adolescents waxes and wanes, as fiscal constraints occur at the federal, state, and local levels. As noted in the previous case study, the grant funding ended. Although the professionals on the interdisciplinary collaborative team may continue to implement System of Care values and principles, new people coming into child serving agencies do not necessarily have the same knowledge and commitment to System of Care. Implementation of System of Care interventions may not remain at the same level in terms of quality care, which points to the need for ongoing in-service education, even without grant funding. The following case study depicts the challenges that the child and adolescent psychiatrist must face to overcome the barriers in maintaining quality programs for children and adolescents.

Case Study 4

The Child and Adolescent Psychiatrist's Role in a Faltering System of Care Program

This case illustrates how the child and adolescent psychiatrist can be a facilitator of System of Care in a situation in which a specific mandate for that role is weak or lacking. In troubled systems, child and adolescent psychiatrists fall quite naturally into a supportive role that mirrors the kind of work they have learned to do with troubled families and individuals. They may be asked in direct and indirect ways to be authoritative and to provide firm guidance. In response, they have the opportunity to advocate for a best practice approach that includes the System of Care method.

In one midwestern county, a wraparound program was developed through the commitment of various community leaders with a combination of local, state, federal, and private funding. A child and adolescent psychiatrist with System of Care experience in another community was hired by the local mental health center for a position that combined delivery of clinical services for children with a role as facilitator for the wraparound program. As the team psychiatrist for the county wraparound team, the child and adolescent psychiatrist was involved in case discussions and treatment planning and was given a role on the plan review team that discussed families that had reached an impasse or required additional time from wraparound facilitators to reach their goals.

The child and adolescent psychiatrist also participated as a clinician member of the wraparound team for specific cases. At the clinical level, child and adolescent psychiatrist contributions included education about diagnosis, prognosis, or medications; the prescription of medication and the ordering of laboratory and other diagnostic tests; referral for general medical, neurologic, genetic, or other subspecialty care; and referral to or recommendations for another level of care within the behavioral health continuum.

The wraparound program was functioning well when the child and adolescent psychiatrist arrived. However, over the next 3 years, a cascading series of fiscal problems led to many cuts in services, especially in the child welfare arena. Collaboration among the child-serving agencies began to break down. Decreased options for interventions led team members to become demoralized. The wraparound team of which the child and adolescent psychiatrist was a part became less interested in didactics and more focused on specific cases, as well as on the future of the team. Funding cuts also affected the child and adolescent psychiatrist's role, as there was increasing pressure to achieve productivity targets in the mental health center.

The child and adolescent psychiatrist's role shifted from being a member of a functioning System of Care program to observing with concern the unraveling of that program while trying to keep up with increasing clinical demands. With a background in systems and group dynamics, the child and adolescent psychiatrist was able to assess the process and provide feedback that helped interagency management and community leaders address obstacles to System of Care.

The child and adolescent psychiatrist noticed that child/family team members were not including representatives of other agencies on a consistent basis. The child and adolescent psychiatrist was able to advocate and to model collaboration, for example, offering to contact a probation officer to speak about an adjudicated juvenile or asking to have a provider team meeting when the child/family team is not working well together.

The community remains committed to the wraparound program and continues its efforts at reimplementation; however, many new people are involved, and the role of child and adolescent psychiatrist as an overall program facilitator is no longer clear. It has been necessary to negotiate participation in community teams and to build credibility through interventions around specific cases that show the benefits of the System of Care method. By a combination of advocacy, consultative support, and relationship building, the child and adolescent psychiatrist's role in advancing the reimplementation process to maintain a quality program has become increasingly effective.

Barriers to Effective Participation by Child and Adolescent Psychiatrists in System of Care

Child and adolescent psychiatrists are limited in many settings by their job descriptions. When their role is defined as someone who does very brief and limited psychiatric evaluations and then prescribes medication, their opportunities to provide education, consultation, and other forms of facilitation can be sharply limited. This problem of a narrow definition of function is part of the larger problem that characterizes our entire health care system. Flexibility of function as well as flexibility in the development of treatment that fits appropriately to each individual case is essential to a health care system that is efficient and cost-effective.

Even if child and adolescent psychiatrists are allowed more flexibility to function within System of Care programs, they will not do so effectively unless they have the appropriate mix of skills and experience. The way that child and adolescent psychiatrists are trained today influences how they function in practice and how their roles are defined.

Schowalter (2003) traced the history of training in child and adolescent psychiatry. Child psychiatry training that had originally taken place primarily in child guidance clinics and was later connected with state and private mental hospitals where many adult psychiatrists received their training ultimately became associated with medical schools that were increasingly located within universities. Thus, child psychiatry gradually separated itself from its companion disciplines of psychology and social work. However, under the influence of "old-timers" in the field, training that emphasized work with other disciplines, including case collaboration, consultation, and experience in community agencies, persisted over the years.

During the past two decades, with a few significant exceptions, child and adolescent psychiatry training programs have focused increasingly on mastering an ever-growing body of knowledge about psychopharmacologic interventions. At the same time, reduction in training funds has forced faculty and trainees to spend hours once devoted to learning to earning money for their cash-strapped training programs. Plus, reduced funding for mental health services has placed a premium on training child and adolescent psychiatrists to do rapid assessment and brief interventions. As hospital stays and outpatient therapies have become increasingly compressed in time, the opportunity for in-depth, long-term contact with seriously disturbed children and their families has been reduced or eliminated from many training programs. Little time remains in most programs to learn the complexities of approaches to families, much less to acquire the skills of participating in a System of Care approach.

Especially as they start their careers, the child and adolescent psychiatrists of today tend to practice as they have been trained, with a heavy emphasis on the role of medical provider. However, some child and adolescent psychiatrists have counteracted the trend toward a narrowly defined medical role for the child and adolescent psychiatrist, as they have gained experience and have seen the importance of the family in the child's recovery. Some have been responsible for developing innovative programs in schools and juvenile courts that emphasize at least dual-system if not multisystem interventions. More recently, some have participated in programs that use a System of Care approach.

Because many of the skills needed for this work have not been covered in their training or early clinical experience, child and adolescent psychiatrists have found themselves reinventing the principles that guided their forebears. Many have turned to the American Academy of Child and Adolescent Psychiatry, as well as other specialty societies, as a resource for development of skills in advocacy, consultation, and System of Care approaches.

The Role of the Child Psychiatrist

The Role of the Specialty Society

In 1953, the leading child psychiatrists of the day established the American Academy of Child Psychiatry on the model of a medical special society. Originally an exclusive organization for distinguished practitioners and academicians, in 1972, the American Academy of Child Psychiatry opened its membership to all who were trained in the field of child psychiatry. To reflect more accurately the training and practice of its members, the American Academy of Child Psychiatry changed its name in 1988 to become the American Academy of Child and Adolescent Psychiatry (AACAP). The AACAP conducts joint projects with both the American Psychiatric Association and the American Academy of Pediatrics (Adams & Fras, 1988).

As it has developed over time, the American Academy of Child and Adolescent Psychiatry has played a vital role in the development of child and adolescent psychiatry and reflects all of the diverse interests and concerns of its members. In addition to creating a venue for scientific exchange, the organization has been a powerful advocate for children both nationally and through local branch organizations. Interested members have participated over the years in testifying, preparing national reports, and even writing legislation related to services for children. Regional organizations have developed programs of advocacy for children in their own communities. Through its complex component structure, the AACAP provides opportunities for members to come together around areas of common interest that range from advocacy to community psychiatry. One such component was the AACAP Workgroup on Community Based Systems of Care formed in 1996 that published *The Handbook of Child and Adolescent Systems of Care* by Pumariega and Winters (2003).

Through participation in the AACAP, child and adolescent psychiatrists who have become interested in such areas as advocacy for children or in community psychiatry and System of Care issues can find the mentoring and encouragement to develop their own skills in these areas. Opportunities also exist for child and adolescent psychiatrists to participate in other organizations such as the American Orthopsychiatric Association, the Child Welfare League, the Children's Defense Fund, and the American Society of Adolescent Psychiatry. In common with the AACAP, these organizations provide opportunities to work with other professionals around issues of advocacy for child mental health, as well as a variety of scientific programs and workshops that can hone the skills needed for working in Systems of Care.

The Choice of Child and Adolescent Psychiatry as a Profession

The need for additional child and adolescent psychiatrists is great. Schowalter (2003) calculated, based on the numbers of children needing psychiatric care, that "there should be two to three times the number of practitioners and researchers, which is approximately 7,000" (p. 1429). In other words, an estimated 14,000 to 21,000 child psychiatrists will be needed in the near future.

Child and adolescent psychiatry offers much to those who choose it as a profession. The study of medicine, psychiatry, and human development is a powerful combination that prepares the professional for mental health and health care contributions at many levels. Child and adolescent psychiatry is a specialty that offers a high degree of flexibility in style of practice and is well suited to combining a variety of interesting and fulfilling activities. Adams and Fras (1988) stated, "The practice of child psychiatry [is] intrinsically gratifying to a service-oriented person [and] to the inquisitive scholar" (p. 579). Whether the child and adolescent psychiatrist chooses teaching, research, clinical practice, administration, advocacy, or some combination of these, opportunities abound for developing a satisfying practice while having a positive impact on our overall system of health care.

Summary and Conclusions

System of Care Approach, Best Practice, and Health Care Reform

What child and adolescent psychiatry has learned about best practice over the past century (and to its sorrow may at times have forgotten and may need to relearn) is that no disturbed child can be treated effectively in isolation. At a minimum, the family and all caregivers need to be active, collaborative participants in the treatment process. It is also clear that in more complex cases it is essential for virtually all participants in the life and care of the child to be included for an intervention to be effective.

We have reviewed contributions from the child guidance movement, the community mental health movement, the alternative services movement, and most recently the System of Care movement. We see that with each successive addition to our understanding, System of Care principles have expanded and become better defined. It is important for these principles to be passed on and the need for rediscovery or reinvention kept to a minimum. The incorporation of System of Care experiences into training programs for all disciplines is one important avenue for reaching this goal. When practitioners are thoroughly trained through experience with complex cases, they are able to streamline their approaches in less difficult circumstances without abandoning the fundamentals of effective care. Best practice becomes the application of just the right kind of care.

The System of Care approach should not be seen as a special type of intervention to be reserved for the very sickest patients. Rather, the principles that underlie System of Care—collaboration among caregivers, empowerment of families, and an approach that is committed, strength-based, flexible, and culturally competent—should be a consideration for every clinical situation. The System of Care model should be viewed as best practice to be fully implemented wherever and whenever appropriate. Clinical interventions with all children with an emotional disorder can benefit from the appropriate introduction of applicable System of Care principles.

Although the System of Care method has been developed and refined to a point where it can function well with appropriate support, the System of Care movement continues to struggle for full recognition, acceptance, and implementation during the managed-care, medication-oriented, quick-fix era. Providing the best practice that System of Care represents is an achievement that requires effort and a commitment to an interdisciplinary, interagency approach. It is difficult to create System of Care capabilities and difficult as well to maintain them. Too often it happens that such capacity is built only to be lost with a change in leadership or funding. The achievement of a well-functioning System of Care program is not something to give up lightly and must be a commitment by all who want to care for needy mentally ill children.

Ultimately, the System of Care approach proves its own value. First, it works. Second, in severely disordered patients and/or complex clinical situations, it will often be the only thing that works. Third, appropriate interventions that are timely and of high quality turn out to be more efficient, more effective, and less costly in the long run.

Hopefully, as savings and good outcomes of best practice continue to be demonstrated, more funding and support for the System of Care approach will be found. However, in our current overstressed and fragmented health care system, established and well-functioning programs are subject to repeated breakdowns as funding evaporates or leadership is lost. It may be that consistent and widespread implementation of the System of Care approach will have to wait on reforms of our entire health care system.

What is being learned from the System of Care method certainly has relevance for efforts at health care reform. The single principle of pursuing best practice in every instance works well for all of health care, and an emphasis on best practice coupled with empowerment of the recipients of care may turn out to be the key to a more efficient and effective health care system in the future.

Activities to Extend Your Learning

- Go to the AACAP website (http://www.aacap.org) and review information on *Workgroup on Community Based Systems of Care.*
- Watch the movie *I Am Sam.*
- Interview or if possible spend time on the job with a child and adolescent psychiatrist who participates in System of Care.
- Read *The Catcher in the Rye* by J.D. Salinger (1945).

List of Professional Organizations

- The American Academy of Child and Adolescent Psychiatry (http://www.aacap.org)
- The American Orthopsychiatric Association (an interdisciplinary mental health organization, including psychiatrists psychologists, nurses, social workers, educators, art/speech/musical/occupational therapists, gerontologists, and others interested in mental health care across the life span) (http://www.amerortho.org)
- The American Psychiatric Association (http://www.psych.org)
- The American Society of Adolescent Psychiatry (http://www.adolpsych.org)
- The Children's Defense Fund (http://www.childrensdefense.org)

References

Adams, P.L., & Fras, I. (1988). *Beginning child psychiatry*. New York: Brunner/Mazel.

Andreasen, N.C., & Black, D.W. (1991). *Introductory textbook of psychiatry*. Washington, DC: The American Psychiatric Association.

Engel, G.L. (1980). The clinical application of the biopsychosocial model. *The American Journal of Psychiatry, 137*, 535–544.

Freud, S. (1925). *Collected papers*. London: Institute for Psychoanalysis and Hogarth Press.

Freud, S. (1955–1972). Analysis of a phobia in a five-year-old boy. In J. Strachey (Ed.), *The standard edition of the complete works of Sigmund Freud* (Vol. 10, pp. 5–149). London: Hogarth Press.

Gesell, A. (1952). In E.G. Boring, H.S. Langfeld, H. Werner, & R.M. Yerkes (Eds.), *History of psychology in autobiography* (Vol. 4, pp. 123–142). Worcester, MA: Clark University Press.

Hall, G.S. (1904). *Adolescence: Its psychology and its relations to physiology, anthropology, sociology, sex, crime, religion, and education*. New York: D. Appleton.

Huffine, C., & Anderson, D. (2003). Family advocacy development in systems of care. In A.J. Pumariega & N.C. Winters (Eds.), *The handbook of child and adolescent systems of care* (pp. 35–65). San Francisco: Jossey-Bass.

Jones, K. (1999). *Taming the troublesome child: American Families, child guidance, and the limits of psychiatric authority*. Cambridge, MA: Harvard University Press.

Knitzer, J. (1982). *Unclaimed children*. Washington, DC: Children's Defense Fund.

Lourie, I.S. (2003). A history of community child mental health. In A.J. Pumariega & N.C. Winters (Eds.), *The handbook of child and adolescent systems of care* (pp. 1–15). San Francisco: Jossey-Bass.

Minuchin, S. (1974). *Families and family therapy.* Cambridge, MA: Harvard University Press.

Musto, D.F. (2002). History of child psychiatry. In M. Lewis (Ed.), *Child and adolescent psychiatry: A comprehensive textbook* (pp. 1447–1449). Philadelphia: Lippincott, Williams & Wilkins.

Porter, G.K., Pearson, G.T., Keenan, S., & Duval-Harvey, J. (2003). School-based mental health services: A necessity, not a luxury. In A.J. Pumariega & N.C. Winters (Eds.), *The handbook of child and adolescent systems of care: The new community psychiatry* (pp. 250–275). San Francisco: Jossey-Bass.

Pumariega, A.J., & Winters, N.C. (Eds.). (2003). *The handbook of child and adolescent systems of care: The new community psychiatry.* San Francisco: Jossey-Bass.

Salinger, J.D. (1945) *The catcher in the rye.* New York: Bantam Books.

Satir, V. (1967). *Conjoint family therapy.* Palo Alto, CA: Science and Behavior Books.

Schowalter, J.E. (2003). Recruitment, training, and certification in child and adolescent psychiatry in the United States. In M. Lewis (Ed.), *Child and adolescent psychiatry: A comprehensive textbook* (pp. 1429–1433). Philadelphia: Lippincott, Williams & Wilkins.

Stroul, B.A. (1996). *Children's mental health: Creating systems of care in a changing society.* Baltimore: Paul H. Brookes Publishing.

Stroul, B.A. (2003). Systems of care: A framework for children's mental health care. In A.J. Pumariega & N.C. Winters (Eds.), *The handbook of child and adolescent systems of care: The new community psychiatry* (pp. 17–33). San Francisco: Jossey-Bass.

Stroul, B.A., & Friedman, R.A. (1986). *A System of Care for children and youth with severe emotional disturbances* (rev. ed.). Washington, DC: Georgetown University, Child Development Center, National Technical Assistance Center for Child Mental Health.

Szurek, S.A. (1952). Some lessons from efforts at psychotherapy with parents. *American Journal of Psychiatry, 109,* 296–310.

Szurek, S.A. (1967). Lecture 5: Psychosis of childhood. In S.A. Szurek & I.N. Berlin (Eds.), *Training in therapeutic work with children: The Langley Porter child psychiatry series* (Vol. 2, pp. 69–90). Palo Alto, CA: Science and Behavior Books.

Szurek, S.A., & Johnson, A.M. (1952). The genesis of antisocial acting-out in children and adults. *The Psychoanalytic Quarterly, 21,* 323–343.

Chapter 8

Building a System of Care in Child Welfare: The Perspective of a Social Worker

Jacalyn A. Claes

Objectives

- Describe the impact of the early history of child welfare on practice with families today.
- Describe the continuum of family involvement in child welfare services and the practices at each stage.
- Identify the stages of family-centered practice and the skills that professionals need at each stage.
- Identify the core elements of a family team meeting.

System of Care practice in child welfare has evolved as a paradigm shift from worker-driven case management to family-centered case management. As family systems become more heterogeneous, there is a greater need for families to participate actively in a plan to ensure child safety.

Historically, child protection measures were established through child-saving agencies. The agency saw its role as guarding the physical and mental safety of children whose parents could not provide for their children's needs and were seen as a possible danger to even their children. Social workers were seen as the guardians of children, and offending parents were perceived as the perpetrators of physical and emotional pain on their children. These historical roots influenced an approach that alienated and discouraged family members.

Since the 1990s, child welfare agencies have acknowledged that in order for families to make significant changes, they need to be at the center of defining those changes and how they will be carried out. Although professionals can be a significant resource for families, "the true power to solve problems faced by families lies with families themselves, and with the communities in which those families live" (McMahon, 2003, p. 3).

The use of System of Care practice revolutionizes child welfare services. The service plan is built around each individual family's strengths and needs, and the family determines the goals that it wants to reach and the mechanisms to reach those goals. The family is moved from an isolationist position, where the parents are solely responsible for the child's well-being, to an extended family/community focus, where the parents bring to the planning meeting important persons who support and influence their family. Extended family members are part of the family team meeting and bring their resources to the table.

Both benefits and barriers exist in applying family-centered practice to child welfare. The benefits to the parents, child, extended family, social worker, and community outweigh the barriers to the proposed change that must be faced in the system. Family team meetings maximize family input and engage the extended family and community in decision making that reduces the isolation of the parents and enlarges the safety net for children.

The Evolution of Family-Centered Practice in Child Protective Services

History of Child Protective Services

The first child protection measures were implemented through the Society for the Prevention of Cruelty Toward Children established in 1874. The focus of this society was on rescuing children and punishing the parents who abused them. The majority of children who were found to be abused in the early 20th century were removed from their homes, and few services were provided to their parents to support the children's return. Many of the children who were removed had parents living in poverty. The view of poverty as sinful and a punishment from God was prevalent, leading child advocates to believe that removal of the child from these parents was morally justified.

After the Great Depression and World War II, many families struggled to provide for their children. This led to a change in public sentiment and welfare programs that were implemented by the federal government to assist families in need. This protective function broadened to include children's physical and emotional safety as the work of the Society for the Prevention of Cruelty Toward Children was taken over by government agencies.

During the early 1970s, physicians began writing about child abuse as an illness. As the attention of the medical community increased on this issue, a number of studies were funded to quantify the extent of abuse on children. The impacts of these studies led Congress to pass the Child Abuse and Prevention Treatment Act in 1974 (PL 93-247). With the passage of Child Abuse and Prevention Treatment Act, states began to enact mandatory reporting laws of child abuse and to maintain a state registry of perpetrators and victims. By the 1990s, the impact of mandatory reporting and public attention to child abuse increased the number of reported cases of child abuse dramatically. In 20 years between 1973 and 1993, the reports of abuse and neglect of children rose 347% (Berg & Kelly, 2000). As caseloads grew, many children were removed from their homes and placed in foster care, which was one of the few alternatives subsidized by the federal government.

As the number of children in foster care increased, attention was drawn to early intervention strategies that might prevent the removal of children from their parents. The intent of the 1980 Adoption Assistance and Child Welfare Act (PL 96-272) was to reunify families and to provide preplacement prevention services. To ensure that children would no longer "be lost in the system," individual states were required to develop a case plan on every child in care that included a plan for permanent placement for the child. This legislation was followed by the 1993 Family Preservation and Support Act (PL 103-66), which was effective in funding an alternative to foster care through the establishment of "in-home services" for families.

Within child welfare, there continues to be a philosophic tug between child rescue and the preservation of the family. The Family

Preservation and Support Act of 1993 provided resources for family preservation; however, the Adoption and Safe Families Act of 1997 (PL 105-89) focused exclusively on the rescue of children. The purpose of this act was to shorten the time that children were in foster care "waiting for their parents to get better." Stricter time lines were established for filing termination of parental rights so that children would be either returned home to their biological parents or eligible for adoption.

Continuum of Family Involvement

The historical roots of child rescue coupled with the influence of the medical model of service delivery have significantly influenced child welfare. Within this model, the social worker is the expert who diagnoses the problems in the family, designs a plan for overcoming the problems, and monitors the family's compliance with that plan. This professional-centered model places the social worker as the expert and the parent as a client to be treated. This hierarchical approach inherently places the social worker in an adversarial role, making compliance by the parents very difficult to achieve. Although the professional-centered model has been used most often in child welfare, there is a continuum of family involvement that has been used in child welfare. The continuum flows from professional-centered services through family-centered services to team-centered services with family involvement increasing at each level (System of Care Institute, 1999).

Services that resulted from the Adoption Assistance and Child Welfare Act were family focused, although the emphasis on partnering with parents was aimed at gaining compliance. Within this model, the professional remained the expert, with the parent as an important ally. Child welfare services moved a step forward on the continuum with implementation of the Family Preservation and Support Act. Family preservation services were designed to be flexible to meet the family's schedule and needs. After an investigation was completed and a treatment plan was developed, a family-preservation team worked intensely in the home (20 to 30 hours per week) with the family to address practical goals that could make a difference in the family's life. These services were family allied, and parents were viewed as equal colleagues in treatment.

Within the last 10 years, traditional Child Protective Services work has been challenged to be more family centered. In adopting a family-centered approach, the family is placed at the heart of the process, with the worker functioning less as an inquisitor and more as a facilitator in getting the family's needs met. This approach works particularly well when children's needs are not being met because of poverty. A strength-based assessment is used to identify the resources and skills in the family's natural environment. Rather than focusing on problems and the mistakes that the family has made in the past, the worker assists that family in focusing on the exceptions to the problems, times when things are going well. The family begins to develop an internal script of success. Families begin to believe in their ability to get things done and have successful outcomes. Bandura (1986) called this belief self-efficacy. Once self-efficacy is developed in a family, the goals that are desired are more easily achieved. The family becomes confident before it begins a task that it is going to be able to master the task (Bandura, Adams, Hardy, & Howells, 1980).

The final model on the continuum is the team-centered approach in which the skills and resources of a team are used for both planning and intervention. In child welfare, this practice is known as family team meetings or family group conferences. "These structured facilitated meetings bring family members together so that with the support of professionals and community resources, they can create a plan that ensures child safety and meets the family's needs" (McMahon, 2003, p. 1).

Applying Family-Centered Practice in Working with Families

Components of Family-Centered Practice

In order to make the shift from traditional practice in child welfare to family-centered practice, the professional needs to be cognizant of the following principles: (1) the focus of attention is on the family as a unit (the safety and well-being of all family members is of paramount concern), (2) the emphasis in family-centered practice is on strengthening the family's capacity for carrying out their responsibilities, (3) the family is central in decision making and goal setting and partners with professionals in designing individualized services to meet the family's needs, and (4) the family is linked with supports and services in the extended family, neighborhood, and community, not just formal services (McMahon, 2002). This approach builds self-efficacy in the family, which leads to more confident decision making in the future.

In order to forge a partnership with families that build self-efficacy, a cognitive map must be used that provides a structure for both professionals and families to turn to when decisions become difficult. One name for this map is a schema, which are "cognitive constructions, or core beliefs, through which people filter their perceptions and structure their experiences" (Nichols & Schwartz, 1998, p. 547). Bass, Dosser, and Powell (2001) recommended a six-step schema for family-centered practice. These steps are illustrated in Figure 8-1.

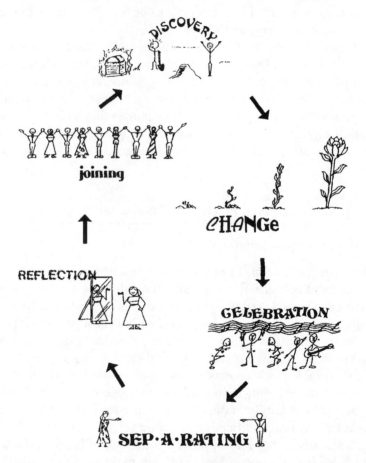

Celebrating Change
A Schema for Family-Centered Practice

Collaborating to help children and families

FIGURE 8-1   A schema for family-centered practice.
Source: Bass et al. (2001). Copyright permission was granted by Haworth Press.

Joining

When a social worker begins working with a family, one of the first things that must happen is to relate to the family's struggles. The family has a story to tell about how their circumstances got to the place where they are, and it is crucial for their future relationship that the worker be respectful of the family's challenges and hardships. Sometimes families do not remember or even realize the coping strategies that they used in overcoming difficulties in the past. This is important information to uncover because remembering these coping strategies can often be the first step in building hope with the family.

Discovery

During the discovery stage, energy is focused on the family uncovering their strengths. The social worker's role in this stage is as a coach helping individual family members and the family as a whole uncover their resources. The role for the professional is not as a central player but rather standing in the wings, for "families ultimately are the architects and constructors of their own growth and change" (Bass et al., 2001, p. 41).

Changing

Persons and systems are most amenable to change during times of crisis (Watzlawick, 1978). In a crisis, the family's defenses are down. The family is in pain and longs for a solution to reduce the pain. It is during this period of destabilization that a family is most open to examining other ways to problem-solve. Often the family is doing the same thing over and over with nonproductive results. These "stuck places" are the catalyst for change.

Goal setting and meeting achievable goals are the activities of this stage. Family members are focusing on this: "What do we need to have a better life?" Once the family begins to list the needs that they have, the social worker can assist the family in delineating a plan to translate those needs into achievable goals.

Once goals have been set, the barriers that get in the way of achieving those goals must be addressed. Barriers to goal achievement are easily recognized on the individual and family levels. However, the social worker can assist the family in developing advocacy skills that address agency attitudes and policies that get in the way of goal achievement.

Celebrating

Celebrations are important rituals of acknowledgment that families can individualize according to their own uniqueness. Some people respond best with individual praise, whereas others enjoy the limelight when extended family gathers to applaud an accomplishment. Celebration is an important part of creating long-lasting changes in a family. It can be an "affirmation of growth, potential, confidence, and hope" (Bass et al., 2001, p. 42).

Separating

As goals are achieved and families celebrate moving toward confidence, the family stories can be rewritten in a more hopeful context (Bass et al., 2001). The social worker can assist the family in uncovering the important lessons learned from struggle that have lead them to accomplishment. The family is no longer trapped in a storyline that leaves them discouraged and without dreams.

Reflection

During the reflection process, the family, the social worker, extended family members, and other professionals reflect on what has happened so far. This provides an opportunity to synthesize the progress that has been made and to uncover the barriers that have impeded desired growth. This process is useful throughout the entire therapeutic process so that acknowledgment and corrections can be made.

Applying Team-Centered Practice in Working with Families

History

The family team meeting was first introduced in child welfare in New Zealand as the family group conferencing model. The model was adopted in response to the growing problem of overrepresentation of Maori children in the child welfare and juvenile justice systems. Maori parents and elders wanted to follow their cultural tradition of clan, tribe, and family decision making with their children. However, they were excluded from such planning by child welfare and the juvenile court when their children's lives necessitated involvement in these systems. Professionals in these systems were comfortable with a professional-centered model of decision making and were anxious about including parents and laypersons in the decision-making process (McMahon, 2003).

The Maori, the indigenous people of New Zealand, elevate the family, the *Whanau*, as the most important institution in society. *Whanau* incorporates not only the nuclear family, but also the extended family members, including those related through marriage. All members of the *Whanau* pledge to uphold the values of "loyalty, unity, mutual interdependence and help mutual responsibility and duty" (Merkel-Holguin, 2001, p. 198). When conflicts in the family arise, a family meeting is held to resolve the conflict and restore harmonious relationships (Walker, 1996).

Because the Maori people already had a strong cultural model for resolving family conflict, Maori activists influenced the Department of Social Welfare to adapt this cultural model in the assessment and treatment of child protective service complaints. The family group conferencing model was piloted in New Zealand, and within a few years, the results were so successful that in 1989 New Zealand enacted the Children, Young Persons, and Their Families Act, which made family group conferencing mandatory for all families with children identified as neglected or abused (Merkel-Holguin, 2001; Pennell, 1999).

In response to the growing concern for alternatives to foster care for children, family group conferencing and its outgrowth of family team meetings became popular in the United States, England, Canada, Sweden, and South Africa. "The evolution of family group conferencing has revolved around two primary realizations or themes: a) children do better when they can maintain strong connections to the primary caregivers and family of origin, including extended family networks, and b) child welfare interventions that assume the primary responsibility for care of children can often be disempowering to a family and do more harm than good" (Merkel-Holguin, 2001, pp. 199, 200).

Structure of Team-Centered Practice

Team-centered practice builds on the values and principles of the family-centered approach while placing more responsibility for decision making on the family team and less on the individual child welfare worker. The structure of the family team meeting is illustrated in Figure 8-2.

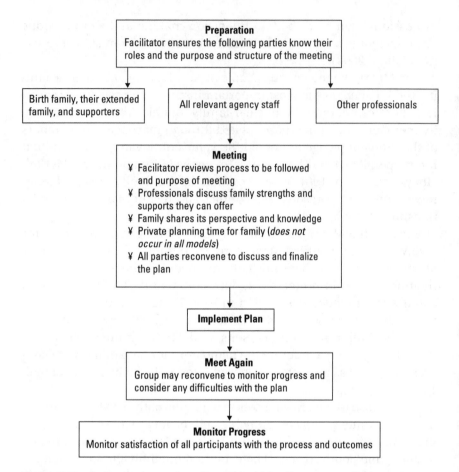

Figure 8-2   A structural overview of a child and family team meeting.

Source: McMahon (2003). Copyright permission was granted by the Jordan Institute of Family-Centered Services, Chapel Hill, NC.

Preparation

The preparation of the family for the family team meeting is an important function of the child welfare worker. The parent(s) plays a central role in deciding attendees to the family team meeting. The advantages and disadvantages of inviting each member of the extended family should be discussed in detail with the parent(s) in terms of their potential for support and/or conflict. A plan for safety should be outlined in case conflict among family members escalates, as may have occurred in previous family encounters. All family members need to be informed of the purpose and structure of the meeting and the acknowledgment of their opinions as experts on their family.

In addition to family members, support persons in the community may be invited. This list may include friends, neighbors, teachers, pastors, coaches, and anyone whose support the family desires.

The final group of attendees will be professionals working with the family. Ideally, this group should be the smallest in number so as not to outnumber the family members. Family and community support members of the team should be the largest in the room, and professionals have the responsibility to encourage participation by everyone. The worker and the family decide who will invite each member of the team and the information that will be provided to them in advance of the meeting, as well as where and what time the meeting will be held. When possible, the location of the meeting should be in a neighborhood setting rather than a professional office. Food is often provided to add to the comfort level of team members.

Meeting

Many settings use a trained facilitator to conduct the family team meeting. The facilitator has no history with the agencies or the family and can facilitate the meeting without bias so that all voices are heard. The meeting begins with the facilitator introducing herself/himself and explaining the process that will be followed and the purpose for calling the meeting. Participants are then invited to introduce themselves and briefly explain their relationship to the family. Then everyone has an opportunity to discuss family strengths while the facilitator writes them for all to see. Issues and concerns are the next agenda item. The family then has an opportunity to discuss their perspective of the current situation. The facilitator urges participants not to discuss previous history, but rather to focus on the current issues that need solution.

In some settings, the family is then left alone to brainstorm privately and come up with a plan that best addresses the present situation from the family's perspective. The settings that use this model believe that more creative solutions will come from family members when they can use their own private language and maintain boundaries around the family system. Other settings do not segregate the family for brainstorming and decision making but rather engage in these processes as an entire team. Regardless of which model is used, all members reconvene to discuss and implement the plan.

An action plan for implementation is agreed on. In each action step, the person responsible for carrying out the step is named, as well as persons that will assist with support in implementation. An implementation date is also agreed on for each goal. The facilitator takes notes during the meeting and provides a written copy of the plan to each team member. Finally, the team decides on a date to reconvene, to monitor progress, and to re-evaluate the plan.

In the case study that follows, a family team meeting was convened to provide team decision making after the birth of a baby to a mom whose other three children were in the custody of the Department of Social Services. The components of the family team meeting are detailed, followed by a discussion of the central elements of the family team meeting.

Case Study of a Family Team Meeting

Mark Morgan, a family team meeting facilitator, provided the case study. All names and identifiers of family members have been changed.

Case Name: Cynthia Ramsey
Social Worker: Ms. Tanya White
Supervisor: Ms. Suzanne Hill
Facilitator: Mr. Mark Morgan

Attendees: Ms. Bonita Poole, Agency Foster Care Social Worker; Ms. Carolyn Ronald, Agency Foster Family Recruitment; Ms. Tanya White, Agency Child Protective Services Social Worker; Calvin Sellers, Father; Sarah Palmer, Family Friend; Cynthia Ramsey, Mother; Denise Ramsey, Maternal Grandmother; Ms. Suzanne Hill, Agency Child Protection Services Supervisor; Jason Myrick, Maternal Step-Grandfather; Virgil Johnson, Paternal Cousin; and Mr. Mark Morgan, Facilitator.

Issues and Concerns: During the week of March 29, 2004, the agency received a report stating that Cynthia Ramsey gave birth to a daughter, Charlotte Ramsey, on March 3, 2004. The Department of Social Service had pursued termination of parental rights of Cynthia over three of her other children; however, Cynthia relinquished her parental rights to the maternal grandparents, Denise Ramsey and Jason Myrick (maternal step-grandfather). According to Ms. White, Cynthia did not successfully comply with her Department of Social Service case plan by not completing (1) the parenting assessment, (2) the offenders of domestic violence program, and (3) the substance abuse assessment.

Calvin Sellers, alleged father of Charlotte, informed the Department of Social Service that he was unsure of being the father of Charlotte and requested a paternity test. In the past, Cynthia and Calvin have engaged in domestic violence episodes, and a year ago, Calvin accrued a criminal charge of assault with a deadly weapon. Calvin immediately pressed criminal charges against Cynthia for "cutting up" his clothes "with a knife." Calvin is currently on unsupervised probation by the court system and reports to his probation officer once per month.

The Department of Social Service has determined that it is necessary to assume legal and physical custody of Charlotte.

Purpose of the Team Meeting: To provide a plan that provides for the safety of Charlotte, Cynthia, and Calvin and to determine the services that are needed for the family.

Strengths:
Calvin loves Charlotte.
Calvin wants to be a father to Charlotte.
Calvin has provided for Charlotte's needs.
Calvin is willing to accept services.
Calvin is willing to work with the agency.
Cynthia wants Charlotte to be with her.
Cynthia loves Charlotte.
Cynthia and Calvin are concerned for Charlotte's safety.
Cynthia's and Calvin's openness.
Family and community support in place.

Team Recommendations:
1. THE AGENCY'S DECISION TO ASSUME LEGAL AND PHYSICAL CUSTODY OF CHARLOTTE WAS REPEALED.
2. Via a voluntary placement plan, developed by Calvin and Cynthia, Charlotte will be placed in the relative home of Denise Ramsey and Jason Myrick, maternal grandparents, effective April 5, 2004.
3. Cynthia and Calvin will explore other potential, relative placement options for Charlotte.
4. Ms. Tanya White will assist Cynthia and Calvin to explore non–Department of Social Service custody placement options for Charlotte within the next 3 months.

5. Cynthia will attend and abide by the recommendations of the offenders of domestic violence program. Cynthia will have registered for the program within 1 week of this meeting.

6. Cynthia will undergo a substance abuse assessment and abide by the recommendations of substance abuse assessment/counseling agency. Cynthia will have made an appointment for a substance abuse assessment within 1 week of this meeting.

7. Cynthia and Calvin will undergo and abide by recommendations of a parenting assessment. Both Cynthia and Calvin will have made an appointment for a parenting assessment within 1 week of this meeting.

8. Calvin will sign an Agency Consent to Release & Obtain Information form, authorizing Ms. Tanya White to attain information from the substance abuse assessment/counseling agency, offenders of domestic violence program, and adult probation services officer. Calvin will sign these forms immediately after this meeting.

9. Ms. Bonita Poole will conduct a home study of the relative home of Jackie Casey, maternal cousin, on April 5, 2004, at 6:00 p.m.

10. Calvin and Cynthia will communicate with Denise and Jason, twice a week by phone, to discuss Charlotte's health and well-being.

11. Calvin and Cynthia will have supervised contact with Charlotte on Sunday afternoons from 12:00 to 2:00 p.m. in the home of Jason and Denise. Either Jason or Denise will be present during this visit. Visits will begin on the Sunday after this meeting.

12. This team will reconvene on May 14, 2004, at 3:00 p.m. in the Westdale Community Center Conference Room.

Discussion of the Case Study

The Ramsey team meeting was an example of a traditional child protection intervention that had atypical results because of the impact of the family team meeting. Cynthia Ramsey was very distrustful of the Department of Social Service because of the previous removal of her three children. When her daughter Charlotte was born and the Department of Social Service became involved once again, Cynthia was noncooperative. When she came to the team meeting, she was resistant to anything that the Department of Social Service suggested. However, in the planning of the team meeting, Cynthia was invited to include supporters from her extended family and friendship networks. Cynthia invited her friend, Sarah; her grandmother, Denise; Calvin, the baby's father; and Calvin's cousin, Virgil. Sarah talked to Cynthia and convinced her that she was capable of getting her baby back and that Sarah would help her do what was needed. Sarah and Denise spoke up for Cynthia at the family team meeting. Denise talked about how important it was in their family for children not to go into foster homes and that she would be willing to care for Charlotte until another family member could be found. Cousin Jackie had phoned the Department of Social Service to express her interest in caring for the baby. As Cynthia felt the support of her family and friends around her during the meeting, she was encouraged. She began to believe that perhaps it was possible for her to have her baby with her again. As she regained hope, it was easier for her to agree to the assessments that would indicate that she was competent to parent.

Summary

Child protective service has had a history of protecting children by taking on the sole responsibility for their care. This practice had the positive intent of safeguarding children but the unintended consequence of depriving the child of the right to grow up in their own home. As parents and community supports were given more responsibility for decision making in the lives of children, the team approach was launched. Through the family team meeting, families are encouraged to take back the right and responsibility to make decisions and implement plans that are in the best interest of their children and family. This is revolutionizing the child welfare system.

Activities to Extend Your Learning

Imagine yourself practicing your profession. How do you see yourself working with children and families experiencing abuse or neglect?

- ▇ Examine your own prejudices or preconceptions about what makes a good family. Does a child need two parents in order to be emotionally healthy? What about the income level of the family? What are the essential needs that you believe must be met in order for a child not to be neglected? What forms of discipline would be acceptable in a "good family"?
- ▇ Examine your beliefs and preconceptions about parents who physically abuse their children. What do you think motivates them? Do they love their child? What would be hardest for you in working with parents who physically abuse their child?

In order to understand family-centered practice more clearly, identify a cri-
sis in your own family when you were growing up. Apply the schema for
family-centered practice to that crisis.

- List the strengths of your family as a whole and also of individual family members. Were these strengths clear to your family at the time of the crisis?
- What were areas of change that were needed by your family at
  that time? What were the barriers that blocked that change
  from occurring?
- How did your family celebrate the successes along the way?
- What beliefs did your family or individual family members
  need to separate from in order to make the necessary change?
- What people or agencies provided support (emotionally, struc-
  turally, or financially) to your family during this time of change?

Describe the essential components of a family team meeting.

- What role(s) might you fill on a family team as a future
  professional?
- What contributions would be essential in your role?
- Attend a family team meeting. Note the strategies that the facilitator uses to encourage all members of the team to participate. Were the ideas from family members listened to as
  respectfully as ideas from professionals and community members? How closely did this family team meeting follow the
  meeting outlined in this chapter? What was your deepest learning in attending the family team meeting?

References

Bandura, A. (1986). *Social foundations of thought and action: A social cogni-*
tive theory. Englewood Cliffs, NJ: Prentice Hall.

Bandura, A., Adams, N.E., Hardy, A.B., & Howells, G.N. (1980). Tests of the
generality of self-efficacy theory. *Cognitive Therapy & Research, 4,* 39–66.

Bass, L., Dosser, D.A., & Powell, J. (2001). Words can be powerful: changing the words of helping to enhance systems of care. *Journal of Family*
Social Work, 5(3), 35–48.

Berg, I.K., & Kelly, S. (2000). *Building solutions in child protective services.* New
York: W.W. Norton & Company.

McMahon, J. (2002). A new direction in child welfare in NC. *Practice Notes,*
7(4), 1–8.

McMahon, J. (2003a). Child and family team meetings in child welfare.
Practice Notes, 8(2), 1–8.

McMahon, J. (2003b). Jordan Institute of Family-Centered Services, Chapel Hill, NC.

Merkel-Holguin, L. (2001). Family group conferencing. In E. Walton, P. Sandau-Beckler, and M. Mannes (Eds.), *Balancing family-centered services and child well-being* (pp. 197–218). New York: Columbia University Press.

Nichols, M.P., & Schwartz, R.C. (1998). *Family therapy: Concepts and methods.* Boston: Allyn and Bacon.

Pennell, J. (1999). *Mainstreaming family group conferencing: building and sustaining partnerships: Real Justice.* Available from: http:www.realjustice. org/Pages/vt99papers/vt-pennell.html.

System of Care Institute. (1999). *Training coordinator orientation.* New Orleans, LA.

Walker, H. (1996). Whanau Hui, family decision-making, and the family group conference: An indigenous Maori view. *Protecting Children, 12*(3), 8–10.

Watzlawick, P. (1978). *The language of change.* New York: Basic Books.

Chapter 9

Integrating Substance Abuse Treatment in Systems of Care

SUSAN TACCHERI

Objectives

- Define substance dependence, substance abuse, and substance-induced disorders.
- Identify the prevalence of substance abuse, including alcohol dependence and coexisting substance use disorder and mental illness.
- Describe a PACT or assertive community treatment team program for adults with a dual diagnosis, which is a case management model for the chronically mentally ill.
- Discuss the reasons that integration of substance abuse treatment with System of Care treatment might be more effective in addressing the needs of families with complex mental health concerns.
- Identify the obstacles to integration.
- Describe a model for integrating interdisciplinary teams to address adolescents who are mentally ill and also abusing substances.
- Discuss the recommendations for integration and care of the client with a dual diagnosis and his or her family.

According to the Diagnostic and Statistical Manual of Mental Disorders–Test Revision (DSM-IV-TR), published by the American Psychiatric Association and used as a diagnostic bible by mental health professionals, substance dependence is a "cluster of cognitive, behavioral, and physiological symptoms indicating that the individual continues use of the substance despite significant substance-use related problems," and substance abuse is "a maladaptive pattern of substance use manifested by recurrent and significant adverse consequences related to the repeated use of substances" (American Psychiatric Association, 2000, pp. 192, 198). Substance use disorders refer to substance abuse and substance dependence. Substance-induced disorders have to do with substance intoxication, withdrawal, and specific syndromes caused from the use of substances, such as delirium, mood disorder, and sleep disorders (American Psychiatric Association, p. 209).

Many families are affected by issues of substance abuse and dependence. According to the Epidemiologic Catchment Area Study data, the lifetime risk in the general population of alcohol abuse and/or dependence was approximately 14%, and the risk of drug abuse and/or dependence was approximately 6% (Anthony & Helzer, 1991; Helzer, Burnam, & McEvoy, 1991). For the families involved with public child-serving agencies, including behavioral health, child welfare, and juvenile justice, and for those whose family members are having problems in school, the risk and prevalence of substance use disorders are higher than for the general population. These families are frequently targeted for treatment by local Systems of Care because of their complex needs and requirements for multisystemic interventions, including treatment for alcohol and drug abuse.

"Growing evidence indicates that genetic factors influence an individual's inherent vulnerability to drug addiction. In humans, such an influence is well established for alcoholism" (Nestler & Self, 1997, p. 792). Other shared risk factors are the ecologic contributions, such as poverty and the use of illicit substances in the family. It is common to see more than one generation having problems with substances (see the case study of RG in Chapter 7). Compounding the seriousness of severe emotional disturbances in children and adolescents is the coexistence of another disorder, such as substance abuse, making the diagnosis and treatment "particularly challenging" for the care providers (O'Malley, 2003, p. 277).

Historical Overview

Historically, the treatment of substance use disorders has been segregated from other behavioral health care. Only one to two decades ago, the client in need of addiction treatment was referred to a community 12-step program. Alcoholics Anonymous and Narcotics Anonymous are spiritual rather than medical programs and have been successful as self-help groups. The group leaders are recovering substance abusers who are role models for other members. They do not subscribe to a particular religion but do believe that the addict is powerless over alcohol and drugs and must learn to turn their problems over to God. Alcoholics Anonymous and Narcotics Anonymous provide a "buddy system" of sponsor and new member; recovery includes healing one's self while helping others.

Psychiatrists waited until addiction issues were stabilized and in remission before medicating co-morbid psychiatric disorders. A co-morbid psychiatric disorder refers primarily to a behavioral health diagnosis that exists with a substance use disorder; dual diagnosis, co-occurring disorders, and co-morbidity all refer to a mental illness and a substance use disorder existing simultaneously. Mental illness and behavioral health diagnosis are interchangable terms. According to Phoenix and Pelish (2004), an epidemiologic survey of 20,000 (conducted by Regier et al., 1990) found that "people with the most severe mental illness had the highest rates of substance abuse and dependence" (p. 508).

Traditionally, 12-step group programs did not support and, in fact, actively discouraged the use of medications for behavioral health issues. This practice has changed, and it is now widely thought that treatment of substance use disorders is more successful if co-occurring psychiatric or behavioral health disorders are treated concurrently.

Case Study 1

An adolescent who is overwhelmed with social anxiety when he or she enters group gatherings starts to use alcohol to feel more comfortable with engaging in the peer group. What starts with one drink "to loosen up" escalates to a number of drinks at every social event. The use then escalates further until the adolescent is drinking daily and soon drinking before school every morning. If the social anxiety is treated with psychiatric medication, the motivation for drinking alcohol can be targeted and decreased; the sober adolescent finds himself or herself more comfortable and without the overwhelming anxiety when entering a social function.

Case Study 2

Another common scenario is the adolescent who is depressed and numbing himself or herself through the use of drugs and alcohol. With treatment of the underlying depression, the urge to be numb through using mind-altering chemicals is reduced. Furthermore, depression often affects concentration, energy level, and motivation, and with treatment, the teenager has more motivation and energy to reconnect with prosocial activities such as sports, can concentrate better on both schoolwork and an after-school job, and can engage in other appropriate developmental activities.

The Evolution Toward Further Integration of Treatment

Over the past one to two decades, there has been a movement toward integrating the treatment of substance use disorders with psychiatric and other behavioral health treatment. The work of Robert Drake, MD, and Kenneth Minkoff, MD, has been instrumental in the integration of care for adults, specifically those who are in need of addiction treatment and have a severe and persistent mental illness (Drake et al., 1998; Minkoff & Drake, 1991). The philosophic underpinnings of the need for integration are that (1) it is more effective for the care-giving community to integrate care rather than to ask the client, who is symptomatic or in crisis, to do the integration of care, and (2) there is more success with remission of both disorders when cotreatment is concurrent.

Over the last ten years, the 12-step community has become more accepting of the use of psychotropic medication. In addition, other community support group models, such as Smart Recovery, have developed, and behavioral health centers offer specific treatment options such as dual intensive outpatient programs for people with co-existing disorders. Furthermore, one community mental health model of care that has developed across the country, the assertive community treatment team, sometimes called PACT, includes the substance abuse counselor as an integral part of the treatment team (Drake et al., 1998). PACT is a case-management model that is community based and closely follows people who are severely and persistently mentally ill (Herrick & Bartlett, 2004). In this model of care, the team takes full responsibility for the treatment, including emergency after-hours availability, as long as the patient can safely stay in the community. (Note: This model excludes hospital care.) PACT programs have documented their success in decreasing the incidence of clients needing to be readmitted to the hospital (Herrick & Bartlett).

In multiple ways simultaneously, on programmatic as well as systemic levels, the integration of care for the dually diagnosed is evolving, and co-occurring treatment is being addressed in research and the literature as well as in community practice.

The substance abuse treatment community has evolved rapidly over the past two decades. The national professional organization for psychiatrists, the American Psychiatric Association, has developed the subspecialty of Addictions Psychiatry and has established a credentialing board to certify the competence of psychiatrists to treat substance use disorders. In order to be examined by the board, the psychiatrist is required to complete a specific subspecialty training for one year in substance use disorders. In the past, the substance abuse treatment staff came from the self-help community, whose members had little or no formal training and had varied credentials.

Addiction service providers in general, as well as those in psychiatry, now have a uniform credentialing process, which includes demonstrating expertise in other behavioral health issues (American Society of Addictive Medicine, 1997).There has been a burgeoning of research in substance use disorders at the federal level in an effort to document successful treatment outcomes that can be easily replicated to guide evidenced-based practice, and to disseminate this information to treatment communities nationwide. (For an example of this effort, see the report by the U.S. Department of Health and Human Services–Substance Abuse and Mental Health Services Administration (SAMSHA)/Center for Substance Abuse Treatment Improvement Protocol Series referred to in the Activities to Extend Your Learning section at the end of the chapter.)

Despite these gains, there is a need to continue to advocate for the integration of substance abuse treatment into behavioral health care, including the participation of substance abuse personnel on the System of Care child/family team. The facts from epidemiologic studies substantiate the need for integration. "Rates of conduct disorder range from 50% to 80% in adolescent patients with substance use disorder," and "the prevalence of depressive disorders ranges from 24% to more than 50%" (Kaminer & Tarter, 1999). Forty-five percent of adults with an alcohol use disorder, and 72% of those with a drug use disorder, will experience one or more psychiatric disorders (Regier et al., 1990). The data strongly point to a correlation between mental illness and substance abuse disorders.

Substance use must be assessed and addressed when treating children and families in System of Care programs. Co-existing diagnoses should always be suspected. The issue may be the elephant in the living room (i.e., it is there but not addressed and is essentially ignored by the family). Overall, therapeutic goals cannot be met if the substance abuse problem is not addressed. The following two case studies are examples of how substance abuse contributed to a child's and family's mental illness.

Case Study 3

Grandfather has an alcohol problem. He drinks to intoxication. While under the influence of alcohol, he sexually and physically abuses members of his family, thus traumatizing them. Consequently, members of the family may suffer from posttraumatic stress disorders. The children perform poorly in school, and the mother suffers from a severe depression. They are all, except for grandfather, being examined by the assessment team in a System of Care program. The System of Care team works toward involving grandfather to get substance abuse treatment while providing mental health care for the rest of the family.

Case Study 4

A mother neglects her children because of her crack cocaine habit. Consequently, the children have had several encounters with the child welfare social workers. Today, they have not seen their mother in a day and a half and are sick with worry about her well-being. They have not eaten in several days, but they are trying to concentrate on their school work. The school reports the mother to the Department of Child Welfare or Social Service. Of course, the children want to stay with their mother and are upset at being placed in a foster home. One child acts aggressively, and the other withdraws. Both are in need of mental health care. The children and mother receive wraparound services, and the professionals work together to assist the mother to get addiction services so that the children can be returned to her care. The Department of Child Welfare or Social Service case manager coordinates the following services: addictions treatment and counseling for the mother; mental health treatment for the children; schooling for the children, including a special classroom setting for the child whose behavior was difficult for the regular teacher to manage; foster care for the children; family preservation services for the family to work toward reunification; and vocational rehabilitation for the mother, who had been unemployed for years, so that she can financially support herself and her children. These types of situations are frequently encountered in treatment settings for children and families.

Addiction issues often are contributing factors in children's antisocial behaviors.

Adolescence is a period when substance use disorders are pervasive (O'Malley, 2003). Illegal behaviors are sometimes the result of wanting to get drugs. Thus, the adolescent will do anything, even steal, to do so. On top of that, substance intoxication impairs judgment and interferes with impulse control, which often leads to the commitment of illegal acts by an otherwise law-abiding youth. Another possible sequelae of substance abuse are high-risk sexual behaviors, which can lead to pregnancy and/or sexually transmitted disease. Once the substance abuse is treated and under control, other problems often naturally recede.

The use of substances deleteriously affects multiple psychosocial domains, such as relationships, work and school, leisure and recreational activities, and physical and mental health. In addition, it may lead to legal problems. Addiction problems frequently lead to chronic unemployment, playing havoc on the financial welfare of the family.

Obstacles to Integration of Substance Abuse Treatment into System of Care

Substance use disorders are commonly a part of the mixture of issues that must be addressed when working with multiproblem families who may be involved with several agencies, and who might be targeted for care by the local System of Care. Nevertheless, the integration of a substance abuse treatment provider on an interdisciplinary System of Care team is frequently missing. Close examination of the obstacles to integration will shed light on the problem. Table 9-1 describes the obstacles that must be overcome in order to integrate substance abuse and mental health care in a System of Care Program.

Table 9-1	Obstacles to Integration

Poor funding for substance use disorders by third-party payers.

A lack of time and flexibility of time for substance abuse providers to participate on System of Care teams.

A disparity of philosophy and backgrounds among service providers, which leads to cultural conflicts between substance abuse programs and behavioral health programs.

Staff resistance based on the historic separation of the programs.

The chronicity of the disease of substance use disorders and feelings of hopelessness on the part of clients, families, and providers.

The historical perspective that psychotropic medication is a crutch and is therefore not therapeutic for the patient who has dual diagnoses.

The main obstacle of integration of the addictions treatment system with the behavioral health system and the System of Care has to do with reimbursement and other fiscal issues. There is a relative lack of funding for addictions treatment, despite the financial burden that substance use disorders cause and the fact that these disorders are a major public health issue. After review of the benefits packages by third-party payers, addictions treatment is the lowest funded of all mental health disorders. Many managed care organizations offer no coverage for alcohol and drug treatment. Intensive outpatient programs are the standard level of care for the patient with a substance use disorder, which recommends that the client attends meetings three times per week for up to 12 weeks. If a managed care organization does cover substance abuse treatment, it may only pay for a few days and is usually less than the standard of care that is recommended.

Because of funding issues, the addictions staff is often overburdened and is without much time flexibility. Another major factor that is related to the lack of participation on an interdisciplinary System of Care child and family team is that the time spent by the addictions counselor attending meetings is not billable time, nor is the time to and from meetings billable. Often System of Care meetings are off-site from where the addictions counselor works, requiring additional driving time.

In the past, disparities in education, qualifications, and philosophic backgrounds have been factors that segregated the addictions staff from the other behavioral health staff. Addictions counselors are usually recovering addicts themselves and come from all walks of life. Many may have no more than a high school education. Meanwhile, the behavioral health staff usually has a mix of bachelor's degrees, master's degrees, or other advanced degrees. Behavioral health staff members are educated in one of these disciplines: nursing, psychology, counseling, social work, or psychiatry. The client/counselor relationships also differ among the treatment models. In the Alcoholics Anonymous/Narcotics Anonymous model, the relationship is based on the "buddy system," where a sponsor is assigned to a member. In the traditional behavioral health model, the relationship is a professional/client relationship and is focused on a one-to-one relationship. The System of Care model proposes that the relationship between client and the professionals should be equal and should be a collaborative partnership with the family and all of the various disciplines who care for the child and family. In other words, the obstacles concerning the disparities between substance abuse programs and behavioral health programs in part have to do with the differences in the philosophic underpinnings of the programs and the educational backgrounds of the staff. However, the principles of inclusion and cultural competence in System of Care may help to overcome some of these obstacles.

The disease itself offers challenges and may present obstacles because it is a chronic, disabling disease and its existence is often denied. Frequently, there is a sense of hopelessness regarding substance use disorders, partially because of unrealistic expectations and hope for a cure. Some diseases, such as acute otitis media (ear infection), are easily cured with one course of antibiotics. Instead, substance use disorders are chronic, relapsing disorders that are more analogous to diabetes mellitus or hypertension or some cancers. These diseases, even with behavioral or lifestyle changes, such as exercise and diet, are long term, may have remissions and exacerbations, and need ongoing and often life-long treatment. Cancers often require more than one intensive intervention before there is a remission. The same may be true for a substance use disorder. Consequently, the chronic nature of the illness provides an obstacle to the integration of substance abuse treatment and traditional models for behavioral health. The System of Care model values a long-term commitment to the child and family, and thus, if other barriers can be overcome, there may be a better fit in terms of integrating System of Care with substance abuse treatment.

Finally, in light of the chronicity and tenacity of the illness, psychotropic medications are a valuable addition to the therapeutic regime. The diagnosis of co-existing disorders is increasingly recognized, and the need for medications and for interdisciplinary teamwork is necessary to provide holistic care for children and families with complex needs who require an array of services, including substance abuse services.

Recommendations

Assessment

Ask questions about substances, and use screening instruments. Be suspicious when other areas are being addressed and the family is still at an impasse. Invite an addictions specialist to a child and family team meeting. "Be sensitive to the range and complexity of co-morbid disorders in youth" (O'Malley, 2003, p. 303). Share your suspicions and reasons for them with the family. Meet with the parents and/or grandparents and bring substance abuse issues to the forefront. It helps to let them know that you think you see an elephant in the living room.

Treatment

The treatment of substance use disorders works. Provide for the treatment of co-occurring psychiatric disorders. Refer to an addiction specialist to get the appropriate level of care that is necessary. (1) Treatment options include individual therapy, psychoeducational groups, an intensive outpatient program; a residential detoxification program and/or rehabilitation program; a medically monitored or managed inpatient program; and a relapse-prevention group. (2) A key component of treatment and aftercare is targeting the way the addicted person spends his or her time. The person with a substance use disorder is helped by the support of a treatment program in promoting the development of prosocial behaviors and learning healthy ways of engaging in the world. The person in recovery must develop new leisure skills that do not involve drugs or alcohol. For many, it has been a number of years since they had fun without using alcohol and/or drugs; at first it seems unnatural. Sometimes it is even surprising to the clients that they can find enjoyment without the use of drugs or alcohol. (3) Community recovery supports include 12-step programs or alternative community support groups. Other community supports include therapeutic communities, religious institutions, and other community programs, such as Big Brothers and Big Sisters Programs, after-school programs, and extracurricular activities of various sorts. (4) Developing friendships with other people who are in recovery or even in one's own family will provide social support to the recovering addict. Developing an informal support system that an abstinent community has to offer is not only helpful but is also fundamental to recovery. (5) All levels of care of addictions treatment involve cognitive behavioral therapy. This model addresses how people think and how their thinking affects their feelings and their behaviors. The assumption is that cognitive structures that are derived from constitutional and experiential factors determine how a person reacts to any given situation or to environmental stressors. The focus is on helping people to rethink ways of coping and to assist them in reframing their perceptions of their problems so they may see them in a different light and thus feel differently about them (Andreason & Black, 1991). Its focus is on changing behavior as well as on getting some distance from and then challenging one's cognitions or thoughts.

In conclusion, recovery often involves a fundamental lifestyle change, which is more likely to succeed with the expertise and support of treatment providers trained in substance use disorders. The recovery process may require a number of different interventions, including medications, addiction-specific treatment programs that use cognitive behavior therapy, and support from family, friends, service providers, and the community.

Integration and Its Advantages

Substance abuse treatment providers and other recovery support persons who are important to the client should be participating members of child and family teams. Integration allows for an early intervention when a "slip" occurs or a relapse begins. Collaboration among providers fosters the ability to monitor all members of the family's progress toward healthy behaviors. With early intervention, one can abort the progression of symptoms into a full-blown relapse. A relapse may lead to further legal, school, or work-related difficulties, problematic relationships, and/or physical and mental health sequelae. By having various health, mental health, and other service systems already in place, recovery interventions can be mobilized more readily, whether these are formal supports, such as a treatment program, or informal or community support systems.

Models of Integration

Integration of the staff can be accomplished through different means. Some programs focus on cross-training staff, for instance, training other behavioral health providers in substance use disorders. The limitation of this model is that it can take years to train the staff. Other programs, such as the assertive community treatment teams model discussed earlier in this chapter, involve providers who are separately trained in either mental health or substance abuse, who are integrated into a collaborative team. Building a collaborative team may be a good place for an agency to begin the integration process and can even be done in collaboration with staff from an outside agency.

Multisystemic Therapy (MST) is another model of care that successfully integrates substance abuse with behavioral health treatment. This model was designed by Scott Henggeler, PhD, at the Medical University of South Carolina, in order to treat conduct-disordered and substance-abusing adolescents. The treatment involves intensive case management and ecologic family therapy, and, as the name suggests, the intervention supports and treats the family and its own network of relationships with the involved or relevant systems. Recent work has shown promising results integrating multisystemic therapy with an empirically supported intervention for substance use disorders—the community reinforcement approach. Multisystemic therapy is intensive, and the therapist has a limited caseload and works outside the 9-to 5-o'clock framework. It is community based, strength based, and family centered—three of the basic tenets of the System of Care philosophy. Multisystemic therapy has a strong evidence base and offers a specific program for implementation, including criteria for supervision (Henggeler, Clingempeel, Brondino, & Pickrel, 2002; Henggeler, Schoenwald, Borduin, Rowland, & Cunningham, 1998; Randall, Henggeler, Cunningham, Rowland, & Swenson, 2001).

System of Care

System of Care is a philosophical umbrella, rather than a model, that comprises specific values and concepts. It is a process that emphasizes an interdisciplinary and usually multisystemic team of providers collaborating for and with a family (see Chapters 1 and 2). One basic tenet of these principles of care is the integration of the family, the professionals, and other relevant community members on a team—a child/family team. Significant others, such as friends and extended family members, are also included on the team. Each family member's strengths are examined in order to build on them, and care is delivered with respect and dignity. Another basic tenet of System of Care is that it is culturally competent, and ideally, the team reflects the cultural needs and cultural makeup of the community. The substance abuse specialist has not always been included at the table, and it is essential to do so. Most substance abusers have lost their self-respect as people and as parents. The System of Care empowerment model helps family members to enhance their self-esteem as important and equal members and partners on the interdisciplinary team. "The family-provider collaboration is a central component" to System of Care (Simpson, Koroloff, Friesen, & Gac, 1999, p. 9).

According to Friesen and Walker (2004), "Partnering successfully [with families, and community members, mental health professionals and substance abuse providers] requires not only a philosophical commitment to the value, but also intentional, specific steps to redesign services and reallocate resources, so as to remove logistical and interpersonal barriers" (p. 3). The commonalities among these models of integration are that they are holistic, family oriented, and focused on building the child and family's self-esteem and prosocial behaviors so that they can cope with life's stressors without the use of chemicals, and by using the expertise of all members of the interdisciplinary team. There may be barriers or obstacles that impede integration, but it can be done. Obstacles should not be viewed as barriers but as challenges.

Some examples of practices that support collaboration and integration are as follow:

- Family groups: This includes families in any treatment of substance use disorders. Addiction programs regularly have family groups, and all involved need to be well informed of this and invited. Families can assist each other in the recovery process, and families find important support from these groups.
- Collaboration (illustrated here with juvenile justice): Call probation officers when sitting with a youth on probation, and share updated information with the youth in the room. Put the probation officer on a speakerphone; sometimes it is helpful to make sure that everyone has the same information.
- Consider needed support services (illustrated here for mothers and mothers-to-be in recovery): Provide daycare and transportation for mothers or mothers-to-be in treatment. It is also important to keep in close contact with child welfare services when that system is involved, as well as primary care providers (such as obstetricians, gynecologists, and pediatricians); a quick phone call is often sufficient to keep other members of the team informed. Provide shelters for homeless mothers who are in re-

covery (see the information about the Second Chance House in Chapter 6) or consider admission to a therapeutic community.

- Integration of services: Invite the substance abuse treatment providers to the child/family team meeting or to the therapy sessions or to the medication management/psychiatric follow-up sessions. If the provider is not able to be present for the meeting or for the entire meeting, consider using a speakerphone for the time the provider is available by phone or have that provider present for at least part of the meeting.

Conclusion

The benefits of the System of Care approach includes the emphasis on family-centered care that is community based, strength based, and culturally competent, and is provided by an interdisciplinary collaborative team. This approach promotes the integration of care, thereby reducing redundancies in services. Thus, the interventions are more holistic, efficient, and effective. Addiction issues can be more fully addressed when care is provided from a holistic and multigenerational perspective so that the focus is not just on one family member, the client, or the child; instead, it is on the entire family.

Activities to Extend Your Learning

■ Read the following:
  ■ Lowinson, J., Ruiz, P., Millman, R., & Langrod, J. (1997). *Substance abuse: A comprehensive textbook* (3rd ed.). Baltimore, MD: Williams & Wilkins.
  ■ Galanter, M., & Kleber, H. (1999). *Textbook of substance abuse treatment* (2nd ed.). Washington, DC: American Psychiatric Press.
  ■ The treatment improvement protocol series from the U.S. Department of Health and Human Services–Substance Abuse and Mental Health Services Administration (SAMSHA). Contact the National Clearinghouse for Alcohol and Drug Information at (800)729-6656 or (301)468-2600, TDD (for hearing impaired) (800)487-4889. These publications are available without charge.

■ The case example in the article *Adapting Multi-systemic Therapy to Treat Adolescent Substance Abuse More Effectively* (see Randall et al. in the reference list).
■ Attend an Alcoholics Anonymous or Narcotics Anonymous meeting or an alternative community recovery support group in your area.
■ Some of these meetings are closed; others are open.
■ Call your local chapter to find out which meetings are open to the public and when they are held.
■ Examine your own or your family's third-party health care benefits package.
■ Compare the benefits between physical health care and mental health care.
■ Then compare the benefits between mental health care and substance abuse care.
■ Are they comparable, or are there discrepancies?

The author extends appreciation and gratitude to Alberto C. Serrano, MD, who provided editorial support and has greatly informed and inspired my work and the work of many.

Suggested Reading

DuPont, R.L., & McGovern, J.P. (1994). *Bridge to recovery: An introduction to 12-step programs.* Washington, DC: American Psychiatric Press.

Horvath, A.T. (1997). Alternative support groups. In J. H. Lowinson, P. Ruiz, R.B. Millman, & J.G. Langrod (Eds.), *Comprehensive textbook* (3rd ed., pp. 390–396). Baltimore, MD: Williams & Wilkins.

Lowinson, J.G., Ruiz, P., Millman, R.B., & Langrod, J.G. (1997). *Substance abuse: A comprehensive textbook* (3rd ed.). Baltimore, MD: Williams & Wilkins.

Minkoff, K., & Drake, R.E. (1991). *Dual diagnosis of major mental illness and substance disorder.* San Francisco: Jossey-Bass.

Websites for additional resources are as follows: http://www.NIDA.gov and http://www.samhsa.gov.

References

American Psychiatric Association. (2000). *Diagnostic and statistical manual of mental disorders* (4th ed.). Washington, DC: Author.

American Society of Addictive Medicine. (1997). *Patient placement criteria* (2nd ed.). Chevy Chase, MD.

Andreason, N.C., & Black D.W. (1991). *Introductory textbook of psychiatry.* Washington, DC: The American Psychiatric Press.

Anthony, J.C., & Helzer, J.E. (1991). Syndromes of drug abuse and dependence. In L.N. Robins & D.A. Regier (Eds.), *Psychiatric disorders in America: The epidemiologic catchment area study* (p. 84). New York: The Free Press.

Drake, R.E., McHugo, G.J., Clark, R.E., Teague, G.B., Xie, H., & Miles, K. (1998). Assertive community treatment for patients with co-occurring severe mental illness and substance use disorder: A clinical trial. *The American Journal of Orthopsychiatry, 68*(2), 201–215.

Friesen, B., & Walker, J.S. (2004). Partnering with families. *Focal Point: A National Bulletin on Family Support and Children's Mental Health, 18*(1), 3.

Helzer, J.E., Burnam, A., & McEvoy, L.T. (1991). Alcohol abuse and dependence. In L.N. Robins & D.A. Regier (Eds.), *Psychiatric disorders in America: The epidemiologic catchment area study* (p. 84). New York: The Free Press.

Henggeler, S.W., Schoenwald, S.K., Borduin, M.C., Rowland, M.D., & Cunningham, P.B. (1998). *Multisystemic treatment of antisocial behavior in children and adolescents.* New York: The Guilford Press.

Henggeler, S.W., Clingempeel, W.G., Brondino, M.J., & Pickrel, S. (2002). Four-year follow-up of multi-systemic therapy with substance-abusing and substance-dependent juvenile offenders. *Journal of the American Academy of Child and Adolescent Psychiatry, 41*(7), 868–864.

Herrick, C.A., & Bartlett, T.R. (2004). Psychiatric nursing case management: Past, present, and future. *Issues in Mental Health Nursing, 25*(6), 589–602.

Kaminer, Y., & Tarter, R.E. (1999). Adolescent substance abuse. In M. Galanter & H.D. Kleber (Eds.), *Textbook on substance abuse treatment* (2nd ed., pp. 465–474). Washington, DC: American Psychiatric Press.

Minkoff, K., & Drake, R.E. (1991). *Dual diagnosis of major mental illness and substance disorder.* San Francisco: Jossey-Bass.

Nestler, E.J., & Self, D.W. (1997). Neurobiologic aspects of ethanol and other chemical dependencies. In S.C. Yudofsky & R.E. Hales (Eds.), *Textbook of neuropsychiatry* (3rd ed., pp. 773–798). Washington, DC: American Psychiatric Press.

O'Malley, K.D. (2003). Youth and co-morbid disorders. In A.J. Pumariega & N.C. Winters (Eds.), *The handbook of child and adolescent systems of care: The new community psychiatry* (pp. 276–315). San Francisco: Jossey-Bass.

Phoenix, B.J., & Pelish, K. (2004). Coexisting psychiatric and substance use disorders. In C.R. Kneisl, H.S. Wilson, & E. Trigoboff (Eds.), *Contemporary psychiatric-mental health nursing* (pp. 506–523). Upper Saddle River, NJ: Prentice Hall.

Randall, J., Henggeler, S.W., Cunningham, P.B., Rowland, M.D., & Swenson, C.C. (2001). Adapting multi-systemic therapy to treat adolescent substance abuse more effectively. *Cognitive and Behavioral Practice, 8,* 359–366.

Regier, D.A., Farmer, M.E., Rae, D.S., Locke, B.Z., Keith, S.J., & Judd, L.L. (1990). Co-morbidity of mental disorders with alcohol and other drug abuse: Results from the Epidemiologic Catchment Area (ECA study). *Journal of the American Medical Association, 264,* 2511–2518.

Simpson, J.S., Koroloff, N., Friesen, B.F., & Gac, J. (1999). Promising practices in family-provider collaboration. *Systems of care: Promising practices in children's mental health* (1998 Series, Vol. II). Washington, DC: Center for Effective Collaboration and Practice, American Institutes of Research.

Chapter 10

The System of Care with Juvenile Justice Populations: The Interface Between Juvenile Justice and Behavioral Health

GERALDINE S. PEARSON

"How am I ever going to figure out what my son needs after he gets out of detention?" asks a mother of a 14-year-old involved in the juvenile justice system.

Families expect assistance with negotiating the service system. In many states and communities, rapidly expanding children's mental health services are relatively new to a child-serving system that includes education, health, child welfare, and juvenile justice. Each of these arenas includes multiple programs, policies, procedures,

*and professionals. It is not easy to describe this system
to anyone, and it is this complexity that underscores the
need for competent service coordination.*

(Jacobs, 1995, p. 389)

Objectives

▣ Identify the historical development of the juvenile justice system in the
United States and the ways that this influences current issues.
▣ Understand the relationship between delinquent behavior and psychiatric
disturbances.
▣ Describe a model of care that integrates system of care issues with a
juvenile justice population.

Historically, juvenile justice populations have received cursory attention in writings about System of Care needs of children with severe
emotional disturbances. Although juvenile justice populations definitely suffer from comorbid psychiatric and substance abuse disorders, they have, in the past, been seen as "acting out" or "delinquent"
individuals who are beyond the realm of mental health interventions
and more in the management of the correctional system. Shelton
(2001) noted, "The complexity of the emotional and behavioral problems youth experience thwart efforts to develop integrated and coordinated Systems of Care for children and adolescents" (p. 259).
Adolescents involved in the juvenile justice system are found in
schools, emergency rooms, community programs, psychiatric and substance abuse treatment programs, jails, and detention centers.
Professionals working with these individuals must understand the
types of crimes the youth committed that resulted in their involvement
with juvenile justice, their status within the system in terms of active
charges and probation, and their risk factors associated with a reoffense
(McCrone & Shelton, 2001).

Even though most juvenile offenders need mental health assessment and treatment, their needs have historically been ignored
(Cocozza, 1992; Knitzer, 1982). Reasons for this could include the belief
that offenders do not deserve treatment or that behaviors are not related
to psychiatric disturbance (Breda, 2003). Thankfully, this attitude is
undergoing a radical change with increasing recognition from the ju-

venile justice and mental health communities that youngsters involved in the juvenile justice system often have a long history of school failure, family dysfunction, psychiatric disorder, and substance abuse problems. Arrest and involvement in the judicial system create another layer of dysfunction and another set of professionals involved in the youngster's life. The need for a System of Care model to address the myriad of needs and problems presented by this population is essential.

The purpose of this chapter is to identify the historical context of the juvenile justice system in America, to delineate the psychiatric/clinical profile of this population, and to define what aspects of the juvenile justice system must integrate with the broader System of Care model. Understanding *how* to integrate this population within a System of Care framework will result in improved coordination of care and better treatment for co-morbid psychiatric issues and will prevent relapse, reoffending, and reincarceration.

History of Juvenile Justice in America

The formal system of juvenile justice has been in existence in the United States for nearly 200 years. The central focus of the system, from the beginning, has been on delinquency—"an amorphous construct that includes not only 'criminal' behavior but also an array of youthful actions that offend prevailing social mores" (Harris, Welsh, & Gutler, 2000, p. 359). The American juvenile justice system was created on the basis of conflicting value systems: "The diminished responsibility and heightened malleability of youths versus individual culpability and social control of protocriminality. . . . Those most caught up in the system, however, have remained overwhelmingly our most marginalized youths, from immigrants' offspring in the early 20th century to children of color in contemporary society" (Harris et al., p. 359).

The concept of adolescence as a separate social entity did not appear in contemporary American history until the 19th century (Chesney-Lind & Shelden, 2004). Up to that point, young adults were the predominant focus of society, and children had close ties to their families until puberty. Before the 19th century, the deviant behavior of adolescents was handled in an informal manner within the family or community and not within a formal juvenile justice system.

Chesney-Lind and Shelden (2004) noted that the appearance of adolescence as a recognized developmental stage coincided with increasing concern for the regulation of moral behavior. Another influencing factor was the population explosion that occurred in America between 1750 and 1850, with the influx of huge numbers of European immigrants. Cities were populated by increasing numbers of unsupervised children who often engaged in behaviors that were unacceptable to established "polite" society. This resulted in the development of groups such as the Society for Reformation of Juvenile Delinquents, founded in 1823 in New York City (Sutton, 1988). This group worked to start the New York House of Refuge, the first correctional institution for children in the United States. The goal of the House of Refuge was reform. Most of the individuals confined to this institution had not committed a crime but were considered "incorrigible" or "beyond control." "The goal of the SRJD [Society for Reformation of Juvenile Delinquents] and like-minded groups was to identify potential delinquents, isolate them, and then 'reform' them" (Chesney-Lind & Shelden, 2004, p. 162).

The development of the Society for Reformation of Juvenile Delinquents and other like-minded civic institutions to deal with the increasing problem of juvenile delinquency reflected society's traditional concern with instilling law-abiding attitudes and behaviors in its young people. This was particularly true during the 20th century when the term *juvenile justice* was adopted. The early part of the 20th century saw the beginnings of the juvenile court system, the enactment of special laws, and the beginning of rehabilitative services for juvenile offenders. Harris et al. (2000) noted that the juvenile justice system in the United States has concerned itself with delinquency—"an amorphous construct that includes not only 'criminal' behavior but also an array of youthful actions that offend prevailing social mores" (p. 359). The authors note that the American juvenile justice system was founded on "internally conflicting value systems: the diminished responsibility and heightened malleability of youths versus individual culpability and social control of protocriminality" (p. 359). In contemporary society, the term delinquent conjures many images and encompasses a complex array of behavioral, psychiatric, cultural, and normative values that intersect with adolescent criminality. For many, juvenile delinquency is not linked with a comorbid psychiatric disorder or learning disability, but is attributed to a failure within the family to manage the youth and their behavior. The origins of juvenile delinquency are complex and often not well understood and may include family, psychiatric, and substance use issues or a combination of all. It is important to understand the interplay of these factors for the youth when planning service delivery in order to meet the needs of the youth.

Historically, individuals involved in the juvenile justice system in America have included marginalized populations and youths from lower socioeconomic groups. In the early 1900s, they tended to be immigrant children, whereas in contemporary society, the number of children of different races is disproportionately represented (Harris et al., 2000). The 19th century was characterized by the Industrial Revolution, religious reform, and organized efforts to discipline youths who got into trouble (Fox, 1970). The cultural conflicts between the rural, Protestant ethic, and the urban underprivileged environments resulted in efforts to control negative youth by placing them in institutional settings. The efforts to pull youth away from the corruption of their urban immigrant neighborhoods resulted in the first US juvenile court in Cook County, Chicago, Illinois, in 1899. This first juvenile court was designed to meet the clinical and developmental needs of wayward children and adolescents who were thought to be in need of benevolent justice to redirect their development in positive ways (Grisso, 1999).

By 1920, all but two states had court models to handle juvenile offenders, and most had some mechanism to handle the process of child evaluation. The doctrine of *parens patriae* was invoked by American juvenile courts to support judges as they strived to understand the child and respond as a "merciful father." The legal system, along with social service and medical professionals, began to realize that understanding the individual needs of the child could result in an improved, collaborative treatment plan. The increasing focus on juvenile delinquency and aggression in youth resulted in the beginnings of treatment intervention models.

During the first half of the 20th century, juvenile court systems flourished in the United States. By 1967, the same system was being criticized for its inability to rehabilitate delinquent youth, its failure at preventing institutionalization, and increasing rates of juvenile crime. The juvenile rights movement that resulted from these criticisms moved toward protecting the rights of children and moved away from mental health interventions as part of the court process.

In the 1980s, states began passing more punitive laws to deal with juvenile delinquents who committed violent crimes. Many of these laws waived certain violent crimes to adult court where there were harsher consequences for behavior and fixed penalties for juvenile offenders. By the end of the 1990s, nearly every state had enacted laws that transferred juveniles of a certain age to adult criminal justice systems if they committed a violent crime.

There is no uniform juvenile code between states in this country. Thus, human service professionals must identify and understand the juvenile statutes, terminology, and age boundaries particular to the state where they practice. It is imperative that professionals dealing with juvenile justice populations understand the philosophy that shapes management of juvenile offenders, the state views on rehabilitation versus punishment, and the available community resources for this population. Each state has different terminology and philosophy around juvenile offenders, incarceration, diversion programs, and management of mental health needs.

The 1990s have also brought a proliferation of forensic mental health professionals (primarily psychiatrists, nurses, psychologists, and social workers) who specialize in psychiatric assessment of youngsters involved at different points in the juvenile justice system. These practitioners are trained to focus on evaluating the mental health and legal issues and to provide crucial information that will assist judges and attorneys as they consider how to manage the legal decision making around a youthful offender. These assessments can also be crucial in assisting providers planning a System of Care for a youngster and his or her family. Again, professionals are involved with juvenile justice populations in a variety of settings and can intervene in ways that facilitate more effective caregiving.

Service Needs of Juvenile Justice Populations

It is nationally recognized that all child and adolescent populations with severe emotional disturbances and their families struggle with coordinated service delivery and with accessing adequate mental health services. The same is true for children and adolescents with severe emotional disturbances or with moderate to severe emotional disturbance involved with the juvenile justice system. The predominant difference involves the overlay of legal and forensic concerns along with the mental health issues that characterize the population. Juvenile justice youth struggle with accessing social, educational, health, and mental health services, just like youngsters who are not involved in juvenile justice. A significant factor that caregivers must consider is the potential bias against a youngster who has committed a crime, the tendency to see the youth as "bad" or "evil" rather than psychiatrically disturbed. Although a small number of youngsters who commit crimes might not be categorized as having behavioral health issues, the majority has co-morbid (i.e., concurrent) disorders that have directly or indirectly influenced their criminal behavior. It is these disorders and their management that have a profound effect on future functioning and, ultimately, whether a youngster commits another crime. Although multi-determined, the literature generally agrees that youth who receive treatment (Bullis, Yovanoff, Mueller, & Havel, 2002) and community transition services (service coordination, academic support, job placement, and training) are less likely to re-offend, at least in the short term (i.e., within 6 months), than those who receive no rehabilitation or treatment. Bullis et al. also found that if study participants were engaged in work or school at 6 months after release, they tended to stay involved in these positive activities at 12 months after release. This is a significant argument for developing a system of care model that serves the juvenile justice population and is activated at the point a youth is incarcerated.

There is often a disconnected communication loop between the juvenile justice system and the mental health system. Both groups need education to restructure their thinking and to begin partnering around meeting the need for coordinated care in a juvenile justice population. More importantly, the historical view of youngsters who commit crimes as "bad" kids needs revision because so many suffer from co-morbid psychiatric disorders that are often unidentified and untreated. The evolving process ideally brings both juvenile justice and mental health professionals to the treatment planning table with the family in a collaborative effort that creates a seamless care delivery system.

Characteristics of a Juvenile Justice Population

Demographics

The US Department of Justice estimated that nearly 2.5 million juveniles are arrested each year (Snyder, 2000). Of these, more than 100,000 youth are incarcerated each year in the United States (Gallagher, 1999). Approximately 15% of the nearly 109,000 youth younger than 18 years old incarcerated each day are housed in adult facilities that lack juvenile services (Austin, Ajohnson, & Gregoriou, 2000; Sickmund & Wan, 1999).

There has been a consistent overrepresentation of minority groups within juvenile justice populations since the first juvenile court was established. This overrepresentation of African American and Hispanic youth accounts for more than 60% of young offenders in juvenile justice facilities throughout the United States (Snyder & Sickmund, 1999).

The reasons for the disproportionate numbers of youth of different races involved with juvenile justice systems are complex and not clearly delineated. Understanding and changing this racial discrepancy is an ongoing debate.

Wolford (2000) noted that between 12% and 70% of incarcerated youth might carry a special education label. The wide variability of this statistic reflects the varying definitions and interpretations of special education needs across states and communities. Special education labels could apply to youth with developmental difficulties, learning disabilities, or behavior disorders that influence their ability to learn and make use of the classroom environment. When Foley (2001) reviewed over 20 publications on the academic standing of incarcerated youth, most were performing between the fifth- and ninth-grade levels academically. Those with more significant academic deficits were more likely to return to the juvenile corrections system.

In 2000, females accounted for 27% of juvenile arrests, an increase of 22% since the early 1990s (US Department of Justice, 2001). Most researchers agree that the reasons behind female delinquency are different than those of male counterparts. Even so, arrests for violent crimes have increased even though running away from home and larceny (theft) remain the major reasons for female involvement in the juvenile justice system (Chesney-Lind & Shelden, 2004).

Although both male and female juvenile offenders are likely to have been exposed to a traumatic event, when compared with males, female juvenile offenders are more likely to be the victim of violence. Males, in contrast, were more likely to report having witnessed a violent event (Steiner, Garcia, & Mattews, 1997). In another sample of incarcerated youth, girls reported higher levels of sexual abuse and physical punishment and higher levels of psychologic distress than boys (Wood, Foyh, Goguen, Pynoos, & Jamese, 2002).

Clinical Profiles of Youth Involved in Juvenile Justice

The premise that youth involved with the juvenile justice system also have co-morbid or co-occurring psychiatric disorders is not new. Abram, Teplin, McClelland, Dulcan, and Mericle (2004), researchers from Northwestern University, conducted definitive research showing this connection. Teplin, Abram, McClelland, Dulcan, and Mericle (2002) found in their study of detained juveniles that even after excluding conduct disorder (and its associated symptoms with delinquency) nearly 60% of males and 70% of females had a psychiatric disorder. They found that these rates far exceeded similar rates in non-detained community populations.

More specifically, they found that significantly more females (56.5%) than males (45.9%) met diagnostic criteria for two or more disorders from the following group: major depressive, dysthymic, manic, psychotic, panic, separation anxiety, overanxious, generalized anxiety, obsessive compulsive, attention deficit/hyperactivity, conduct, oppositional defiant, alcohol, marijuana, and other substances. In their research, they found that 17.3% of females and 20.4% of males had only one disorder. They found that 14% of females and 11% of males had both a major mental health disorder and a substance use disorder. They concluded that co-morbid psychiatric disorders were a major health problem for detained youth (Abram, Teplin, McClelland, & Dulcan, 2003).

Similarly to the prevalence studies, Abram, Teplin, Charles et al. (2004) studied the rate of posttraumatic stress disorder and trauma in a population of youth in a juvenile detention center in Illinois. Their large-scale study involved 1,829 youth ages 10 to 18 years who were arrested and detained. They found that 92.5% of the sample had experienced at least one trauma and that 84% had experienced more than one trauma. Trauma incidents were defined as witnessing trauma; being attacked, threatened, or forced to do something sexual; being in a car accident, fire, flood, or other natural disaster; seeing someone badly hurt; or being upset by seeing a dead body. There was no significant difference in overall prevalence of trauma across race/ethnicity for males and females. Significantly more females reported being forced to do something sexual, whereas non-Hispanic white males were more likely to have been attacked physically or badly beaten. The researchers concluded that exposure to trauma is a "fact of life for delinquent youth" (Abram et al., 2003, p. 407).

More specifically, the researchers found that 11.2% of detainees had posttraumatic stress disorder during the year before the interview, based on the Diagnostic Interview Schedule for Children interview. Although results were influenced by the choice of instrument, the point where the youth was interviewed (immediately after incarceration versus in stable placement), and ethnicity of the detainees, the results reflect a higher rate of posttraumatic stress disorder in this population than would be noted in the general, nondetained community population (Abram, Teplin, McClelland, & Dulcan, 2004). They recommended research that looks at vulnerability to posttraumatic stress disorder of this high-risk population, the relationship of chronic community violence and posttraumatic stress disorder, and further definition of trauma and the diagnosis of posttraumatic stress disorder. They also recommended improving community services for victims of trauma, improving the detection of posttraumatic stress disorder, and avoiding retraumatizing youth by incarceration procedures in detention (Abram et al., 2004).

Widom (1995) found that people who experience any type of maltreatment during childhood, sexual or physical abuse, or neglect are more likely than people who were not maltreated to experience arrest during their lives. She found that being abused or neglected as a child increased the likelihood of an arrest as a juvenile by 59% and as an adult by 28%. Similarly, Smith and Thornberry (1995) found in the Rochester Youth Development Study that a history of maltreatment significantly increased the risk of arrest for violent, serious, and moderate forms of crime even when controlling for race, sex, social class, family structure, and mobility. The authors emphasize that the majority of maltreated youngsters are not arrested. Nevertheless, the research makes a compelling argument for juvenile delinquency as a potential consequence of childhood maltreatment. It also makes an indirect argument for a service system that identifies children at risk for maltreatment and provides the services necessary to keep them from experiencing this (Siegfried, Ko, & Kelley, 2004).

These statistics apply to a population of incarcerated youth and do not include rates of psychiatric disturbance present in youngsters who are never placed in detention but are still involved with the juvenile justice system through arrests, adjudication, and probation. Abram et al. (2003) made notable recommendations for improving the system that included improving screening, increasing the diversion system and linkage, and reducing barriers to service in the community. They recommended further research on co-morbidity, health disparities, effectiveness of intervention, and the relationships between co-morbid mental and physical disorders. This research and other subsequent studies that have supported the findings make a sound argument for a System of Care model that incorporates knowledge about the population and is applicable to youngsters involved with the juvenile justice system.

Models of Need Assessment with Juvenile Justice Populations

The need to screen youngsters involved with the juvenile justice system has been identified as imperative in planning more extensive psychiatric assessment (Grisso & Underwood, 2003; Grisso, Barnum,

Fletcher, Cauffman, & Peuschold, 2001; Wasserman, McReynolds, Lucas, Fisher, & Santos, 2002). Several studies have looked further into the relationship between screening and assessment, accessing treatment, and treatment response (Lyons, Griffin, Quintenz, Jenuwine, & Shasha, 2003).

Stewart and Trupin (2003) studied whether a screening instrument, the Massachusetts Youth Screening Inventory, 2nd edition, was able to identify delinquent youth with mental health and substance abuse problems. They further examined the relationship between identification of problems via the Massachusetts Youth Screening Inventory and mental health treatment received before and after entering the juvenile justice system. Youth who had more extensive mental health histories before entering the juvenile justice system were more likely to receive longer sentences in more restricted settings, limiting their access to community-based services.

In Illinois, a study was conducted that identified youth with psychotic or affective disorders as they entered the juvenile justice system. They were then linked with the appropriate community resource. The researchers found that of the youth who entered the program, 46% completed it. Of this 46%, a longer-term follow-up revealed a significant decrease in emotional problems and lower rearrest rates (Lyons et al., 2003).

Although many research and practice efforts are directed at identifying the youngsters in juvenile justice who exhibit psychiatric disturbance and require psychiatric treatment, there is little mention of System of Care principles in planning care and integrating evidence-based treatments. It is clear that the problems exhibited by juvenile justice youngsters are multifaceted and require an integrated approach of community caregivers in order to prevent reoffending and the eventual and often inevitable move into the adult corrections system.

Applicability of System of Care Principles to a Juvenile Justice Population

The core values associated with a System of Care model have complete applicability to populations of youngsters within the juvenile justice system. Stroul and Friedman (1986) initially identified these core values as child centered and family focused, community based, and culturally competent. If the services are child centered and family focused, the needs of the youngster and the family drive the service delivery system and services are adapted, within the community, to fit their needs. For youngsters in juvenile justice, this has meant that more services that are home based and community oriented versus more traditional psychiatric care models in clinics or offices. Services provided in the community ideally provide less restrictive, more normative environments. Culturally competent services have enormous importance with this population because so many incarcerated youth are from ethnic minorities. Isaacs and Benjamin (1991) noted that ethnicity shapes beliefs about mental health and disorder, symptoms, and help-seeking behaviors. A culturally competent System of Care is critical to success.

As noted in Chapter 6, System of Care principles are the same across disciplines, but they may be implemented in different ways, depending on the discipline. The System of Care principles can also have differing application depending on the specific needs of the population served. The general principles—namely that services are comprehensive and occur in the least restrictive setting, are strength based, individualized, and normalized, are delivered by an interdisciplinary system, and are seamless—have complete applicability to a juvenile justice population. The use of a case manager to coordinate care and act as a care liaison between agencies and families and to facilitate general empowerment of self-care applies to juvenile justice populations. Nevertheless, particular differences do apply to juvenile justice populations and are described.

Comprehensive

Finkelman (2001) noted that the continuum of care is a variety of services and care settings that are needed by an individual at any point during illness. The service continuum is further defined as the least restrictive setting, including schools, recreational activities, and other community settings focused on prevention. Community-based care such as clinics, community mental health centers, and day programs for emotionally disturbed youth also encompass this continuum. For juvenile justice populations, these programs can also include court-based intervention programs either during or after school that incorporate mental health and juvenile justice components. The goals of all of these programs are to maximize functioning and to prevent use of inpatient settings. For youngsters involved in juvenile justice, the goal is also avoiding rearrest and incarceration.

The most restrictive settings in the continuum of care are hospital-based treatment models or residential treatment centers. For youngsters involved in juvenile justice, the most restrictive setting is the juvenile detention setting or the inpatient setting that might be conducting a court-ordered psychiatric evaluation. As with severely emotionally disturbed youngsters, the goal of care needs to be maximizing functioning while maintaining functioning in the community.

Although educational services and vocational services are essential for all youngsters involved in a System of Care, they are essential for youth in the juvenile justice system. Research has shown that staying involved in a regular school program is the best prevention for avoiding incarceration. Vocational training assists in getting a job, which in turn makes it less likely for a youngster to reoffend.

Throughout this text we note the absolute need for linkages between agencies and programs in order to plan, develop, and coordinate services that will meet the individual and family needs. With youngsters involved in juvenile justice, this is even more essential and must involve the juvenile justice system, including probation officers, court-based clinical coordinators, court-based psychiatric evaluators, and attorneys. Without these linkages, the care becomes fragmented and lost until the youngster reoffends and emerges again in a detention center, requiring services.

The Least Restrictive Alternative

In a System of Care model, the care coordinator works with the family and individual to choose the best health care and mental health service setting that meets the individual and family needs. Unfortunately, there are often long waiting lists for outpatient mental health services, especially if the youth and family use public services of health care and have Medicaid as payment. This often limits choices for care.

Going without services is likely to result in rearrest, worsening of symptoms, and a lack of developmental progress (Bullis et al., 2002). Choosing the least restrictive setting for care is essential to a System of Care model but must also be tailored to the community and personal resources held by the youngster involved with the juvenile justice system.

Individualized

The most important aspect of individualized care for a juvenile justice population involves understanding the youngster's personal strengths, including personal, family, and community. It also involves tailoring care with an awareness of the youngster's status in the juvenile justice system. Is the youth on the verge of a court-ordered placement outside of the community? How much supervision is required after school? Are there school issues that are unresolved and require intervention to maintain the school placement?

The youngster's history of psychiatric problems, the duration of the problems, and their severity will also influence care planning. Similarly, his or her history of involvement in the juvenile justice system and the severity of charges will also influence planning individualized care.

Normalized

Normalized care is defined as care that occurs in an environment supportive of the family, their strengths, and their lifestyle. It must be culturally sensitive and can occur in traditional and nontraditional ways. It involves using available community resources in a creative, positive manner that enhances the family's functioning. For populations in the juvenile justice system, this might include involvement in a neighborhood family advocacy group or a Big Brother/mentor program. By normalizing the services, the family and youth are most likely to make use of it.

Interdisciplinary

Interdisciplinary care is organized across a continuum of agencies providing different but necessary clinical services to a youngster and family. The plan of care emerges from the input of several agencies, family members, and caregivers. It takes into consideration the status of the youngster within the juvenile justice system. Is the youth on probation? If so, how long is probation? Are current charges pending in both adult and juvenile court? What prior evaluations and treatment influence the planning of current care?

Seamless

An integrated System of Care design allows families easy access to services that are "wrapped" around the youth and family to avoid their getting lost in the system. One of the greatest risks of a fragmented health care system involves the family dropping out of treatment and avoiding services that might keep their youngster away from reoffending within the juvenile justice system. Handron, Dosser, McCammon, and Powell (1998) noted that a wraparound program provides comprehensive services across the health care continuum, is individualized, and is intensive.

For youngsters involved in juvenile justice, this means a seamless transition from the detention center into the community, to school, and to work. It also means activation of the System of Care even when a youngster offends and is placed in a detention setting. Planning for discharge from the juvenile justice setting, assisting the family in managing the legal system, and negotiating services for the youngster are essential to a System of Care.

Coordinated by a Care Coordinator or Case Manager

It is essential for youth in the juvenile justice system that a person or agency be identified to coordinate all of the individuals and family members involved in care issues. This will include the juvenile justice staff, that is, probation officers, detention staff, nurses in detention settings, psychiatric providers, attorneys, and even judges. The care coordinator must have an understanding of all of the players in a youngster's life and must be able to decipher the effect that legal charges will have on care provision. A youngster might be court-ordered by a judge to adhere to treatment. This is likely to influence whether the youngster and family follow through with treatment, especially if the alternative if further incarceration.

Role of Nursing in System of Care with Juvenile Justice Populations

Nurses are in a unique position to intervene with juvenile justice populations in many arenas where they receive physical and behavioral health care. Shelton (2001) noted that nurses who work with adolescent populations within the nonmedical structure of the juvenile justice system require specialized knowledge and skills for meeting the special needs of the population. She noted that nurses must be tolerant of the uncertainties associated with the unique juvenile justice environment. Shelton also noted that mental treatment of juvenile offenders requires an understanding of the overall societal need for security and the needs of the individual.

Nurses encounter juvenile justice populations in a variety of practice settings that provide physical and behavioral health care. The point of entry into a detention center almost always involves nursing assessment of physical health care needs, the need for ongoing medication, and assessment of health teaching needs. This is generally provided by a generalist registered nurse but may be under the responsibility of a pediatric nurse practitioner who manages the care of detainees.

Once discharged from detention settings, nurses working in health care clinics also encounter this population as they provide in a physical health care setting or in a behavioral health care delivery context either as a registered nurse doing generalist care or as a nurse in an advanced practice role. Advanced practice nurses may function in many of the ways noted in previous chapters, as clinicians, health educators, case managers, or prescribing practitioners. Whatever the nursing role, it is essential that any nurse encountering a youngster involved with the juvenile justice system understands that he or she is likely to be psychiatrically vulnerable, experiencing associated physical health issues and substance abuse issues, and in critical need of responsible case management and community System of Care involvement.

Summary

This chapter builds on previous chapters in this text and deals specifically with juvenile justice populations and the ways that System of Care can be applied to this vulnerable and psychiatrically complex group of youngsters that frequently go untreated.

The chapter detailed the historical development of the juvenile justice system within America over the past century and discussed the clinical profile of youngsters in juvenile justice. Gender and cultural differences were also discussed. Juvenile justice populations require the same System of Care as other severely emotionally disturbed youngsters. Caregivers need to maintain an awareness and acknowledgment of the court, probation, and legal systems that strongly influence care planning and often directly or indirectly influence treatment.

The HomeCare Program: Community-Based Psychiatric Services for Juvenile Justice Youth in Connecticut

The following is a program description of an innovative treatment model that provides a bridging service to youngsters being released from detention who need follow-up care for their psychotropic medication. The HomeCare Program, currently operative in Connecticut, provides outpatient psychiatric medication management services until a longer-term provider is identified and accessed. This program is an example of one aspect of a System of Care that can be provided to a juvenile justice population.

The HomeCare Program, under the auspices of the Department of Children and Families/University of Connecticut Health Center Joint Institute for Public Psychiatry, was developed within a system of community-based psychiatric services with alliances with the state's federally qualified health centers.

Under this initiative, the HomeCare Program director works with the Connecticut Court Support Services Division's probation staff to identify and track youngsters in detention as they are screened and evaluated in preparation for disposition and care. Children whose disposition plan includes home- and community-based services and who need short-term psychiatric care, including medication management, while they wait for other services are eligible for the program. The HomeCare Program was established as a *bridging program* until more long-term psychiatric services are established in the community. Families may choose to continue their care at the federally qualified health centers, but most will have active referrals with other psychiatric providers and are treated in HomeCare Program clinics while waiting for these psychiatric services to begin.

The basic services offered by the HomeCare Program and the federally qualified health centers include psychiatric assessment and medication management, as well as clinical supportive services that help ensure adherence to the care. These supportive services might include more traditional case management, individual and family treatment, group treatment, and less traditional services such as transportation and child care. Uninsured clients may have their clinical services and psychotropic medication covered under the program. Supportive services are delineated in the individual plan of care and must be approved by the HomeCare Program director.

Once referred to the HomeCare Program, the program director arranges for psychiatric and supportive clinical services through a federally qualified health center as close as possible to the child's home. As services are provided, the program director works directly with the probation officer who is responsible for care management of the child and family. All care provided under this initiative, including a crisis intervention plan, will be provided in the context of the child and family's individualized plan of care.

Program staff include the program director, a PhD-prepared advanced practice registered nurse, who is responsible for the overall management of the program, the development of policies and proce-dures, the development of a performance data tracking system, and responsibility for the myriad of communication systems involved with Department of Children and Families, court staff, and federally qualified health centers. Systematic monitoring of service delivery regularly occurs. An administrative assistant supports the program director and maintains operational and clinical record systems and the administrative management of participating clinicians. Each week a treating child psychiatrist evaluates and treats the youngsters referred for care. These psychiatrists work collaboratively with the program director.

Finally, through contractual agreements with the federally qualified health centers, the services of midlevel clinicians (nurses, social workers, mental health technicians, etc.) are made available to provide supportive services to ensure compliance to psychiatric treatment. The specific arrangement for these services is unique to each clinic and involves a range of services.

The HomeCare Program embraces a system of care model, and the program director is actively involved with all other systems providing treatment for the child. Clinical ownership of the youngster and family varies and may rest with a System of Care coordinator, as illustrated by the case study. For other youngsters, the program director organizes and arranges the System of Care services required in order for the youngster to avoid re-offending and a return to a detention center.

The services are culturally sensitive and if needed involve language translation, Spanish-translated forms, and specific contacts with Spanish-speaking providers. Each clinic where the HomeCare Program is located has an array of culturally sensitive services that are implemented based on the individual and family need.

Case Study

Jose is a 14-year-old Hispanic male who lives in the inner city with his mother and two younger sisters, ages 6 and 4 years. His birth father is incarcerated on drug-trafficking charges and is unlikely to be released from prison before several more years of incarceration. His mother's boyfriend of several years lives with the family and is the biological father of Jose's sisters.

Jose was born when his mother was 15 years old and his father was 16 years old. He spent his early years in his maternal grandmother's care. His birth was unremarkable, and his mother denied drug or alcohol use during her pregnancy even though she had been incarcerated for 2 years when Jose was age 3 for drug trafficking. When she was released from prison, she resumed Jose's care, later met her male partner, and had Jose's two sisters.

The family resides in an upstairs apartment, and both parents are employed as housekeepers at a local hospital. Jose has a history of school difficulties dating to kindergarten; he repeated first grade. He was diagnosed with attention deficit hyperactivity disorder at 6 years old and was treated briefly using play therapy at a local outpatient clinic by a social worker. He was also prescribed Ritalin, but his mother only gave it to him for 1 week because she believed that it was "overdosing" him. He received no medication until sent to detention.

Jose spent many of his latency-aged years struggling in school, getting into low-level difficulties with friends. He was first arrested at 11 years old for stealing candy from a local grocery store. He had three more arrests in a 3-year period—the most recent and the one that resulted in his detention stay involved stealing a car where the keys had been left in the ignition. He crashed the car and was unhurt but was arrested with three peers for this act.

While in detention, he made vague references to gang involvement, talked about wanting to hurt himself, and noted that he had witnessed his best friend be shot on the streets 6 months before the detention stay.

Jose's charges were settled within the court system, and he was given extended probation and was court-ordered to participate in outpatient psychiatric treatment. He was referred to the HomeCare Program for short-term medication management because while in detention he was prescribed Adderall XR 10 mg at 8 a.m. and 1 p.m. to treat his symptoms of attention deficit hyperactivity disorder, combined type.

At the time of referral to the HomeCare Program, Jose and his mother were also assigned to a System of Care social worker in a local outpatient child guidance clinic. Within 1 week of discharge from detention, his worker had called a System of Care meeting in which all the professionals involved in Jose's life met with Jose and his mother to outline an aftercare plan that would ensure success outside of the detention center. The involved professionals included his probation officer, the guidance counselor at the local high school, the director of the HomeCare Program (an advanced practice registered nurse), his worker in the child welfare department, the System of Care social worker who would coordinate and monitor his care, and the pastor from the family's church. Also invited, with his mother's permission, was Jose's grandmother, a powerful and important member of this matriarchal family.

The following plan of care was developed and implemented after the meeting.

Jose would receive

1. Outpatient counseling and after-school monitoring through a court-monitoring program that also included his mother and siblings in weekly family sessions.
2. Short-term medication management at the HomeCare Program with a concurrent referral to the child guidance clinic waiting list for longer-term medication and psychiatric management.
3. Mentoring services through a church-sponsored program coordinated by his pastor.
4. Probation services, to include weekly contact with the probation officer who was monitoring his probation.

Jose and his mother were pleased with this plan, and it was implemented. The System of Care worker quickly formed a strong relationship with Jose and his mother and "owned" the management of his care plan. She either made a weekly home visit or had frequent phone contact with both Jose and his mother as Jose transitioned back to the community from the detention center.

The plan was for this service to last 3 months with a gradual withdrawal of the System of Care services and a transfer of care to the child guidance clinic, *if Jose was stable and functioning in school and in the community*. At the end of 2 months, another System of Care meeting was held with all providers and the family members to discuss progress and to finalize the long-term plan. At this meeting, it was clear that Jose was benefiting from the services, especially the mentoring program through his church. As planned, the child guidance clinic would assume responsibility for his out-patient care, including medication, within 1 month of the meeting. His pro-bation would continue for 15 more months with biweekly monitoring from the probation officer. The System of Care worker would continue with the family for 4 months in a less intense capacity. After that, services would be provided as needed. Jose was regularly attending school, had not been re-arrested, had no other offenses and appeared stable on stimulant medica-tion. A seamless transition occurred between the HomeCare Program and the child guidance clinic with a transfer of records and several phone calls be-tween providers.

Some questions for discussion are as follows:

1. What would have happened to Jose if there had been no System of Care worker involved with him and his family?

2. Were his problems strictly ones involving a conduct disorder or "willful" acting-out behaviors?
3. At what points in his care, beginning with his admission in detention, could nurses have intervened in providing services?

Activities to Extend Your Learning

■ Identify the historical development of the juvenile justice system in the United States and the ways that this influences current issues.
　■ Identify the prominent issues in juvenile justice in the past 25 years in your geographic locale by doing a search of newspaper archives and meeting with juvenile court staff.
　■ Define the current legal structure of juvenile justice in the state where you will have your professional practice. Identify the differences between probation, parole, adjudication, trial, and arrest.
　■ Ask to spend a day with a juvenile probation officer, following them through their contacts with juveniles, the court process, meetings with families, and meetings with youth.
■ Understand the interplay between delinquent behavior and psychiatric disturbances.
　■ Identify the juvenile court clinics providing psychiatric services that might exist within your state's juvenile justice system.
　■ Visit the court clinic and ascertain the types of services that are offered and how this translates into community care.
　■ Contact the intake worker at a local community mental health clinic that provides children's services and inquire about the numbers of individuals referred from the juvenile justice system. Do they have a specific protocol for managing these youngsters? Is their care different from individuals who enter the clinic through more traditional routes?
　■ Review the literature on juvenile delinquency and comorbid psychiatric disorders.
　■ Visit juvenile court and obtain permission to observe a court hearing. Note whether psychiatric issues are identified and discussed as part of the hearing.

■ Describe a model of care that integrates System of Care issues with a juvenile justice population.

   ■ Identify the System of Care that exists for juvenile justice youngsters in your state and community.

   ■ Conduct a literature search on System of Care issues with juvenile justice populations.

   ■ Identify the potential role of the discipline you may select as a potential profession in your future in the juvenile justice system, either in detention settings or in the community.

References

Abram, K.M., Teplin, L.A., McClelland, G.M., & Dulcan, M.K. (2003). Comorbid psychiatric disorders in youth in juvenile detention. *Archives of General Psychiatry, 60,* 1097–1108.

Abram, K.M., Teplin, L.A., Charles, D.R., Longworth, S.L., McClelland, G.M., & Dulcan, M.K. (2004). Posttraumatic stress disorder and trauma in youth in juvenile detention. *Archives of General Psychiatry, 61,*403–410.

Austin, J., Ajohnson, K.D., & Gregoriou, M. (2000). *Juveniles in adult prisons and jails: A national assessment (NCJ 182503).* Washington, DC: Bureau of Justice Assistance.

Breda, C.S. (2003). Offender ethnicity and mental health service referrals from juvenile courts. *Criminal Justice and Behavior, 30*(6), 644–667.

Bullis, I.M., Yovanoff, P., Mueller, G., & Havel, E. (2002). Life on the "outs": Examination of the facility-to-community transition of incarcerated youth. *Exceptional Children, 69,* 7–22.

Chesney-Lind, M., & Shelden, R.G. (2004). *Girls, delinquency, and juvenile justice.* Stamford, CT: Wadsworth Publishing.

Cocozza, J.J. (1992). Introduction. In J. Cocozza (Ed.), *Responding to the mental health needs of youth in the juvenile justice system* (pp. 1–6). Seattle: The National Coalition for the Mentally Ill in the Criminal Justice System.

Finkelman, A.W. (2001). *Managed care: A nursing perspective.* Upper Saddle River, NJ: Prentice Hall.

Foley, C. (2001). Academic characteristics of incarcerated youth and correctional education programs: A literature review. *Journal of Emotional and Behavioral Disorders, 9,* 248–259.

Fox, S.J. (1970). Juvenile justice reform: An historical perspective. *Stanford Law Review, 22,* 1187–1239.

Gallagher, C.A. (1999). *Juvenile offenders in residential placement, 1997: OJJDP Fact Sheet.* Washington, DC: Office of Juvenile Justice and Delinquency Prevention.

Grisso, T. (1999). Juvenile offenders and mental illness. *Psychiatry, Psychology, and Law, 6*(2), 143–151.

Grisso, T., & Underwood, L. (2003). Screening and assessing mental health and substance use disorders among youth in the juvenile justice system. *National Center for Mental Health and Juvenile Justice Research and Program Brief.*

Grisso, T., Barnum, R., Fletcher, K.E., Cauffman, E., & Peuschold, D. (2001). Massachusetts youth screening instrument for mental health needs of juvenile justice youths. *Journal of the American Academy of Child and Adolescent Psychiatry, 40*(5), 541–548.

Handron, D.S., Dosser J.R., McCammon, S.L., & Powell, J.Y. (1998). "Wraparound" the wave of the future: Theoretical and professional practice implications. *Journal of Family Nursing, 4*(1), 65–86.

Harris, P.W., Welsh, W.N., & Gutler, F. (2000). A century of juvenile justice. *The nature of crime: Continuity and change* (pp. 359–425). Washington, DC: US Department of Justice Office of Justice Programs.

Isaacs, M., & Benjamin, M. (1991). *Towards a culturally competent system of care: Vol. II: Programs which use culturally competent services.* Washington, DC: Georgetown University Child Development Center, CASSP Technical Assistance Center.

Jacobs, F.J. (1995). States' policy response to the need for case management. In B.J. Friesen & J. Poertner (Eds.), *From case management to service coordination for children with emotional, behavioral, or mental disorders: Building on family strengths* (pp. 373–400). Baltimore, MD: Paul H. Brookes Publishing.

Knitzer, J. (1982). *Unclaimed children: The failure of public responsibility to children and adolescents in need of mental health services.* Washington, DC: Children's Defense Fund.

Lyons, J.S., Griffin, G., Quintenz, S., Jenuwine, M., & Shasha, M. (2003). Clinical and forensic outcomes from the Illinois mental health juvenile justice initiative. *Psychiatric Services, 54*(12), 1629–1634.

McCrone, S., & Shelton, D. (2001). An overview of forensic psychiatric care of the adolescent. *Issues in Mental Health Nursing, 22,* 125–135.

Shelton, D. (2001). Emotional disorders in young offenders. *Journal of Nursing Scholarship, 33,* 259–263.

Sickmund, M., & Wan, Y. (1999). *Census of juveniles in residential placement datebook: Detailed offense profile by sex for United States, 1999.* Available from: http://www.ojjdp.ncjrs.org/ojstatabb/cjrp.

Siegfried, C.B., Ko, S.J., & Kelley, A. (2004). Victimization and juvenile offending. Los Angeles: National Child Traumatic Stress Network. Available from: htpp://www.NCTSNet.org.

Smith, C., & Thornberry, T.P. (1995). The relationship between childhood maltreatment and adolescent involvement in delinquency. *Criminology, 33*(4), 451–481.

Snyder, H.N. (2000). *Juvenile arrests 1999.* Washington, DC: Office of Juvenile Justice and Delinquency Prevention.

Snyder, H.N., & Sickmund, M. (1999). *Juvenile offenders and victims: 1999 National report.* Washington, DC: Office of Juvenile Justice and Delinquency Prevention.

Steiner, H., Garcia, I.G., & Mattews, Z. (1997). Posttraumatic stress disorder in incarcerated juvenile delinquents. *Journal of the American Academy of Child and Adolescent Psychiatry, 36*(3), 357–365.

Stewart, D.G., & Trupin, E.W. (2003). Clinical utility and policy implications of a statewide mental health screening process for juvenile offenders. *Psychiatric Services, 54*, 377–382.

Stroul, B.A., & Friedman, R.M. (1986). *A system of care of children and youth with severe emotional disturbances* (rev. ed.). Washington, DC: Georgetown University Child Development Center, National Technical Assistance Center for Child Mental Health.

Sutton, J.R. (1988). *Stubborn children: Controlling delinquency in the United States, 1640–1981*. Berkeley, CA: University of California Press.

Teplin, L.A., Abram, K.M., McClelland, G.M., Dulcan, M.K., & Mericle, A.A. (2002). Psychiatric disorders in youth in juvenile detention. *Archives of General Psychiatry, 59*, 1133–1143.

US Department of Justice (2001). *Sourcebook of criminal justice statistics 2001.* Available from: htpp://www.albany.edu/sourcebook.

Wasserman, G.A., McReynolds, L.S., Lucas, C.P., Fisher, P., & Santos, L. (2002). The voice DISC-IV with incarcerated male youths: Prevalence of disorder. *Journal of the American Academy of Child and Adolescent Psychiatry, 41*, 314–321.

Widom, C.S. (1995). Victims of childhood sexual abuse: Later criminal consequences. *National Institute of Justice: Research in brief.* Washington, DC: US Department of Justice, Office of Justice Programs.

Wolford, B. (2000). Youth education in the juvenile justice system. *Corrections Today, 62*, 128–130.

Wood, J., Foyh, D., Goguen, C., Pynoos, R., & Jamese, C. B. (2002). Violence exposure and posttraumatic stress disorder among delinquent girls. *Journal of Aggression, Maltreatment and Trauma, 6*(1), 109–126.

Chapter 11

Healthy Lifestyles
Through Inclusive Recreation

STUART J. SCHLEIEN, KIMBERLY D. MILLER,
PAULA BROOKE, AND GREY COCKERHAM

Objectives

- Define the values and principles of therapeutic recreation practice and their relationship to System of Care.
- Describe the advantages of an inclusive versus segregated model of therapeutic recreation service delivery.
- Understand the importance of collaborative therapeutic recreation programming that includes practitioners, family members, advocates, and friends.
- Apply the six-component process of inclusive volunteering to support successful volunteering as a leisure activity.
- Recognize the myriad of benefits that are accrued by individuals of varying abilities when they participate in inclusive community recreation/leisure activities within typical settings.

Recreation/leisure is one aspect of service delivery that has the potential to make significant contributions in the lives of individuals with disabilities and their family members. The US Department of

Health and Human Services has recommended that recreation efforts and services address the myriad of needs of individuals of varying abilities and that they be provided in a variety of settings, including community recreation agencies (Groff, Spencer, & McCammon, 2004; Park et al., 2001). Others have challenged the service delivery system to devise strategies that successfully include and engage people with disabilities in normative recreational activities. A critical component of these interventions is the preparation of group leaders, individuals with disabilities, and their caregivers, as well as individuals without disabilities and their caregivers (Marcenko, Keller, & Delaney, 2001).

When identifying key components of the System of Care for children and adolescents with severe emotional disabilities, recreational services, including relationships with significant others, and participation in after-school programs, summer camps, and special recreational projects, have been noted (Epstein, Kutashik, & Duchnowski 1998; Stroul & Friedman, 1994). In recognition that a majority of services received by individuals with disabilities are delivered in educational and/or vocational settings. Groff et al. (2004) reported that a president of the National Recreational Park Association called for inclusion and more diversity in recreation and parks, not as an annual goal, but rather as an ongoing initiative requiring education, involvement, and commitment (Donahue, 2004). As we learn about more effective variations on these practices, these authors no longer promote models but processes that must be individualized and community specific (VanDenBerg & Grealish, 1996).

Within the last two decades, human service professionals have been providing services to individuals with disabilities in community settings with greater frequency. The least restrictive environment is commonly used to describe this service emphasis. As we apply recreation/leisure and discretionary time use to the least restrictive environment doctrine, it is defined as the acquisition and performance of recreation/leisure skills by individuals with disabilities in typical and the most normative community environments and situations. The use of the adjectives *typical* and *normalized* is critical because many human service professionals provide programs not in the community, but in segregated, restrictive, and contrived settings. Also, a common mistake within these segregated settings is the provision of services on behalf of individuals with disabilities that do not take into account peoples' interests, strengths, and chronological ages.

Therapeutic recreation preference has been shifting from providing specialized and separate recreation/leisure services to include people with disabilities in already existing community programs and activities.

We strongly believe that community activities within which people with disabilities participate should not be different or separated from the activities and settings that community members without disabilities access on a regular basis. How people spend their discretionary time and the settings to which they have access should not be decisions based on their labels and diagnoses.

These trends indicate that several underlying principles be incorporated in every process guiding the development of inclusive recreation services and leisure participation.

- Recreation activities and programs designed for people with disabilities must be suitable to one's chronological age and based on an individual's strengths and personal interests and not on one's diagnosis or label.
- Programs preparing people for inclusive recreation participation must occur within their home communities and must not be in restrictive, highly contrived, or irrelevant environments.
- Communication and coordination among participants, family members, friends, and recreation professionals must occur if inclusive services are to be initiated, successful, and sustainable.
- Participants with and without disabilities, their family members, advocates, and recreation practitioners must take a shared-responsibility approach to ensure that every community member's leisure and social needs and interests are being met, including the needs of entire families.

The entire community benefits from including people with disabilities in typical recreation activities and programs. Through exposure to and ongoing interaction with people with disabilities, individuals without disabilities gain knowledge about and become more sensitive to individual differences, develop more accepting attitudes, feel better about themselves, and broaden their own opportunities for friendship.

The purpose of this chapter is to describe and illustrate best practices of the therapeutic recreation discipline that are consistent with the values and principles of System of Care. It is only when programmers conduct careful assessments of the strengths and personal interests of participants and then use this information to help individuals select appropriate recreation/leisure activities and settings that individuals with disabilities become active, socially connected, and viable members within their communities. In addition to strengths-based and personal interests-based assessments, it is essential that the recreational and social environments be carefully prepared or engineered so that all of the participants, with and without disabilities, can be successful to the greatest extent possible. Neither the assessment nor the environmental engineering processes are possible without the coordination and full participation of family members, advocates, and friends. Social inclusion in the community results only when individuals are engaged as active participants in activities with the provision of necessary advocacy, supports, and coordination.

After a review of best practices in therapeutic recreation, an inclusive volunteering program will be described. This program will help to illustrate the principles and practices used to facilitate active and healthy leisure lifestyles. An inclusive volunteering process is depicted and illustrated by two case studies describing individuals constructively using their free time as volunteers in their respective communities. The leisure experiences of two volunteers—one youth and one adult and each with a disability—are described to highlight inclusive practices and outcomes obtained by both volunteers and agencies.

Therapeutic Recreation and the System of Care

Principle 1: Recreation activities and programs designed for people with disabilities must be suitable to one's chronological age and based on an individual's strengths and personal interests, and not on one's diagnosis or label.

The acquisition of and engagement in recreation/leisure that is (1) functional (i.e., naturally occurring, frequently demanded, and has a specific purpose), (2) age appropriate and personally preferred (i.e., activities typically performed by persons in the same age group and chosen autonomously), and (3) referenced by their peers' recreation/leisure present powerful tools to include individuals with disabilities in typical community environments. The selection of skills and activities should reflect this potential benefit, in that only those skills or activities that can be performed in interaction with their peers without disabilities should be encouraged and supported. Anything short of this goal will do little to mitigate the (unnecessary) segregation and sheltering of individuals with disabilities.

Principle 2: Programs preparing people for inclusive recreation participation must occur within their home communities and not in restrictive, highly contrived, or irrelevant environments.

Although the normalization principle and social value concept have been guiding forces behind efforts to include people with disabilities, adherence to this philosophy does not guarantee that people with disabilities who live in the community will be less socially isolated than if they were living in less natural, more restrictive environments. Providing opportunities for people with disabilities to live in neighborhoods alongside residents without disabilities, to work, or to go to neighborhood schools is consistent with normalization, but such opportunities alone do not ensure that social inclusion will occur. Too often, people with disabilities who reside in communities have minimal social contact with people without disabilities in their neighborhoods (Hayden, Lakin, Hill, Bruininks, & Copher, 1992). Also, people with disabilities generally spend much less time working, playing, and living in community environments and may actually decrease their involvement in community activities over time (Hayden, Soulen, Schleien, & Tabourne, 1996).

Socially valued services have been gaining momentum throughout the past two decades, and inclusive community recreation programming has been emerging. This period also saw the beginning of empirical research to develop best practices that promote more welcoming and accommodating recreation and sports services. With the development of new instructional strategies, innovative research is demonstrating that people of varying abilities can acquire age-appropriate leisure, physical activity, and social skills in inclusive community environments. Leisure skills instruction and participation in inclusive settings have been found to promote social interaction between participants with and without disabilities, encourage positive attitudes, and facilitate friendships (Anderson & Kress, 2003; Schleien, Ray, & Green, 1997).

The extent of social inclusion in a community may be measured by how people with disabilities are viewed by their peers who do not have disabilities, physical proximity during an activity, and how much they participate in the same kinds of activities and social interactions as their peers without disabilities (Green, Schleien, Mactavish, & Benepe, 1995). True social inclusion is achieved when friendly and ongoing interactions take place between community residents of varying abilities.

Principle 3: Communication and coordination among participants, family members, friends, and recreation professionals must occur if inclusive services are to be initiated, successful, and sustainable.

It is believed that community recreation agencies and other leisure service providers, along with family members, are mostly responsible for the continued proliferation of segregated recreation programs and limited access to opportunities for social inclusion. Recreation providers continue to offer segregated programs because this type of programming has been the accepted way of delivering services over the years. These methods and models are likely viewed as the norm among our community agencies and citizens. Previous surveys showed that many practitioners and consumers believe that it is the responsibility of special advocacy associations and organizations (e.g., Arc, formerly known as the Association for Retarded Citizens) to serve people with disabilities. Others attribute the failure to offer inclusive services to a scarcity of requests for such programs by consumers with disabilities and their families, and for still others, the barrier to developing and implementing inclusive programs is the inefficiency of agency staff who have had little to no experience working with people with disabilities (Schleien et al., 1997).

The reluctance of program staff to share responsibility for including and engaging individuals with disabilities can be understood because of the overreliance placed on trained specialists, such as special education teachers and therapeutic recreation specialists. It is recommended that therapeutic recreation specialists, general recreation professionals, and family members attempt to erase the mystique surrounding people with disabilities by de-emphasizing their need for special programs and facilities and encouraging the use of general services and providers. Together, through communication on a regular basis, those professionals and care providers can figure out what adjustments need to be made to an already existing program to make it more manageable, effective, and successful. When we use the voices and expertise of many key players, including those of individuals with disabilities, family members, advocates, and friends, our services and programs will become more responsive, welcoming, and inclusive. Meaningful collaboration and dialogue are the foundation on which inclusive recreation will be built.

The responsibility for failing to have a truly inclusive community must also be shared by people with disabilities and their family members. Several studies have shown that people with disabilities generally do not choose to use community programs or to be active members of their communities. The professional literature also lists a variety of issues that hinder the inclusion of people with disabilities in community leisure services, including: voluntary service organizations that provide separate and segregated programs are hesitant to relinquish their participants to agencies that had previously ignored them; parents of children without disabilities may oppose inclusive programs; people with disabilities and their parents or care providers do not communicate their desires for general programs to the right people; people with disabilities may fail to participate in general programs for a variety of reasons, such as not believing that the community agency has the appropriate expertise to serve them adequately; and recreation practitioners who previously had been led to believe that they did not possess the expertise to work effectively with people with disabilities may question their abilities to conduct inclusive programs and accommodate people in their existing agencies.

Principle 4: Participants with and without disabilities, their family members, advocates, and recreation practitioners must take a shared-responsibility approach to ensure that all community members' leisure and social needs and interests are being met, including the needs of entire families.

If the goal of fully inclusive recreation services is to be realized, programs must not only be readily available, but also accessible and welcoming to individual participants and their families. The involvement of individuals with disabilities in community recreation activities is largely contingent on family support (Schleien, Green, & Heyne, 1993). Mactavish and Schleien (2004) conducted an investigation to address the issue of the recreation participation of families that include members with disabilities. Parents were asked questions about the impact of family recreation in their lives and the impact on their children both with and without disabilities. Parents spoke at length about the many benefits of family recreation, and the most popular conclusion was that it was a "way of re-establishing what is important in life." However, many parents noted that shared family experiences were limited when their children's abilities varied significantly. One recurring constraint was the receipt of ambiguous or unwelcoming messages from recreation service providers. When asked to identify social services that were most important to children with severe emotional disturbance and their families, recreational and after-school activities were rated the highest priority (94%) by the respondents. Ninety percent of the respondents identified the summer camping experience as a necessary opportunity for their children (Marcenko et al., 2001).

Families are fundamentally important to their children's recreation experiences. In a sense, they are the first recreation service providers that include and involve their children in the community. Families serve as "gatekeepers" to the recreation and social experiences of their children. Also, families are the primary recipients of a family-centered approach to services. Therefore, it appears logical that the onus should be on recreation service providers to involve entire families in the planning of activities, as this should increase the likelihood that any decisions are acceptable to the participants and their family members

(Bailey, McWilliam, & Winton, 1992). Parents and other family members are invaluable sources of knowledge and creativity. They know their children's needs and abilities and have the skills and resources to make things happen. One parent said, "I always laugh when they (service providers) talk about 'adaptive recreation' and the like, being sort of a new idea or at least something that you people (practitioners) are into these days. . . . We've been adapting and integrating within our own family for years now."

Parents have a responsibility as their children's advocates to collaborate with recreation/leisure service providers. They can share their goals and concerns with agency staff. They can be involved with the identification of their children's needs and preferences and help design necessary modifications to equipment, programs, and environments. Parents have formed and served on advisory boards as a vehicle to provide honest and immediate feedback to agency administrators and program staff. Through this kind of advocacy and with a family-centered rather than a child-focused approach, parents can ensure the sustainability of successful inclusive recreation options. Understanding families and their recreation needs and interests is the key to building bridges between family and community recreation options.

Volunteering as a Recreational Activity

Partnership F.I.V.E. (Fostering Inclusive Volunteer Efforts) is a program that fosters inclusive volunteer efforts to ensure that individuals with disabilities are recognized as valuable assets to their community and afforded their right to full community involvement (http://www.uncg.edu/rpt/five). Inclusive volunteering is defined as volunteer opportunities that allow individuals with and without disabilities to work together to improve their community through voluntary service.

Partnership F.I.V.E. uses the following "6-component process to inclusive volunteering," which is consistent with the principles of System of Care:

1. *Recruitment and preparation:* Individuals with disabilities, family members, care providers, volunteer coordinators, volunteer partners (those without disabilities), and nonprofit agency staff are recruited and prepared for inclusive volunteering. Many individuals with disabilities, most often viewed as the recipients of services instead of the givers of volunteer services, have simply not been asked to volunteer in their communities in the past and may have limited knowledge on what it means to be a volunteer.

Depending on their current level of knowledge regarding volunteering (e.g., what it is, why people volunteer, what they do, how they can benefit from volunteering, responsibilities of being a volunteer), individuals with disabilities may need to be educated on the subject. Once individuals with disabilities are provided information regarding volunteering, they are then offered the opportunity to express interest in participating, and often, this is the first time that they have been asked to volunteer. Parents and care providers are provided with information on why they should support inclusive volunteering and how best to provide support in these endeavors. Volunteer coordinators and other nonprofit agency staff are provided with training on how to engage volunteers of varying abilities successfully. Individuals without disabilities that may volunteer side by side with those with disabilities who are recruited and prepared to support their partners in their volunteer roles.

2. *Assessment:* Individuals with disabilities are assessed for preferences, abilities, and needed supports. It is crucial that volunteers are performing volunteer tasks that interest them and match their skill and age levels appropriately in order to experience volunteering as a recreational or leisure activity. In some instances, an individual's recreation interests can be converted into a volunteer opportunity. For example, someone who enjoys sewing can make baby blankets for newborns who are born to drug-addicted mothers. An individual who likes to sing can perform for residents of a skilled nursing unit. Someone who enjoys watching plays can distribute programs or take tickets at a community theater and possibly enjoy the show afterward. Information on an individual's interests should be gathered from not only the potential volunteer, but also from other individuals involved in their quality of life (e.g., family members, teachers, advocates, friends).

3. *Matching:* Based on the preferences and abilities identified in the assessment, individuals are matched with volunteer tasks that meet community needs. Many communities have volunteer centers, sometimes independent of and other times part of the United Way, whose mission is to mobilize resources to meet community needs. They often have a listing of volunteer opportunities and community needs that can be accessed so that a viable match can be made for the individual placement. Other possible resources for identifying volunteer opportunities include the United Way 2-1-1 system, the local professional association of volunteer

administrators, newspaper listings, and online sites such as Volunteer Match (http://www.volunteermatch.org) and Network for Good (http://www.networkforgood.org). If the individual has very specific or unique interests or skills, nonprofit agencies that may be able to that ability are contacted directly. When individuals are very direct about their abilities and how they may be engaged in a positive manner, volunteer coordinators tend to be much more receptive in comparison to when volunteer coordinators are expected to assess individuals' interests independently and match them to their current volunteer roles.

4. *Building supports:* Necessary supports for a successful volunteer experience are identified and implemented. Emphasis is placed on ensuring these supports are as natural and nonintrusive as possible so as not to interfere with opportunities for volunteers to develop social connections or call attention to their limitations. These supports may take many shapes and forms, including adaptations of equipment and/or tasks, alternative training formats, transportation strategies, and identification of a mentor or peer partner, just to name a few. For example:

- A volunteer who needs prompts to remind her of what she is to do next is given a card with pictures representing the series of tasks she is to complete. The card is small enough and laminated in order for the volunteer to easily slide the card out of sight once she identifies her next task.

- A volunteer in a children's museum who has difficulty dealing with unavoidable down time between visitors is matched with a peer partner. Together, they serve the museum guests, but during down time between guests, they play a game of cards.

- A volunteer who can read but struggles with the spatial order of the alphabet is provided with an alphabet card in order to shelve books in the library. She loves books and enjoys exploring the books as she puts them away. Again, the alphabet card is small and durable so that it is unobtrusive.

- A volunteer who uses a motorized wheelchair controlled by head movements, has his legs and arms strapped down to control spasticity, and has limited verbal articulation abilities wishes to participate with volunteers raking leaves of older adults' yards. A rake is taped to the individual's wheelchair so that the rake will drag behind him while he moves across the yard, pulling leaves with it. The rake is taped to his wheelchair in such a manner that he can push down on the end of the handle to lift the rake blades sufficiently above the grass blades to release the trapped leaves and then reposition his chair for the next pull. This simple solution is chosen over a highly technical, complicated, and expensive piece of adaptive equipment so that the activity remains as typical as possible among his peers without disabilities.

5. *Communication:* Communication is facilitated and maintained between the volunteer, volunteer partner (if applicable), volunteer coordinator, family members, and other professionals (e.g., teacher and case manager). A volunteer may not know how to discuss with the volunteer coordinator her dissatisfaction with a peer partner or that she has outgrown or tired of her current volunteer role. A family member may observe that the individual appears agitated during or after volunteering, which may signify that a change in volunteer task or environment is warranted. A volunteer coordinator may have to discuss the need for a change in behavior (e.g., personal hygiene) with the volunteer and may need assistance in doing so. Communication is essential so that these issues can be resolved before becoming problematic, and it must include all individuals involved in the volunteer's life.

6. *Evaluation:* Feedback is gathered from all key players to determine whether alterations to the volunteer experience should be made. Factors that are assessed include the following: Is the volunteer enjoying his or her placement (because this is a leisure pursuit), establishing social connections or making new friends, feeling valued, and learning new skills? Are family members feeling pleased with the volunteer experience? Does the volunteer coordinator believe that the volunteer is an asset to the agency? Is the agency staff feeling comfortable working with the volunteer? Is the volunteer partner feeling valued and comfortable? Adjustments to the volunteer experience are made accordingly to ensure a positive recreational experience.

Case Study: Trey's Story

Trey is an intelligent and active 14-year-old. He lives with his mother, father, and older sister (Figure 11-1). Both parents are employed full-time, but as a youth minister, his father has flexibility in his work schedule.

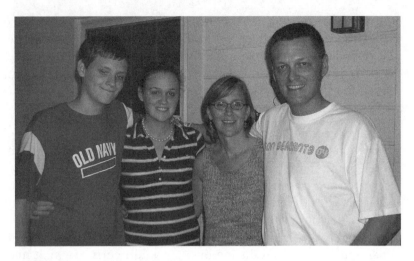

FIGURE 11-1 Trey and his family

Trey has been attending a private school for the past few years, and his parents have been very happy with his success there. With teachers, parents, and students working hand in hand at school, he receives the support that is necessary to be educated in the mainstream, despite having Asperger's syndrome, or autistic psychopathy, which is a pervasive developmental disorder that is characterized by severe and sustained impairment in social interactions and the development of restricted and repetitive patterns of behavior, interests, and activities. These characteristics result in significant impairments in social, occupational, or other important areas of functioning (ERIC Clearinghouse on Disabilities and Gifted Education, 2002).

Trey's love of movies and music brings his conversation to life. He readily remembers scenes and even script parts from many of the latest films that he has seen, and he considers one of his strengths to be his ability to "voice act" or perform voice imitations. He also enjoys video games, reading, walking, and playing golf. His attention to detail, easygoing attitude, and inquisitiveness are also identified as strengths.

His carefree and upfront conversation with adults should not cause one to believe he has a completely functional social life. Among peers, Trey struggles. He has been teased by peers to the point that he often avoids interacting with them. In addition, Trey has difficulty with boredom, sometimes becomes overfocused, and easily becomes frustrated when his attention is being requested from more than one direction. Conflicting requests of Trey's time and attention cause the greatest difficulty as he struggles to prioritize where to place his attention.

With summer quickly approaching, Trey and his parents searched for something to enable Trey to have a productive, yet enjoyable, summer. Many of Trey's peers would be spending their time volunteering. Although Trey had successfully volunteered with his family and with church groups in the past, he had never even thought of volunteering independently. His parents were unsure of how to begin a search for a volunteer position, especially one in which they could approach a volunteer coordinator concerning Trey's unique learning style, behaviors, and social needs. They learned of Partnership F.I.V.E. from a friend and made contact to see what options for volunteering Trey may have.

A trainer advocate from Partnership F.I.V.E. met with Trey and his parents (and his dog). Trey's strengths, interests, and preferences were discussed, along with his needed supports for success. When discussing various volunteer roles that were available in the community, Trey displayed an immediate positive reaction to those relating to animals. He quickly identified his responsibility for the family pet, a golden retriever named Van.

Trey chose two potential volunteer roles. The first role was with a natural science museum that had a petting barn, a herpetology laboratory, and a sea creature laboratory. The volunteer role would be to handle the small animals so that visitors could interact with the animals in a safe manner and to educate the visitors about the animals and their ecologic role and survival needs.

The second volunteer role was to assist staff at a therapeutic horseback riding facility with the cleanliness and maintenance of the facility and horses. Trey had actually been served by this agency when he was 7 years old, and thus, he was aware of the impact that this agency was having on individuals with disabilities in his community.

The Partnership F.I.V.E. trainer advocate knew that many teens volunteered at both of these agencies, especially during the summer months, and thus, both would be age-appropriate. The trainer advocate contacted both volunteer coordinators. She presented the assets that Trey could bring to their respective agencies, supports necessary for success, and how those supports could be provided. A meeting was scheduled so that Trey could visit both places, meet with the volunteer coordinators, and decide where he wished to volunteer. His mother and the trainer advocate accompanied him on these visits.

The choice was easy for Trey. He would do both. He decided to volunteer at the natural science museum for 4 hours each Saturday and at the therapeutic riding center 2 days per week for 3 to 4 hours each time. Because of the flexibility in his father's work schedule, Trey would have transportation to both sites, and his father would be able to communicate (if necessary) with the volunteer coordinators between the time Trey was dropped off and picked up.

At the natural science museum, the volunteer coordinator initially assigned Trey to work with a fellow adult volunteer as a mentor. This would enable Trey to learn about the responsibilities of his volunteer position at his own pace and in the presence of an adult, where he was most comfortable. After several sessions with the adult mentor, Trey was paired with a peer mentor, also a teen volunteer, to continue his training. The peer mentor was asked to be ready to step in for assistance if more than one person was demanding Trey's attention or requesting to see more than one animal at a time. With visitors coming and going and asking to see different animals, Trey rarely got bored or had the time to focus too intently on any one task.

At the therapeutic riding center, the trainer advocate from Partnership F.I.V.E. was Trey's adult mentor, accompanying him during his first few weeks. The agency's volunteer coordinator provided Trey with a list of tasks to complete each day. The list was prioritized for Trey so that he could focus on one task at a time. Having the "to-do" list also prevented Trey from becoming intensely focused on any one task, as he had a daily goal to complete the entire list of tasks before leaving. In addition, the trainer advocate assisted Trey with establishing a routine for each of the commonly assigned tasks (Figure 11-2).

While accompanying Trey, the trainer advocate identified another teen volunteer that Trey could connect with socially. The volunteer coordinator agreed that this other teen volunteer would have "empathy but not sympathy" for Trey and would possibly make for a good partner. The teen volunteer agreed to work in close proximity to Trey. In other words, they would both be working on different volunteer tasks but be near each other. For example, while Trey was sweeping the tack room, the fellow teen volunteer would be cleaning the tack. Trey now had someone with whom to share his love of movies and music and to entertain with his voice impersonations.

Trey's mother stated that she could count on one hand the number of experiences in which Trey had been so happy. "We are so encouraged by his success this summer. It gives us hope and helps us as we continue to plan for his future. We are so proud of his will-

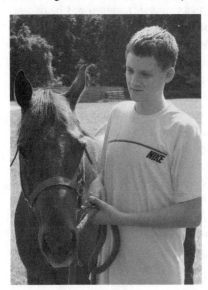

FIGURE 11-2   Trey volunteering

ingness to help others and the dedication and responsibility he has shown in both areas."

Success for Trey in these leisure experiences is directly linked to two key factors: First, the emphasis that is placed on his strengths and personal interests, and second, the communication is established and maintained between Trey, his family, volunteer coordinators, peer and adult volunteers, and trainer advocates so that appropriate accommodations and supports could be established and modified as needed.

Case Study: Grey's Story

Grey Cockerham, born and raised in Greensboro, North Carolina, a city of 300,000, is an assertive advocate and valued community volunteer. He attributes his personal growth to his varied and rich support network and leisure participation in the community. Two years before his 41st birthday, he became involved with Partnership F.I.V.E. through the local Arc.

When describing his disability, Grey says he is a slow learner (professionally diagnosed with mental retardation) and acknowledges taking medication to remedy attention deficit disorder, anxiety, depression, and high blood pressure. He graduated from a segregated special education high school at the required graduation age of 21 years. Reflecting on his education, he does not feel he would have done well in a mainstream high school, as he thinks other students would have made fun of him. He lives with his mom and feels closer to her than his two brothers and sister, although he and his siblings see each other occasionally. Grey disliked the 4-year period of his life when he was subjected to placement in the sheltered workshop for little pay. Neither Grey nor his support network thought they had a say in the matter, especially because other employers told him that they could not hire him because he was mentally retarded.

Many years later, American society was finally beginning to treat individuals with disabilities more like true American citizens. Grey's network of support expanded in both size and power. For Grey, the increased advocating, assertiveness, and inclusion have led to many life enhancements. The following case study focuses on the positive developments credited to his leisure lifestyle.

Grey offered to serve as a Partnership F.I.V.E. representative and has consequently volunteered to co-present at several conferences, participate in a college course, work alongside high school students with disabilities on long-term municipal parks and recreation inclusive volunteer projects, and engage in many inclusive community volunteer events.

Grey's strengths run the full gamut—from gardening and designing flower arrangements to organizing parties and making others feel good about themselves (Figure 11-3). Because of a strong network of support, Grey's abilities have not gone untapped. His involvements have increased dramatically because community programs such as Partnership F.I.V.E. have embraced the concept of inclusion and recognized individuals with disabilities as contributors to society.

Much credit is due to Grey for seizing the opportunities that the community offered. His home town is the beneficiary of Grey's active participation, and the result is the initiation of a positive cycle. Grey has gained self-assurance, and this newfound confidence has enabled him to seek activities that develop additional skills and enhance existing abilities. For example, Grey is an extrovert and enjoys social interactions. A couple of years ago he would not have dreamed of having the courage to stand in front of a room full of professionals to inform them about his community experiences and how he has used his interests and strengths to become a valuable volunteer. During the presentation, he spoke to a love of gardening and creating flower arrangements and how that led to a unique volunteer role. A nonprofit agency recognized Grey's talent and requested his expertise in the arrangement of flower centerpieces for fundraising events.

Not only has he educated hundreds of people about the matching process integral to successful volunteering, he has captured the hearts of many attendees. A majority of the session evaluations exclaimed praises, including the following: "Grey did a wonderful job." "I was inspired by this presentation." ". . . discussed material that will be helpful for me to utilize in the future." "Having him present made this the best presentation of the entire conference!" The feasibility of this feat can be attributed to both Grey's determination and a good deal of coaching and support from his advocates. Now he is discovering conferences to which the Partnership F.I.V.E. team submits proposals.

The director of Partnership F.I.V.E. (and senior author of this chapter) and Grey have developed a strong relationship, and the close friendship has extensive benefits for each party. Dr. Schleien is a

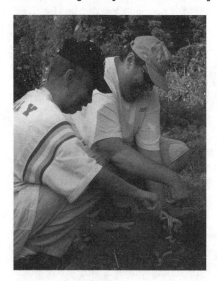

FIGURE 11-3 Grey volunteering at a community garden

source of support vital to Grey's goal setting and goal achieving; age-appropriate goals are imperative to life so that a person has a real sense of belonging to the community (Figure 11-4).

Grey has received a variety of Arc services over the years. Six years ago, his job coach assisted him in obtaining an employment position with dining services at the local university. Employment has been a prominent aspect of Grey's "normalization" and has increased his independence level significantly. Grey has not yet learned to drive a car, although it is now on his list of attainable goals, along with living in his own apartment. Currently, his mother provides much of his transportation, as well as his abode, and she supports Grey in all of his autonomous endeavors.

Another instrumental player in Grey's inclusive volunteering success has been his church. His friend proclaimed that his church has "always rallied around him," probably partly because "everyone loves Grey." Grey attends computer skills classes and Sunday school and has learned a lot from the volunteer-run church programs in which he participates.

The Arc facilitated a program called "Partners" (akin to Big Brothers/Big Sisters), whereupon a volunteer and a member of the Arc become "partners" and participate in community recreation events together. Grey and his partner hit it off and are great friends to this day, three years later, even though the program had to cease because of a lack of funding shortly after their connection. They often join forces to volunteer as part of their shared leisure repertoire.

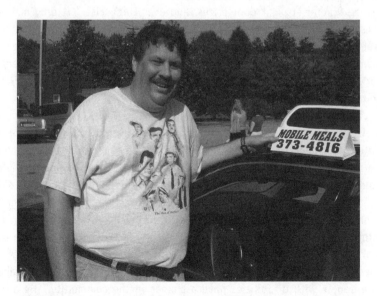

FIGURE 11-4   Grey volunteering with Mobile Meals

The executive director of the local Arc is a close friend of Grey's, and her "life is better because he's been in it." Over the years, she has seen a transformation in Grey and feels that it is attributed to his own conviction to be the best person he can be, living the life that he really wants to live. With a sibling-close friendship, she speaks to his difficult start in life growing up as an individual with mental retardation in an unaccepting environment. The positive input from Grey's natural system of care has made activities such as his membership to a self-advocacy group possible. She stated that for as long as she has known him he has been striving for a normal life, and fortunately, his support system facilitated his inclusion into society. Consequently, society has received an upstanding citizen by the name of Grey Cockerham.

The executive director of the Arc founded a recreational club for individuals with disabilities. Grey was right there with her and became an active Sunshine Club member, as it enabled him to attend social events with his peers. Over the years, his role evolved from being a program participant to becoming a spokesperson, leader, advocate, and role model for other club members. Grey still gets to enjoy being a "social butterfly" but understands the importance of simultaneously giving and providing others with support so that they, too, can become leaders. Grey's system of care strives for the development of his confidence and his empowerment, as they are elements essential to his proven positive outcomes.

Grey states that he feels accepted in his community: "I have been living in this town all my life. It is my hometown forever." He is the co-chair for his neighborhood watch and says, "I'm the co-chair person; I help organize fundraisers, get door prizes, and everything else." It only makes sense that his leisure activities take place within his community, and he feels "lucky that we have so much of an opportunity to volunteer here in town." The entire community shares the responsibility of including everybody in the mission of meeting their age-appropriate recreation needs in a normalized, accepted, and positive way.

It is apparent the Arc has played a key role in Grey's life, as he has in theirs. He volunteers for all of their fundraising events because he appreciates their services: "Two years ago the Arc . . . asked me to be on the Good Morning show in front of about 1,000 people (to promote one of their fundraisers); so I had to get up at 5 o'clock in the morning, and they did a live interview with me." Partnership F.I.V.E. rolled the news clip during a conference presentation, and Grey gave a disclaimer to his starring role; he informed the audience that it was far too early in the morning for him to look his best. Everyone agreed he did a great job. "I did it 'cause the Arc does so much for people with disabilities. They go out of their way to make sure people with disabilities have a chance in the community." He also made an impressive appearance on the local university's television station, as he relayed to viewers the message that Partnership F.I.V.E.'s actions are facilitating a necessary societal change.

None of Grey's actions stand alone. Imperative links exist between those most involved in his life to ensure his maturity into a productive and content adult who has real meaning in his life. These connections are open communication avenues in which these key players all manage to coordinate their participation in Grey's life. Each member of an individual's system of care should strive to understand much of what is going on in the individual's life, simply because only then can each member best meet the individual's current needs.

Grey had been the benefactor/recipient of services for many years. Through support from family, the Arc, Partnership F.I.V.E., friends, church, employer, and opportunities to become an integral member in the community, he has become increasingly self-confident. "It has made me feel a lot stronger in the community, which I think everybody, if they get a chance, I think everybody should volunteer." He advocates, recreates, and contributes, and successfully lives life as a person with a disability in a community among individuals with and without disabilities. Because of the supporting nature of Grey's community, he is now in the position to offer services to others to make the community a better place and to empower other individuals with disabilities to become valuable members of society.

Summary

What everyone should understand is that success stories such as Trey's and Grey's should be common, not exemplary, and that the community should not help individuals with disabilities *exist*. Instead, it should empower them to really *live*. It is up to individuals with disabilities and system of care key players to create these win–win situations.

Every individual has the ability and right to recreate, as a healthy leisure lifestyle is a necessary ingredient for a full and meaningful life. People deserve to be happy and engaged. If you did not have activities and friends to look forward to, would you really continue to go through the motions day in and day out? Probably not!

In this fast-paced age, few people take a moment to "stop and smell the roses." The discipline of therapeutic recreation is so important because it reminds and helps people to participate in meaningful activities they enjoy. Can you picture yourself as an older adult regretting not finishing that last stack of paperwork in lieu of witnessing your daughter's very first home run or dance recital?

Therapeutic recreation goes much deeper than simply facilitating enjoyment—it can be very beneficial and has a unique ability to address both functional and substantive goals. When the outcomes are functional, one can assume that the goals address improvements akin to the following: increasing physical fitness levels, decreasing depression, and enhancing memory (physical and mental abilities). The substantive goals, such as raising self-esteem, making friends, and gaining a sense of belonging and purpose, are reasons to get up in the morning. All goals aim to improve the participant's quality of life.

The mediums capable of meeting such goals for persons of all abilities are inclusive recreation and sports services and leisure participation. The healthiest leisure lifestyle adheres to system of care values and principles. If one's leisure is based on individual preferences, is age appropriate, occurs in the natural community environment, and actively involves his or her entire support network, then one's leisure can meet its full potential and provide endless benefits.

It is not difficult to incorporate system of care principles into recreation and sports services, as proven by the inclusive volunteering program examples. A client-centered approach is the foundation of the Partnership F.I.V.E. program, and this has led to the development of the "6-component process to inclusive volunteering." For both Trey and Grey, suitable volunteer matches were made possible via their preferences, strengths, and support assessments. The necessary supports were examined throughout their case studies, along with the essential communication, systematic evaluations, and programmatic adjustments. Most importantly, Trey and Grey have taught us that their own efforts must be united with the coordinated efforts of system of care key players to ensure success. The outcomes speak for themselves.

In order for individuals of varying abilities to participate successfully in recreational and physical activities, the community must provide a cohesive, supportive, and welcoming environment. Everyone needs to play and remain active and engaged!

Activities to Extend Your Learning

■ Think of someone close to you who never has time to do anything for him or herself. Now, as a member of that individual's support network, what could you do to assist that individual achieve a healthy leisure lifestyle?

■ As a professional and advocate, you want to include a child with autism and severe behavioral problems into a community recreation program. You arrange a meeting with the center director. The director listens carefully to your suggestion but rejects your idea, arguing that the center's programs are not designed to serve children "like that." She suggests that you take your idea to a recreation center designed specifically for "these types of kids." Describe and justify the steps that you would take to gain access to the generic community recreation program for this child.

■ Ask people that you know who volunteer why they do so (i.e., what motivates them) and what they get out of being a volunteer (i.e., the outcomes). Based on these conversations, outline how these motives and outcomes make volunteering an important leisure activity. Of the outcomes that you outline, identify those that are of particular relevance to individuals served through system of care services and your rationale for their relevance.

■ Refer back to this chapter's case study addressing Trey's volunteering. What were the system of care principles used in successfully connecting Trey with volunteer opportunities during his leisure time?

The development and dissemination of this chapter was partially supported by Cooperative Agreement No. H128J020074 funded by the Rehabilitative Services Administration, US Department of Education. The content and opinions expressed herein do not necessarily reflect the position or policy of the US Department of Education, and no official endorsement should be inferred.

References

Anderson, L., & Kress, C. (2003). *Inclusion: Including people with disabilities in parks and recreation opportunities.* State College, PA: Venture.

Bailey, D., McWilliam, P., & Winton, P. (1992). Building family-centered practices in early intervention: A team-based model for change. *Infants and Young Children, 5*(1), 73–82.

Donahue, J. (2004). Diversity and inclusion in parks and recreation. *Parks and Recreation, 39*(5), 2.

Epstein, M., Kutashik, K., & Duchnowski, A. (1998). *Outcomes for children and youth with emotional and behavioral disorders and their families.* Austin, TX: Pro-Ed.

ERIC Clearinghouse on Disabilities and Gifted Education. (2002). *Asperger's syndrome.* Retrieved July 7, 2004, from: http://ericec.org/faq/asperger.html.

Green, F., Schleien, S., Mactavish, J., & Benepe, S. (1995). Nondisabled adults' perceptions of relationships in the early stages of arranged partnerships with peers with mental retardation. *Education and Training in Mental Retardation and Developmental Disabilities, 30,* 91–108.

Groff, D., Spencer, S., & McCammon, S. (2004). Building a system of care: Partnering with public agencies to provide recreational therapy to children with emotional and behavioral problems and their families. In M. Devine (Ed.), *Trends in therapeutic recreation: Ideas, concepts, and applications* (pp. 177–200). Ashburn, VA: National Recreation & Park Association.

Hayden, M., Lakin, K., Hill, B., Bruininks, R., & Copher, J. (1992). Social and leisure integration of people with mental retardation in foster homes and small group homes. *Education and Training in Mental Retardation, 27,* 187–198.

Hayden, M., Soulen, T., Schleien, S., & Tabourne, C. (1996). A matched, comparative study of the recreation integration of adults with mental retardation who moved into the community and those who remained at the institution. *Therapeutic Recreation Journal, 30*(1), 41–63.

Mactavish, J., & Schleien, S. (2004). Re-injecting spontaneity and balance in family life: Parents' perspectives on recreation in families that include children with developmental disability. *Journal of Intellectual Disability Research, 48,* 123–141.

Marcenko, M., Keller, T., & Delaney, M.A. (2001). Children with SED and their families in an urban public mental health system: Characteristics, needs, and expectations. *Journal of Child and Family Studies, 10*(2), 213–226.

Park, M., Macdonald, T., Ozer, E., Burg, S., Millstein, S., Brindis, C., & Irwin, C. (2001). *Investing in clinical preventive health services for adolescents.* San Francisco: University of California, San Francisco, Policy Information and Analysis Center for Middle Childhood and Adolescence, and National Adolescent Health Information Center.

Schleien, S., Green, F., & Heyne, L. (1993). Integrated community recreation. In M. Snell (Ed.), *Instruction of students with severe disabilities* (4th ed., pp. 526–555). New York: Merrill.

Schleien, S., Ray, M.T., & Green, F. (1997). *Community recreation and people with disabilities: Strategies for inclusion* (2nd ed.). Baltimore: Paul H. Brookes.

Stroul, B.A., & Friedman, R.M. (1994). *A system of care for children and youth with severe emotional disturbances.* Washington, DC: Georgetown University Child Development Center, CASSP Technical Assistance Center.

VanDenBerg, J., & Grealish, E.M. (1996). Individualized services and supports through the wraparound process: Philosophy and procedures. *Journal of Child and Family Studies, 5*(1), 7–21.

Chapter 12

Integrating System of Care Philosophy and Practices into Schools: The Perspectives of Special Education and General Education

STEPHANIE KURTTS, GERALD PONDER, AND JEWELL COOPER

Objectives

■ To describe the foundation for school-based implementation of System of Care philosophy in recent and relevant legislation and policy frameworks.
■ To examine the relationships between schools, families, and communities in implementing System of Care principles and practices.
■ To explore the ways that teachers and other educators can provide a sound and supportive educational environment for children and families with complex needs.

The mission of public education is complex. It must assure that the next generation of workers and citizens are literate, knowledgeable, and capable of the kinds of analytic and inventive thinking that sustain

America's place in the global economy. It must instill in children and youth the values and habits of mind that advance democracy and promote social justice. It must educate in a way that provides opportunity for success for an increasingly diverse population. It must meet the needs of individuals and promote their healthy intellectual, psychological, social, and emotional development.

In the past two decades, continuing efforts to accommodate and accomplish these complex missions have led education policymakers and practitioners to frame directions for schools within two broad conceptualizations: *systems thinking* and a *results orientation* (Fullan, 2002; Sparks & Hirsh, 1997). The broad purposes of these frameworks for thinking about school practice are to create ways of enhancing student engagement in school life and work and thereby to increase the likelihood of student success. The System of Care philosophy and wraparound orientation, with their emphases on collaborative, interagency, and interprofessional teams that view families as partners and act in culturally competent ways, fit into this larger context of emerging school practice.

The most notable manifestation of the results orientation is the set of accountability standards under which schools and teachers operate. Testing programs that measure student progress and provide sanctions for schools and teachers who do not meet expected standards of performance are throughout the teacher education system and school performance systems. As examples, new teachers are licensed under the standards of the Interstate New Teacher Assessment and Support Consortium or the Council for Exceptional Children, and many experienced teachers of quality aspire to certification by the National Board for Professional Teaching Standards. Schools of Education adhere to the standards of the National Council for Accreditation of Teacher Education, and all public schools and districts receiving federal money must comply with the standards of the No Child Left Behind legislation and its requirement for annual yearly progress for all populations in a school.

Systems thinking has led to continuing efforts to link productively all parts of education and other human service systems (Brabeck, Walsh, & Latta, 2003). Professional development schools (Teitel, 2003) now link university-based teacher education programs with schools and children. Community-based schools (Epstein & Salinas, 2004), full-service schools (Dryfoos, 1994), and school mental health projects (http://smhp.psych.ucla.edu) provide structures for interdisciplinary and interagency collaboration on behalf of families and children. The wraparound process has grown from the System of Care concept, a community-based approach to providing comprehensive, integrated services through interprofessional collaboration, and collaborations with families (Eber, Sugai, Smith, & Scott, 2002). Although the System of Care concept and the wraparound process are most frequently targeted for children who display severe behavioral and emotional disorders and their families, the principles and practices engendered by System of Care and wraparound provide a means for schools to link more productively with families and providers for *all* children and youth in *all* classrooms.

Legislation and Policy Foundations for Educational Services for Children with Emotional and Behavioral Disorders: Links to System of Care and Wraparound

Educational services for children with behavioral and emotional disorders have been mandated since the mid-1970s with the passage of the original legislation of Public Law 94-142. This legislation established six principles that continue to provide the foundation for educational services to students with disabilities: (1) zero rejection of children with disabilities from school, (2) appropriate educational services to meet the student's individual educational needs, (3) procedural due process, (4) parental involvement, (5) least restrictive environment, and (6) nondiscriminatory evaluation (Turnbull, Turnbull, Shank, & Leal, 1999).

Even with these principles supporting the last three decades of policy and legislation, children with emotional and behavioral disorders have not fared well in the public schools (Eber et al., 2002). Historically, these students have experienced disproportionately higher dropout rates and academic failure than their peers without disabilities and students with other less disruptive disabilities. They also have a greater likelihood of being arrested, living in poverty, being unemployed, becoming involved with illegal drug use, and becoming teen parents (Carson, Sitlington, & Frank, 1995; Kauffman, 1999; Nelson & Pearson, 1994; US Department of Education, 1998). For the most part, despite legislation, students with emotional and behavioral disorders have been educated in restrictive and exclusionary environments, a far cry from the move toward more inclusive educational practices for children with disabilities (US Department of Education, 1998).

With the 1997 reauthorization of the Individuals with Disabilities Education Act (1997), there continues to be a significant need to understand better the curriculum and instructional practices used to educate students who receive special education services under the category of *emotionally disturbed*. It is also important to continue to explore proactive interventions that address collaborative, comprehensive, integrated services through multiple professionals and agencies, with families being at the center of the Systems of Care (Burns & Goldman, 1999; Stroul, 1993).

As schools focus on more effective ways to assist families and children with complex behavioral and emotional needs, the wraparound process that has emerged from the System of Care philosophy supports a move toward behavioral intervention procedures that focus on (1) the child's challenging behaviors, (2) teaching replacement behaviors, and (3) systematic reinforcement of desired behaviors as alternatives to using punishment-based strategies (Scott et al., 2002). Wraparound practices can create collaborative systems in local communities and a positive change for children and their families. These practices also support and assist the development of school and community partnerships that can identify predictable problem contexts, develop proactive and preventative solutions, and teach and reinforce behaviors that predict student success (Nelson & Colvin, 1996).

As such, the wraparound process has clearly influenced the increased use of positive behavioral support systems as effective for students with emotional and behavioral disorders. Positive behavioral support can best be described as a school-wide system to teach, model, and reinforce social behaviors as part of a student's educational experience in order to establish a learning climate in which appropriate behavior is the norm (National Technical Assistance Center on Positive Behavioral Interventions and Support, n.d.). Positive behavioral support systems divert at-risk behaviors and keep families at the center of intervention practices (Eber et al., 2002; Walker & Sprague, 1999). Positive behavioral support systems are part of a cluster of initiatives by schools and educators (other initiatives in the cluster include character education and assets development) designed to focus on positive behavior modification and teaching productive alternatives to disruptive behavior (School Mental Health Project/Center for Mental Health in Schools, 2004).

Positive behavioral support systems theory stands in stark contrast to punishment-based interventions that have tried—and failed—to use negative behavior modification to reduce disruptive and disengaged behavior in schools. Although analysts and advocates urge educators to go "beyond positive behavior support initiatives" and increase their attention to re-engaging students through broader approaches that

work on intrinsic motivation and "reduce negative and increase positive feelings, thoughts, and coping strategies with respect to learning,"
the procedures and practices of positive behavior support systems
clearly represent a change in direction from the emotional, behavioral, and psychological damage of punishment-based social control
practices (School Mental Health Project/Center for Mental Health in
Schools, 2004, p. 6). Positive behavioral support systems offer opportunities for the student's voice to be heard, as part of the PBS team, in
creating strategies that will be effective in producing positive social and
academic skills. As such, creative and realistic problem solving becomes a reality for child and the family.

Teacher Education Standards: A Foundation for Wraparound and Systems of Care in Schools and Teaching

Standards for certification and accreditation have become the structure
for teacher education curriculum. Preservice and inservice teacher certification candidates not only have to be competent in specific academic
content, they also must show evidence that their pedagogy is sound
and that improving the quality of their teaching is an ongoing professional process (Kozleski, Pugach, & Yinger, 2002). This reform in teacher
education is supported by standards from several organizations: (1) the
National Council for the Association of Teacher Education, the accrediting body for colleges and universities that prepares teachers and other
professional personnel for preschool through 12th-grade schools
(National Council for Accreditation of Teacher Education, n.d.); (2) the
Interstate New Teacher Assessment and Support Consortium principles, which represent "a common core of teaching knowledge and skills"
that new teachers should know and be able to do (Interstate New
Teacher Assessment and Support Consortium, 1992); (3) the National
Board for Professional Teaching Standards, which presents five core
propositions that seek "to identify and recognize teachers who effectively enhance student learning and demonstrate a high level of knowledge, skills, abilities, and commitments" (National Board for Professional
Teaching Standards, n.d., p. 3); (4) the Council for Exceptional Children,
which provides standards for the preparation and licensure of special education teachers (Council for Exceptional Children, n.d.).

In schools, given the growing numbers of culturally and linguistically diverse students who are taught by monolingual white teachers,
it has become essential for preservice teachers to recognize the
strengths of the family and community as active partners in the

process of educating all children. Both preservice and inservice teachers should accept the values of culturally competent and culturally responsive pedagogy. Each organization's standards for teacher preparation recognize not only content area competence and pedagogical skills, but they also insist on the importance of the involvement of parents, community members, and the collaboration of agencies and programs in the educational process. All of the standards from the several certification organizations cite the positive benefits of the collaboration of schools, parents, and community in the schooling of children and youth. Table 12-1 shows the family and community collaboration emphasis in each group of teacher preparation standards.

Table 12-1	Alignment of Professional Teaching Standards Related to Collaboration with Families, Communities, and Professional Agencies
National Council for the Accreditation of Teacher Education Unit Standards	Standard 4: Diversity The unit designs, implements, and evaluates curriculum and experiences for candidates to acquire and apply the knowledge, skills, and dispositions necessary to help all students learn. These experiences include working with diverse higher education and school faculty, diverse candidates, and diverse students in preschool through 12th-grade schools.
National Board for Professional Teaching Standards	Proposition 5: Teachers work collaboratively with parents. Teachers take advantage of community resources.
Interstate New Teacher Assessment and Support Consortium Principles	Principle 10: The teacher fosters relationships with school colleagues, parents, and agencies in the larger community to support students' learning and well-being.
Council for Exceptional Children Performance-Based Standards	Standard 10: Special educators routinely and effectively collaborate with families, other educators, related service providers, and personnel from community agencies in culturally responsive ways. Individualized general curriculum knowledge–parent education programs and behavior management guides that address severe behavior problems and facilitate communication for individuals with disabilities.

According to the National Council for the Accreditation of Teacher Education, candidates should understand the influence of culture on education and should be able to translate that understanding into meaningful, contextual learning experiences for their students. In doing so, Standard 4—Diversity of the National Council for the Accreditation of Teacher Education Unit Standards—encourages candidates not only to interact with culturally diverse faculty members and students at their institutions of higher education, but also to work in their clinical experiences with "exceptional students and students from different ethnic, racial, gender, socioeconomic, language, and religious groups" (p. 31). These interactions include those with students' families and other community members and agencies (http://www.ncate.org).

The National Board of Professional Teaching Standards—Proposition 5 acknowledges that parents also are educators of their children. Therefore, teachers seek information and support from parents to guide them as they teach their children. Furthermore, teachers consider the school's community as another vital resource to extend and contextualize learning in significant ways for students.

Interstate New Teacher Assessment and Support Consortium Principle 10 states that new teachers should understand how the intersection of students' lives beyond school affects their learning. Therefore, new teachers seek assistance and cooperation from family and community members as well as from personnel from professional agencies.

Finally, Standard 10 of the Council for Exceptional Children Performance-Based Principles notes the intentional collaboration of special education teachers, parents, community members, and professional agencies in the teaching and learning process as necessary and beneficial, and that it must be done in culturally responsive ways.

Community-Based Education Principles as a Foundation for System of Care and Wraparound Practices in Schools

Although the beginning of formal education is when students enter kindergarten classes, the actual foundation for their education occurs at home, with parents or guardians as a child's first teachers. According to Nicholas Hobbs, parents are "the true experts on their children" (Muscott, 2002). Where children with special needs are concerned, parent voices were long silenced (Turnbull & Turnbull, 2001). However, with the enactment of Public Law 94-142 and its 1997 reauthorization, parent voices have been acknowledged as vital contributors and hopefully equal partners (Johns, Crowley, & Guetzloe, 2001) in providing an education for their children that is equal to that of their nondisabled peers.

Teachers should recognize the importance of the family and the community in the education of all children, especially those with special needs. Good teacher education programs increasingly place preservice teachers in schools with highly diverse populations. Diversity—including multicultural student populations, linguistically different students, students of poverty, and students who are physically, mentally, and emotionally challenged—sets conditions under which teachers have both greater opportunity and greater motivation to better understand children, their families, and the communities from which they come. Community-based learning is critical for teachers in urban schools especially, when teachers often live outside the neighborhoods and communities served by the school (Boyle-Baise & Sleeter, 1998; Sleeter, 2000).

There are advantages to instituting community-based preservice teacher education programs. First, community-based teacher education helps teachers to realize that their students are cultural beings (Boyle-Baise, 2002). Preservice and in-service teachers may not be familiar with the family and community and the frames of reference that children bring with them to school, or children's ways of understanding and acting within their cultural backgrounds, such as their verbal responses and behaviors. These responses may often be misunderstood and thus misinterpreted. Being in the community of their learners offers teachers an avenue to share experiences with their students and make connections about their learning. It may also provide a means for a better understanding of the child, based on community context in ways not afforded them, when they only see the child in the classroom. Second, teachers can become acquainted with important community landmarks such as churches and community centers that are influential in students' lives. It is in these places where students may demonstrate strengths not evident in schools but that can be related to their academic potential. Connecting learning with students' personal interests can help teachers get to know their students in order to develop culturally relevant and culturally competent pedagogy (Johnson, 2002). Furthermore, by spending time in the communities of their students and listening and observing—but not judging—teachers have greater opportunities to understand the language, behaviors, traditions, and values that families and communities share. Such knowledge—seeking strengths in the community and its families—can help teachers to make their instruction more culturally relevant and responsive (Gay, 2001; Ladson-Billings, 1994, 2001).

Another advantage of community-based learning is its "potential to help teachers learn to contextualize marginalized communities within systems of unequal power" (Boyle-Baise & Sleeter, 1998, p. 7). Preservice and inservice teachers can confront personal and societal issues of "able-ism" with visible evidence of parents and communities actually working together for the learning and quality of life for children with disabilities. By going into the homes and communities of their students, teachers are better able to view the characteristics, interactions, functions, and life-cycle issues of the family (Turnbull & Turnbull, 2001) as sources of strengths, not deficits (Boyle-Baise & Sleeter). Thus, the family's individuality can be valued, and collaboration can be much more effective.

Furthermore, going beyond families and into the general communities of students with special needs allows teachers to enter the context of the worlds of their students and to speak to them as real and valuable parts of their lives. Teachers can also experience and better understand nonverbal and verbal communication skills that are taught through community interaction and learned through social constructivism. Finally, teachers can gain greater understanding of the community and its influence on the skills used by their students, including various discourse styles (Gee, 1989; Payne, 2001). They can also note the coping, survival, and problem-solving skills that students use when they are faced with difficult situations (Turnbull & Turnbull, 2001).

Community-based learning is a broad framework that includes such pedagogies as service learning and experiential learning (Owens & Wang, 1996). All promote the personal benefits of community-based learning, an approach grounded in the skills that teachers can learn and hone while engaging in the communities of their students. Teachers can strengthen interpersonal communication skills, become more active listeners, become more self-aware, exercise more flexibility, and be more willing to take risks because they have greater understandings of the cultures and communities of their students and their families. This is particularly important because teachers use a more family-centered approach to working with students with special needs.

Community-based learning can help teachers in their social and citizenship education. Their intercultural and multicultural competencies can broaden and grow. An intergenerational connectedness can be strengthened at a time when traditional nuclear family compositions are not always the norm. Teachers can adopt a sense of heightened civic and community responsibility as well as develop valuable leadership skills. In the age of the No Child Left Behind "highly qualified teacher," community-based learning can encourage teachers to deepen their understanding of their content area and to use skills and techniques in problem solving and decision making (Benefits of Community-Based Learning, n.d.; Owens & Wang, 1996). Table 12-2 describes themes, attitudes, and examples of indicators that would maximize collaborative family-centered school partnerships. It illustrates a framework for collaborating with families and also examines the benefits of building collaborative relationships between families and teachers.

In Practice: Positive Behavioral Support and School-Wide, Family-Centered Interventions

The use of positive behavioral support has emerged in recent years as an effective and productive system to decrease problem behaviors of students and to provide professionals and families with a clearer focus for intervention with students with complex needs for support. Recent legislation impacting reauthorization of the Individuals with Disabilities Education Act (IDEA) continues to support strongly the use of positive behavioral interventions that involve collaborative problem solving with families and professionals (Smith & McGinley, 2004). Therefore, effective models that support the inclusion of students with emotional and behavioral challenges in general education classrooms should be examined closely.

A model of positive behavioral support for schools can be constructed with emphasis on (1) a proactive continuum of positive behaviors supports, (2) more individualized and intensified interventions, as needed, when problem behaviors and needs become more complex, (3) a family-centered, team-based planning process, and (4) comprehensive planning that takes into consideration the strengths and needs of the student, the family, the teacher, and other supports for the child and family (Eber et al., 2002). Table 12-3 provides a model for decision making that professionals and families can use in creating the collaboration needed for a positive behavioral support system in school. The key here is working toward change that will positively impact the student and family. Table 12-3 addresses critical decisions important to student-centered interventions.

Minimal Intrusive Interventions—Including Students with Behavioral and Emotional Disorders in General Education

A key to meeting the educational needs of students with emotional and behavioral disorders in inclusive learning environments is to pay close

Table 12-2 A Framework for Collaborating with Families and Others for the Benefit of Children and Youth
Collaborative Family–Professional Partnerships Themes and Indicators

Themes	*Attributes*	*Examples of Indicators*
Communication	Quality: positive, understandable, and respectful of all members.	Being clear, honest, tactful, and open Listening Sharing resources Communicating frequently Coordinating information
	Quantity: enables efficient and effective coordination and understanding of all members.	
Commitment	Members share assurance of each other's (1) devotion and loyalty to student and family and (2) belief in importance of goals being pursued.	Being consistent, accessible, sensitive, and flexible Regarding work as more than a job and the student and family as more than a case.
Equality	Members feel equity in decision making and service implementation and work to help others feel equally empowered.	Being willing to explore all options Fostering harmony Avoiding turfism Allowing reciprocity Validating others Advocating for student or family with other professionals.
Skills	Members perceive others as competent in fulfilling their roles.	Being willing to learn Expecting student progress Taking action Considering the whole student or family

continues

Table 12-2   Continued

Themes	Attributes	Examples of Indicators
Trust	Members view other members as reliable and dependable.	Following through on commitments Being discreet Keeping the student safe
Respect	Members regard each other with esteem and demonstrate that esteem through communication and actions.	Being nonjudgmental and courteous Valuing the student Exercising nondiscrimination Avoiding intrusion

Source: Blue-Banning, Summers, Frankland, Nelson, and Beegle (2004, p.174).

Table 12-3   Critical Data-Based Decision Points in Student-Centered Behavior Intervention Planning

General Questions	Key Decision Questions	Source(s)	Outcomes
Level I: What problems are predictable?	1. What is a problem: operational definition, effect on environment? 2. What environmental conditions predict behavior?	School-wide discipline data and staff experiences	Determination whether any action at all is necessary
Level II: How might problem behavior be prevented school-wide?	1. What teachable expectations are necessary? 2. What routines can be arranged to predict success? 3. What is the simplest course of action?	School-wide discipline data analysis, staff discussion and consensus of logical and realistic strategies	Plan for school-wide prevention of predictable problems and student failure
Level III: Is individualized intervention warranted?	1. What is the extent of the problem? 2. Is the behavior dangerous? 3. What is the simplest course of action?	School-wide discipline data for individual student, perceptions of staff, parent, and others	Determination whether individualized assessment is necessary
Level IV: Is development of a student-centered planning team warranted?	1. Have simple interventions proven unsuccessful, or is the behavior dangerous? 2. Who should sit on the team?	Teacher data from classroom, school-wide discipline data, data collected by specialists (e.g., functional behavioral assessments), discussion among all involved	Behavior referred to appropriate course of actions: more complex teams and interventions for more complex problems

continues

Table 12-3 Continued

General Questions	Key Decision Questions	Source(s)	Outcomes
	3. How does assessment data inform intervention: predictors, function, replacement behavior? 4. How will intervention be implemented?		
Level V: Is intervention effective?	1. What is the criterion for success? 2. Is the student making sufficient progress? 3. How can the data inform intervention changes?	Data representing current level of functioning, individual monitoring data, discussion among all involved	Evaluation of the success of intervention and plan for changes as necessary

Source: Scott (2003).

attention to using interventions to manage surface behaviors that could escalate if the teacher's response is inappropriate. Some of these interventions include (1) catching the student being "good," (2) planned ignoring of an inappropriate behavior that is not disrupting and can be tolerated, (3) providing opportunity for physical movement and release, (4) managing the physical environment of the classroom, (5) demonstrating personal interest in the student, (6) easing tension in the classroom through humor but not sarcasm, (7) appealing to the student's sense of values and beliefs, (8) modeling appropriate behaviors, and (9) helping students to build a positive self-image by identifying their strengths and helping them to understand that they are valued and valuable.

Assessment of Students with Emotional and Behavioral Disorders

In understanding complex and challenging behaviors exhibited by children with emotional and behavioral disorders, educators turn to functional behavioral assessments to assist in making decisions concerning behavior. When these students face disciplinary action such as suspension from school, a team of professionals and parents completes a *manifestation determination* before permitting significant behavioral interventions. The Individuals with Disabilities Education Act and many state regulations require the completion of the functional behavioral assessment before these interventions can be implemented.

The functional behavioral assessment forms the foundation for interventions that support positive change in behavior. The results of a functional behavioral assessment can lay the groundwork for a plan that will be most effective for students with behavioral challenges. The team that completes the functional behavioral assessment works to reduce or eliminate challenging behavior.

A functional behavioral assessment is composed of the following components: (1) clearly described challenging behaviors, including behaviors that occur together; (2) identification of the events, times, and situations that predict when the challenging behaviors will and will not occur across the range of daily activities and routines; (3) identification of consequences that maintain the challenging behaviors; (4) the development of one or more statements or hypotheses that describes specific behaviors, specific types of situations in which they occur, and reinforcers that maintain the behaviors in that situation; and (5) a collection of data from observations that directly support the behavioral statements. From the functional behavioral assessment an intervention plan can emerge that will provide steps to an effective and positive change in behavior for the student (O'Neil et al., 1997).

Summary and Conclusion

This chapter described conceptual frameworks, policies, legislation, standards, and practices that provide the foundation or support for the integration of System of Care and wraparound principles, philosophies, and practices in special education and general education school settings. Multiple influences have impacted the development of System of Care practices in educational settings. A confluence of systems thinking and result-oriented frameworks, preservice, and inservice teacher education standards, legislation, and policies regarding children with complex needs, partnership, and collaborative pressures and structures among schools, communities and agencies, professionals, and higher education institutions has provided a broad basis for restructuring schooling and service delivery for children—especially children with complex needs—and their families. The policies, conceptual frameworks, and emerging partnership and collaborative structures place families firmly in the center of decision making.

In addition, practices based on positive behavioral support systems and the use of data gleaned from behavioral and academic assessments have become increasingly prevalent models of good, if not best, practice in special education and to a lesser, but still notable, extent in general education.

Although the structural foundations for integrating System of Care and wraparound principles and practices in special and general education are there, much work remains in order to "reculture" (Fullan, 2001) the work of schools and the practices of teachers. Teachers and schools do not routinely adopt a diagnostic bent toward student behavior, motivation, and academic engagement, in which teachers and schools routinely think in collaborative "together we can" ways about families and communities; in which strengths, rather than deficits, form the presumptive basis for assessment. The goal is that in the future schools and teachers will incorporate System of Care principles and values readily and willingly, and will preferentially empower parents and families in the school-based education of their children. We may not be there yet, but these practices are beginning. The enterprise of schooling is far too large and too complex, with too many as-yet misaligned or unaligned systems to change easily or swiftly. However, the beginnings of a more comprehensive, integrated system of services in collaboration with families are here, and the lessons are growing.

Case Study: The Case of Sophie

Sophie is a Hispanic female who is in the sixth grade. She lives with her mother, father, grandparents, and three of her four other brothers and sisters (two girls and two boys). Sophie is the third of the five children in her family. Her grandparents immigrated to the United States from Mexico when they were in their early 20s and still speak mostly Spanish in the home. Sophie, her parents, and her siblings were all born in the United States and are bilingual in English and Spanish. However, they rarely speak to anyone except their grandparents in Spanish. In fact, most people do not know that Sophie speaks Spanish at all. If someone outside of her family speaks to her in Spanish, she will pretend that she does not understand them. Sophie's parents and grandparents miss the rest of the family, a tight-knit group of uncles, aunts, and cousins, who are all still in Mexico—a trip that Sophie and her family take at least once a year. Sophie's father works in a textile factory, and her mother is a secretary. Neither attended college primarily as a result of limited financial resources but value education greatly. Recently, Sophie's favorite aunt has been diagnosed with bone cancer. The entire family is worried, and Sophie's mother is trying to find a way to get her to the United States for medical treatment. She has not been successful so far.

Sophie attended a small elementary school in which the same children were together at each grade level. Her elementary school teachers and records indicate that she was a consistent *B* or *C* student who usually stayed out of trouble. She was not particularly popular in elementary school, but did have a few close friends. She was involved in just one fight in elementary school when a group of boys were teasing one of her close friends. She mostly stayed out of people's way and for the most part was motivated to complete work, with only the occasional missed homework assignment. Sophie was not referred to the school student support assistance team while in elementary school.

However, Sophie's family moved over the summer, and she is now starting middle school with an entirely new group of children. She has lost contact with the few friends she had in elementary school. Sophie is in Ms. Miller's 6th-grade home base and language arts class. Ms. Miller reports that Sophie has few, if any, friends, does not participate in class, is disorganized, completes less than half of her class and homework assignments, and is argumentative with her peers. At the beginning of the year, Ms. Miller assumed that Sophie was an "English as a second language" student. She mistakenly asked Sophie about it in front of the entire class one day, and Sophie defensively shouted back to the teacher, "I don't know one word of Spanish." Since then, the other children know that this upsets her and use it to pick on her frequently. Although it is not yet October, Sophie has already gotten into four fights as a result of these taunts. She does not seem to be able to ignore or walk away when the others try to push her buttons. However, Sophie is usually more defiant with her teachers, rather than rude or aggressive.

Sophie's parents have met with Ms. Miller for conferences twice and are very concerned about her. They are afraid she will be suspended from school. They say that she hates school now and has to be forced to go every morning. They try to force her to do her homework, but even when she does complete it, she will leave it at home or just not turn it in. They are worried that her grades are slipping. This is a critical issue for them because of how important they consider education to the future of their children. They report that her older brother is in college on a scholarship and that her older sister is a junior in high school and doing well. They do not understand the change that has occurred in Sophie this year and desperately want help in knowing what to do.

Problem Solving Worksheet for the Case of Sophie

Each of the following components of the case will help you to resolve the issues presented in Sophie's case. Remember that there will never be one absolutely correct solution—several alternatives may be available, but you will need to determine what solution should be tried first.

Who are the individuals involved in the case?

Describe the problem presented in the case.

What are some of the details of the case that help you determine the problem?

1. _____

2. _____

3. _____

4. _____

Alternative Solutions	Possible Consequences	Priority

Use the chart to determine alternative solutions that will emphasize a family-centered approach to intervention and the consequences of the solution.

Which of these solutions will you try first? What will be your implementation plan? How will you monitor the progress of the plan? What might be your criteria for determining the success of the plan?

Discussion Questions/Exercises

1. Observe in an inclusive classroom with children identified as having emotional or behavioral disabilities. What are the behaviors of the children in the class? What are the behaviors of the teacher and other adults?

2. Self-assess parent communication skills, strategies, and methods. What strengths or assets do they show for helping their child?

3. Arrange a visit to a neighborhood or community where some of the children with complex needs live. Go with a parent or community agency staff member who understands the strengths-based approach to assessment. Ask your guide about the important places and people in the community, the kinds of experiences that school-age children have in the community, the local names for sites, and the local meanings of words and sayings, as a means for understanding the community. Ask also about the strengths or assets the community has to support the healthy education and development of children and youth.

Recommended Resources

- Center for Mental Health in Schools/School Mental Health Project (http://smhp/psych.ucla.edu). This center and its website deal with a wide range of policy, practice, and reform issues that are related to students with complex needs and their experience in schools. The center is co-directed by Howard Edelman and Linda Taylor at UCLA, and it offers a convenient quick-find service for topics related to mental health and special needs in schools.
- National Alliance for the Mentally Ill (www.nami.org). Find support: state and local National Alliance for the Mentally Ill, educational programs, consumer services, child and adolescent mental health consumer groups, self-help groups, multicultural groups, and online communication and discussion groups.
- National Mental Health Consumer Self-Help Clearing House.
- Oppositional Defiant Disorder Support Group (http://www.conductdisorders.com/). This site is a companion site to a wonderful message board filled with personal stories.
- Partnerships Against Violence Network (http://www.pavent.org). This is a "virtual library" of information about violence and youth at risk, representing data from seven different federal agencies. It is a "one-stop," searchable, information resource to help reduce redundancy in information management and provide clear and comprehensive access to information for States and local communities.
- Safe and Drug-Free Schools Programs Office (http://www.ed.gov/offices/OESE/SDFS/). This is the federal government's primary vehicle for reducing violence and drug, alcohol, and tobacco use through education and prevention activities in our nation's schools. The program supports initiatives to meet the seventh National Education Goals, which state that by the year 2000 all schools will be free of drugs and violence and the unauthorized presence of firearms and alcohol, and offer a disciplined environment conducive to learning. These initiatives are designed to prevent violence in and around schools, strengthen programs that prevent illegal use of substances, involve parents, and are coordinated with related federal, state, and community efforts and resources.
- Social Development Research Group (http://weber.u.washington/edu/ ~ sdrg/). Research focuses on the prevention and treatment of health and behavior problems among young people. Drug abuse, delinquency, risky sexual behavior, violence, and school dropout rates are among the problems addressed. J. David

Hawkins, director, and Richard F. Catalano, associate director, began in 1979 to develop the social development strategy, which provides the theoretical basis for risk- and protective-focused prevention that underlies much of the group's research.

- Tough Love International (http://www.toughlove.org). The TOUGHLOVE Parent Support Group is a self-help, active, parent support group for parents who are troubled by their children's behavior. Many are parents of teen-aged children, but there are also parents of preteens, parents of adult children, and grandparents. Over 500 parent support groups are affiliated with TOUGHLOVE International, a nonprofit educational organization.

References

Benefits of community-based learning (n.d.). Retrieved July 14, 2004, from: http://www.cclc.umn.edu/crimson/dependancies/multimedia/cofaab4ae911836f624ead8a_230d5933.pdf.

Blue-Banning, M., Summers, J.A., Frankland, H.C., Nelson, L.L., & Beegle, G. (2004). Dimensions of family and professional partnerships: Constructive guidelines for collaboration. *Exceptional Children, 70,* 167–184.

Boyle-Baise, M. (2002). *Multicultural service learning: Education teachers in diverse communities.* New York: Teachers College Press.

Boyle-Baise, M., & Sleeter, C.E. (1998). *Community service learning for multicultural teacher education.* Washington, DC: US Department of Education Educational Resources Information Center. (ERIC Document Reproduction Service No. ED 429 925). Washington, DC.

Brabeck, M.M., Walsh, M.E., & Latta, R. (Eds.). (2003). *Meeting at the hyphen: Schools-universities-communities-professions in collaborations for student achievement and well being.* NSSE Yearbook 102, Part II. Chicago: National Society for the Study of Education.

Burns, B.J., & Goldman, S.K. (Eds.). (1999). *Promising practices in wraparound for children with serious emotional disturbance and their families* (1998 Series, Vol. 4). Washington, DC: Center for Effective Collaboration and Practice, American Institute for Research.

Carson, R.R., Sitlington, P.L., & Frank, A.R. (1995). Young adulthood for individuals with behavioral disorders: What does it hold? *Behavioral Disorders, 20,* 127–135.

Council for Exceptional Children (n.d.). *CEC performance-based standards.* Retrieved July 24, 2004, from: http://www.cec.sped.org/ps/perf_based_stds/standards.html.

Dryfoos, J.G. (1994). *Full service schools: A revolution in health and social services for children, youth, and families.* San Francisco: Jossey-Bass.

Eber, L., Sugai, G., Smith, C.R., & Scott, T.M. (2002). Wraparound and positive behavioral interventions and supports in schools. *Journal of Emotional and Behavioral Disorders, 10*(3), 171–180.

Epstein, J.E., & Salinas, K.C. (2004). Partnering with families and communities. *Educational Leadership, 61*(8), 12–18.

Fullan, M. (2001). *The new meaning of educational change* (3rd ed.). New York: Teachers College Press.

Fullan, M. (2002). *Change forces with a vengeance.* New York: Falmer Press.

Gay, G. (2001). *Culturally responsive teaching.* New York: Teachers College Press.

Gee, J.P. (1989). Literacy, discourse, and linguistics: Introduction. *Journal of Education, 171,* 5–17.

Individuals with Disabilities Education Act. (1997). Public Law No. 105-17.

Interstate New Teacher Assessment and Support Consortium. (1992). *Models standards for beginning teacher licensing, assessment and development: A resource for state dialogue.* Retrieved July 19, 2004, from: http://www.ccsso.org/content/pdfs/corestd.pdf.

Johnson, E.B. (2002). *Contextual teaching and learning: What it is and why it's here to stay.* Thousand Oaks, CA: Corwin.

Johns, B.H., Crowley, E.P., & Guetzloe, E. (2001). *Effective curriculum for students with emotional and behavioral disorders: Reaching them through teaching them.* Denver, CO: Love Publishing.

Kauffman, J.M. (1999). The role of science in behavior disorders. *Behavioral Disorders, 24,* 265–272.

Kozleski, B., Pugach, M., & Yinger, R. (2002, February). *Preparing teachers to work with students with disabilities: Possibilities and challenges for special and general teacher education: A white paper.* (ERIC Document Reproduction Service No. ED 468 743). Washington, DC: American Association of Colleges for Teacher Education.

Ladson-Billings, G. (1994). *The dreamkeepers: Successful teachers of African American children.* New York: John Wiley & Sons.

Ladson-Billings, G. (2001). Multicultural teacher education: Research, practice, and policy. In J. Banks & C.M. Banks (Eds.), *Handbook of research on multicultural education* (pp. 747–759). San Francisco: Jossey-Bass.

Muscott, H.S. (2002). Exceptional partnerships: Listening to the voices of families. *Preventing School Failure, 46*(2), 66–69.

National Board for Professional Teaching Standards. (n.d.). *What teachers should know and be able to do.* Retrieved July 19, 2004, from: http:www.nbpts.org/pdf/coreprops.pdf.

National Council for Accreditation of Teacher Education. (n.d.). *NCATE unit standards.* Retrieved July 19, 2004, from: http://www.ncate.org/standard/m_stds.htm.

National Technical Assistance Center on Positive Behavioral Interventions and Support, n.d.). School-wide PBS. Retrieved March 28, 2004, from http://www.pbis.org/schoolwide.htm#PositiveSocialBehavior.

Nelson, J.R., & Colvin, G. (1996). Designing supportive schools environments. In R.J. Illback & C.M. Nelson (Eds.), *Emerging school-based approaches for children with emotional and behavioral problems: Research and practice in service integration* (pp. 225–249). New York: Haworth Press.

Nelson, C.M., & Pearson, C.A. (1994). Juvenile delinquency in the context of culture and community. In R.L. Peterson & S. Ishii-Jordan (Eds.),

Cultural and community contexts for emotional or behavioral disorders (pp. 78–90). Boston: Brookline Press.

O'Neil, R.E., Horner, R.H., Albin, R.W., Sprague, J.R., Storey, K., & Newton, N.S. (1997). *Functional assessment and program development for problem behavior: A practical handbook.* Pacific Grove, CA: Brooks/Cole.

Owens, T.R., & Wang, C. (1996). *Community-based learning: A foundation for meaningful educational reform.* Retrieved July 14, 2004, from: http://www.nwrel.org/scpd/sirs/10/t008.html.

Payne, R.K. (2001). *A framework for understanding poverty.* Highlands, TX: Process.

School Mental Health Project/Center for Mental Health in Schools. (2004). Beyond positive behavior support initiatives. *Addressing Barriers to Learning, 9*(3), 1–3, 6–7.

Scott, T.M. (2003). Making behavior intervention decisions in a school-wide system of positive behavior support. *Focus on Exceptional Children, 36(1),* 1–18.

Scott, T.M., Nelson, C.M., Liaupsin, C.J., Jolivette, K., Christle, C.A., & Riney, M. (2002). Addressing the needs of at-risk and adjudicated youth through positive behavior support: Effective prevention practices. *Education and Treatment of Children, 25,* 532–551.

Sleeter, C. (2000). Strengthening multicultural education with community-based service learning. In C.R. O'Grady (Ed.), *Integrating service learning and multicultural education in colleges and universities* (pp. 263–276). Mahwah, NJ: Lawrence Erlbaum Associates.

Smith, D., & McGinley, K. (2004). *Side-by-side comparison of Senate bill 1248 (as passed on May 13, 2004) and House bill 1350 (as passed on April 30, 2003) with parts A and B of the IDEA (current law).* Washington, DC: National Association of Protection & Advocacy Systems. Retrieved July 23, 2004, from: http://www.wrightslaw.com/law/idea/sidebyside.06.04.pdf.

Sparks, D., & Hirsh, S. (1997). *A new vision for staff development.* Alexandria, VA: Association for Supervision and Curriculum Development.

Stroul, B.A. (1993, September). *Systems of care for children and adolescents with severe emotional disturbances: What are the results?* Washington, DC: CASSP Technical Assistance Center, Center for Child Health and Mental Health Policy, and Georgetown University Child Development Center.

Teitel, L. (2003). *The professional development schools handbook.* Thousand Oaks, CA: Corwin Press.

Turnbull, A.P., & Turnbull, H.R. (2001). *Families, professionals and exceptionality: A special partnership* (4th ed.). Upper Saddle River, NJ: Merrill.

Turnbull, A.P., Turnbull, H.R., Shank, M., & Leal, D. (1999). *Exceptional lives: Special education in today's schools* (2nd ed.). Upper Saddle River, NJ: Prentice Hall.

US Department of Education. (1998). *Twentieth annual report to Congress on the implementation of IDEA: Individuals with Disabilities Education Act.* Washington, DC: US Government Printing Office.

Walker, H.M., & Sprague, J.R. (1999). Longitudinal research and functional behavior assessment issues. *Behavioral Disorders, 24,* 335–337.

Chapter 13

Integrating System of Care into Music and Arts Education

Randy Kohlenberg

Objectives

- Comprehend the importance of music and the arts as necessary to healthy living for people of all ages, children through adults.
- Identify the four themes for learning music and the arts.
- Discuss the importance of music participation and why involvement in performance can enhance an individual's self-esteem as well as improve feelings of self-worth, especially for children who have special needs.
- List System of Care values and principles and their relationship to music and arts education.
- Apply System of Care principles and values as a framework for teaching music and the arts to children.
- Apply System of Care values and principles as a framework for teaching music and the arts to children with special needs.
- Describe how involvement of the family can enhance the child's musical experience.
- Explain how musical experiences for children can be made culturally sensitive and responsive.

▓ Describe how every individual has the intrinsic ability to understand and appreciate the artistic experience as a foundation for learning, thus reinforcing a child's strengths.

▓ Discuss how music and all art activities can serve as a catalyst for learning to function successfully in other educational domains.

▓ Identify the successes and challenges in building a music program based on a System of Care framework involving one university's experience in teaching music in public schools.

During the last approximately 20 years, the value of the arts in education has been studied extensively, and the benefits have been documented substantially. Although many of the studies have focused on music and the education of young children, the implications of these investigations can be extended through all of the arts because of their creative commonalities. These findings can be translated to a broader population, including individuals who are considered to be at risk for behavioral or learning problems. Although many of the studies have not been longitudinal nor have they encompassed a broad population, the consistent results from study after study reinforce the notion that involvement in the arts impacts significantly on productive learning. Without question, the arts provide experiences that are difficult to duplicate through any other medium.

The various areas in the applied arts, including visual art, music, dance, theatre arts, and others, all support the underlying principles on which a System of Care is constructed. Those principles include the following:

- Implementing a family-centered approach to services
- Employing an approach that builds on individual strengths
- Establishing full partnerships with families and professionals
- Using community-based services, both formal and informal
- Providing culturally responsive services
- Establishing an interagency collaboration that focuses on wraparound services and that encompasses the child and family.

Although all values and principles are significant in the consideration of a System of Care, the inclusion of the arts in educating children who are "at risk" is paramount in one area: identifying individual strengths and building on them.

Although the focus and examples throughout this chapter are based on music, the ideas presented may be extended to a variety of the arts, including visual art, dance, theatre arts, and others. Thus, the approaches and achievements that can be attained through the arts can reach far beyond what is included here. General references to the musician are intended to encompass all areas of creative activities and not just the traditional musical performer.

This chapter primarily focuses on ways that music can be used as an intervention strategy within the System of Care for persons with special needs. The study of music and personal involvement in music, both listening and participation, is considered. The field of music therapy has evolved into a sophisticated approach using music in treating a variety of physiologic and psychologic disorders. The emphasis focuses on how music improves the quality of living and the ability of an individual and family to function successfully. The arts always have been a component in the daily living activities of humankind and are reflected in the culture. The strength of music for everyone is the foundation on which this chapter is based.

The use of music in a System of Care is propagated by a principle tenet based on the personal strengths model. Categorized by Huber (2000), this model was developed in the 1980s to de-emphasize individual limitations and impairments. The purpose is to provide a framework whereby individuals can achieve personal goals, thus helping them to identify, secure, and sustain resources needed to live, work, and play independently within the community. The basic assumption is that people can be successful if they are able to develop their own potential and are able to access appropriate resources to meet their needs. The exploration of creativity and the development of artistic potential within students can lay the foundation for building skills that result in successful achievement and healthy living.

Themes to Promote Effective Learning

Traditional academic skills are not a prerequisite for involvement in the arts. Many individuals may not have reached required standards in reading, writing, or mathematical skills and may be unsuccessful in activities that require those skills. A substantial number of these same individuals, however, are able to become successful in the arts because the skills are taught from the most basic concept and do not require many of the traditional academic skills.

Bruner (1960), a clinical psychologist and protégé of Piaget, in his *Structure of Education*, presented four basic themes considered to be essential for optimal learning to occur: structure, motivation, readiness, and intuition. The four themes are paramount in any learning situation but are especially important in the nurturing of an individual who may have academic deficits but may be successful in musical activities and the arts.

Structure is an essential element in the learning situation and determines how the environment is designed to promote optimal learning. Within arts education, the learning environment will be teacher- or learner-centered and is determined day by day. Although the balance of the approach may vary substantially each day, and even within the instructional time, arts instruction necessarily migrates ultimately to the point where the learner, and in essence the one who is creating the art, is in the position of making the primary decisions. The teacher, of course, provides the necessary instruction and critique to ensure that the person who is involved in the creative process has enough expertise to accomplish whatever the task or product may be. Ultimately, artists must reach a point where they can make the driving decisions that result in a creative presentation. Thus, the ever-evolving structure not only places an emphasis on individual achievement, but also allows the artist essentially to take full credit for the presentation or product. The art, therefore, is person-centered. Using a System of Care framework, the individual achievement is self-enhancing, providing the child with an empowering experience.

Motivation is tantamount to the artistic experience. In many situations, motivation is more external than self-directed. External motivation is a necessary component of any learning situation, but the ultimate goal is for the learner to become self-directed, especially in the development of an artist. Consequently, there is a quest for productivity, efficiency in the process, and excellence in the achievement. Thus, self-motivation is the desired and optimal type of motivation that is fostered intrinsically though involvement in the arts. Within the System of Care, the ability of an individual to learn to make judicious decisions as a result of self-motivation can be exercised substantially as the student learns to be self-directed through participation in arts activities, both presentations and products.

Readiness is based on the premise that any individual can learn any concept as long as it is presented at its most basic level. Thus, a kindergarten student can study physics if the most basic concept is presented. From the most basic, more sophisticated concepts are built on and developed. Within the learning situation, a review of the primary concepts is the foundation for more advanced ideas. In virtually all types of instructional teaching plans, this review is integral to the learning process, and in the instruction of arts, building on several basic concepts is a central key to learning. In most of the arts areas, all activities or processes can be narrowed to several basic concepts that are essential to every activity. Thus, the curriculum emanates from the idea that the objectives for learning continually reflect the basic concepts even as the learner begins to comprehend and incorporate increasingly advanced ideas.

Intuition is an idea that is particularly valuable in the area of arts education where an individual learns to assimilate knowledge in one area and can transfer it to another situation. Although most problem solving follows the scientific method in which each step leads systematically to the next, intuition is more like "educated guessing." When a problem has been addressed and resolved and a similar problem is confronted, rather than going through every step in the scientific process, the individual proceeds from the initial challenge directly to the solution, resolution, or product. Although steps in the process may be skipped, the result is essentially the same because the individual understands the problem and its resolution. In the study of the arts, components of the process can often be skipped to achieve an effective and successful end result. For example, in the case of music performance, intuition is particularly appropriate in performing different works of music that are in the same style. A performer is able to transfer the ideas learned in one composition to another in the same or a similar style.

Objectives for Integrating Music and Arts Instruction into the System of Care

Instruction in music and the arts involves a variety of learning activities that are interrelated and ultimately incorporated into a comprehensible experience or product. Specific objectives that can be employed in almost any type of creative learning experience are especially appropriate when working with a student who is being served within the concepts of the values and principles of the System of Care. These objectives, developed initially through the Manhattanville Music Curriculum Project during the late 1960s and early 1970s, focused on the creativity of the learner and the expressive aspects of music (Thomas, n.d.). In contrast to the competitive and punitive methods used in the many music-learning situations that once predominated, this approach focused on individual achievement, promoting individual excellence and encouraging self-expression. Furthermore, the Manhattanville Music Curriculum Project was guided by the steadfast notion that involvement in creative activities is central in the development of every child and, indeed, every human being. Four general objectives regarding the delivery of music instruction emerged: (1) acquisition of knowledge, (2) development of skills—aural, translative, and dexterous, (3) promotion of a positive attitude toward self and healthy living, and (4) enhancing the aesthetic experience.

In every learning experience, the *acquisition of knowledge* assumes primary importance. In music and the arts, however, many of the areas and levels of achievement measured by standardized tests are not prerequisites for study. Thus, knowledge is presented as it relates to specific instruction and assumes the student has reached a prescribed level. Knowledge, in the instance of music and arts instruction, is empowerment for achievement rather than remediation of skills to which many at-risk students or special learners are exposed in academic pursuits. Thus, in every instructional activity, explanations are presented to the learner from the most basic concept to ensure comprehension and maximum achievement.

Skill development is another area within music and arts instruction that assumes little prior experience other than the initial exposure afforded through the home, school, and recreational activities of childhood. Of primary importance, aural skills are developed through everyday listening that occurs from birth and continues throughout life.

Translative skills are enhanced through problem-solving activities that are the foundation of every creative experience. Extending dexterous or kinesthetic skills involves the fine tuning of basic motor skills, becoming comfortable with body posture and stature, and learning how humans use such basic everyday functions such as eye–hand coordination, breathing, and many others to develop artistic creativity.

The importance of developing, fostering, and maintaining a *positive attitude* is a primary focus in the study of the arts, and thus, its importance cannot be underestimated for students within the System of Care. As in the personal strengths model, students through the study of music and the arts build self-esteem and confidence. The positive reinforcement inherent in every successful performance or creative activity enables the student to experience a feeling of accomplishment and satisfaction. Through these types of experiences and feelings, the student develops a can-do approach, a feeling of self-worth, and a positive attitude toward pursuing activities that promote happy and healthy living.

Although the first three general objectives appear to be more applicable to the System of Care, the fourth, *aesthetic awareness and enhancement*, plays an important role in musical achievement and indeed self-awareness. Although the aesthetic experience is mentioned rarely within the context of teaching because it cannot be tested or observed objectively, the importance cannot be ignored. All humans experience music and the arts with aspects of their being beyond intellectual and emotional consciousness. Students with special needs and those who are considered to be at risk likewise appreciate the creativity that spawns this intense experience. Even though instruction does not focus specifically on the aesthetic, the study of music and the arts is assumed to play a significant role in the enhancement of the experience and thus contributes positively to the well-being of the individual.

System of Care as a Framework for Music and Arts Instruction: One University's Experience

Through an interdisciplinary, collaborative project at the University of North Carolina at Greensboro begun in 1995, the area of music was integrated by university faculty and students into a System of Care initiative (established in Guilford County, North Carolina) for children with serious emotional disturbances. The four-year project was accomplished by university faculty members and university student teachers enrolled in music education classes and private music instruction. University student teachers ranged from the first- through fourth-year undergraduate to master's and doctoral graduate students. Students enrolled in the Guilford County System of Care initiative at the Mental Health Center were served through music classes and in one-on-one instructional settings. The school-aged students were identified by public school personnel as having behavioral challenges. As in the concept of wraparound, the university student teachers were involved in the music component of the project and worked collaboratively with the interdisciplinary team of specialists, each of whom provided expertise geared toward the well-being of the public school students.

Importance of Music and Arts Instruction for Students with Special Needs

The university student teachers working with the public school students enrolled in the System of Care did not diagnose conditions or identify problems, nor did they participate in therapeutic treatment. The emphasis was on the personal development of the student's potential for creative achievement. In consultation with teachers and counselors in the public schools, parents or caregivers, and other professionals, university student teachers focused on a number of students who had been assessed to have special needs. Traditionally, music instruction has been provided to those students who have been categorized as being intellectually gifted or artistically talented, or to students who have never endured some type of limitation that might require intervention to accommodate learning. The focus of this project, however, was to encourage the involvement of students with special needs. Students who were overcoming physical, emotional, social, learning, and other challenges were involved and encouraged to participate in the music instruction. Accommodations were made for students with psychosocial or physical challenges. Emphasis was placed on the idea that all students can be involved successfully in music at some level. The underlying principle that music is essential to the healthy development of every individual was emphasized in every instructional approach. Achievement in music is crucial to the measurement of musical success; however, success and the level of accomplishment can be assessed at many levels. Some of the students were able to effect substantial changes quickly, whereas others required more extensive instruction and time. The amount of instructional effort, pacing, and length of time required, however, was never the measure for success. Success was measured by the completion of creative accomplishments by the public school students at an appropriate level.

Music Instruction Within the Classroom Setting

Classroom instruction was led by a university student teacher and involved students from the elementary through secondary levels. At all levels, classroom music instruction was geared toward a larger group of students with the intention of providing experiences that included presenting knowledge, listening to music, and participating. At the secondary levels, beginning in the sixth and seventh grades, classroom instruction became more highly specialized and individualized.

Creating music as an ensemble while maintaining individuality became a focus, and a systematized method of teaching music reading was employed. In the case of vocal music, students learned to read parts that corresponded with their vocal quality (soprano, alto, tenor baritone, bass, etc.). Instrumental music was presented to students in a heterogeneous group setting that included traditional wind and percussion or string instruments but not keyboard instruments, which were used only to accompany vocal students or in vocal or instrumental ensembles. This aspect of the project did not focus specifically on individual students who were in the System of Care. Rather, instruction was presented to students with the primary goal being to instill a feeling of accomplishment and success in their experience and ultimately to provide a positive activity that reinforced the self-worth for each individual.

The Delivery of Music Instruction in an Individualized Setting

Another component of the project involved private, individualized performance instruction. University student teachers, who were responsible for all aspects of instruction, were paired with public school students involved in the System of Care. A set of guidelines and a general timetable were presented to the university student teachers in an initial orientation. A mandatory weekly meeting was set aside for instruction, discussion, and collaboration with the university faculty. University student teachers also studied a musical instrument in a performance studies course, which was taught by a university faculty member during a weekly private lesson. Specific instructional approaches that could be used by the student teacher were role modeled by the university instructor and were a focus in each of the private lessons taught by the university professor.

University student teachers were responsible for the initial contact with the school teachers, parents, and public school students. A brochure describing the goals and objectives of the music instruction, along with an outline of teacher and parent/student responsibilities, was presented to each family. A business card was included in the material that listed the name of the student teacher, a telephone number, an e-mail address, and the location for the lesson. Those students who came to the university to take their lessons were given parking instructions and told that the student teacher would be waiting at the front door of the building. Before the initial lesson, the parents or caregivers, along with their child, were encouraged to attend a meeting at the university. Both public school teachers as well as family members were encouraged to attend the orientation. Held at the university, the family members and the students received a guided tour of the music building, were introduced to other students and faculty members, and visited the music library. Parents of students whose lessons were at the public school also were invited to the orientation. In those instances in which parents could not attend, the university student teachers met individually with parents either after school or in the home. In cases when the parent was unable to attend or participate in the orientation or the lessons, the school music teacher may have functioned in a supportive role as a substitute parent.

Weekly contact before the lesson and the follow-up after the lesson were also emphasized. The university student teachers determined the instructional time and setting; some lessons were taught at a school, whereas others were presented at the university. Some of the public school students who were participants in the System of Care program possessed neither instruments nor instructional materials; the university student teachers were required to resolve all of those issues to ensure that instruction could progress successfully. In several cases, individuals in the community donated instruments, and others were provided through local music stores. Music instructional materials were obtained from the schools, the university library, and even the university student teachers' and the university performance instructors' own collections.

Musical instruction was presented based on the four themes for learning: structure, readiness, motivation, and intuition. University student teachers structured lessons that focused on development of the fundamentals of music. After an initial assessment of a student's capacity for accepting instruction and the level of musical development, a weekly plan was developed to project outcomes. Adjustments before the lesson and during the instructional period were continual. Music instruction was presented at the appropriate level for the student's abilities. Musical concepts were presented either starting at the basic level or according to the background and experience of the student. Because some type of music is taught in virtually every elementary school, all students had some prior musical experience. The university student teacher was cognizant that early musical experience plays a significant role in how formalized instruction is perceived and progress occurs. Transfer of musical understanding from past experience played a central role in how the student accepted suggestion and instruction. Finally, every event in the lesson was designed to encourage the student toward individual achievement. The university student teacher planned and presented the lessons so that the student understood the concepts, could replicate the ideas and suggestions in practice sessions at home or school, and was confident and excited about what could be achieved.

In most cases, the university student teachers worked with the students for a set number of 13 to 16 weeks, corresponding to the traditional academic semester. Most of the instruction continued through the fall and spring semesters, although many of the students continued to study with the university student teacher through the summer months. Some students participated for 1 year, whereas others participated during the entire System of Care project (4 years). Opportunities were provided for students and their families to have free admission to university concerts and recitals, access to the library, invitations to participate in special events held on campus, the use of university practice and performance facilities, and other opportunities.

Collaborative Relationships: Children and Parents, Public School Music Teachers, University Faculty, and Student Teachers

Collaborative relationships with public school music teachers, students, parents, and the university professors and students were established at the beginning, which is another principle in the System of Care philosophic framework. Interdisciplinary collaborative relationships are essential to the Systems of Care framework. In the public school setting, the working team included the students, the parents, the music teachers, the public school administrators, the university faculty member, and the university student teachers.

Parents were involved in all lessons whenever possible, and the public school teachers were informed regularly about the progress of the students. When possible, university student teachers visited the students in the school and their homes by appointment. All instructional responsibilities were shouldered by the university student teacher in consultation with the teacher and counselor in the school, the university professor, and the parent or caregiver.

The Core Values as Applied to Music Instruction

The System of Care core values essential to the overall framework are family-centered, community-based, and culturally competent and were essential in the delivery of musical instruction to students in the project. Thus, the System of Care core values were embedded in the music instruction and were emphasized.

Interventions That Were Family Centered

The university student teachers focused on delivering instruction that involved the family. Parents or caregivers were invited and welcomed to the private lessons. Progress reports were delivered in person and in writing, and students were encouraged to present home demonstrations of their learning and musical accomplishments. The university student teachers emphasized to both parents and students the importance of the family spending time daily either making and/or listening to music together, even if only for a limited amount of time. As stated, to help establish positive and trusting relationships, the university student teachers visited the students and their parents in the home.

The university student teachers also communicated regularly with the music teachers in the schools where each music student was enrolled. The university student teacher shared with the public school teacher the student's acquisition of performance skills, issues of attendance and involvement, student attitudes, personal achievements, parental involvement, and other issues that came to their attention. Also, the public school teacher shared the student's progress within the context of the group or the ensemble. Reports of how each student was progressing were presented to the parents or caregivers by the student teacher.

Community-Based Interventions:
Integration of Technology into Music Instruction

Although the community focus was on the public schools, during the second year of the project, university teachers began to use technology for communicating with the students and to teach and reinforce musical concepts. The university student teacher helped each student, in consultation with the parent or caregiver, the teacher in the school, or the director of a community center or library, to identify a computer where the student could access the Internet. Some students were able to access computers in their homes, although most could not, and initially, schools and libraries were used.

During this phase of the project, the university student teachers helped the students to learn basic computer processes, including startup and accessing programs. In many instances, the university student teacher went to the setting or home in person to explain the basic technology needs for the music student and provide initial assistance. Every university student teacher worked with a music student and parents or caregivers during the process of acquiring and providing playback equipment that could be attached to the computer. In many instances, useable equipment was already located in the home, and only a connection was needed. For students who had access to a computer but no Internet service, free dial-up Web access was researched, and e-mail accounts were set up. The music students were asked to access e-mail every day to receive messages from the university student teacher and were asked to respond. The frequent daily communication between the university student teacher and the music student provided reinforcement of ideas and an avenue to motivate students to play, practice, and listen to music daily. Some of the students were unable to access music-specific programs at public sites because of policies prohibiting program installation. Others were unable to play their instruments in public sites to avoid disturbing other patrons. The use of computers, however, fostered a stronger link between the music student and university student teacher. Telephone contact was also a link to communication with students; however, the availability of telephone service, the student and teacher schedules, and the use of the telephone by other family members limited the frequency of contact.

The use of technology was significant in facilitating communication between the music student and the university student teacher and was particularly successful in motivating the students. During subsequent stages of the project, plans were developed (1) to identify computers and playback equipment that could be located in the music student's home where sound could be generated, and (2) to provide computer and playback access for the university student teacher to use during the lessons. Several corporations in the area were contacted to provide assistance. Many of the computers that were contributed had been replaced by newer models and typically would have been sold in large lots at a low cost. Also, individuals in the community who learned about project needs donated computers and playback equipment. The computers donated to the project were installed in the music students' homes. If the student did not have telephone access or Internet capability in the home, the computer was placed elsewhere but in a place where the student had personal access to the equipment. The donated computers and playback equipment ultimately became the property of the student and family. The computer and other equipment were set up in the home of the music student by the university student teacher.

To provide a portable accommodation for the university student teachers to use instructional technology in private lessons, a grant from the Advancement of Teaching and Learning at the University of

North Carolina at Greensboro was awarded to the project. The funding provided a laptop computer, playback equipment, a portable case securely containing all of the equipment, and the purchase of interactive music software. At this time, most lessons were taught at the university in a room that offered high-speed Internet access. For special presentations, the portable unit could be moved to any location and set up in moments. Specifically, the unit contained a laptop computer with the maximum amount of random access memory, a CD-ROM drive, a floppy disk drive, an expanded hard drive, an internal modem, and an Ethernet card. Attached were two high-quality, self-powered speakers that allowed playback without the use of an amplifier. Later in the project, a detachable CD burner was acquired. The primary software programs used were free, basic demonstration programs that were provided by software makers who developed highly sophisticated versions for purchase. Thus, identical programs could be installed on the student's home computer without copyright infringement. The software program purchased for use in the lessons included a microphone to capture the student's musical performance. The musical line captured by the computer then instantaneously generated the playback of a musical accompaniment that followed the tempo of the solo line using an early version of SmartMusic, produced by Coda Music, later renamed "Make Music!"

Because the interactive accompaniments were developed for students at every level from the most basic to the most advanced, all students could perform with a keyboard and, in some instances, a band, orchestra, or jazz ensemble accompaniment. This software was used only in the lesson, which motivated the student to play and practice the assigned music materials. Also, opportunities for students to play in a recital setting with accompaniment became a reality. Although not a component in the original plan, the integration of electronic technology into the project became a cohesive and essential factor in the musical achievement and personal success of many students.

Culturally Competent Education

The university student teachers were involved in discussions that focused on the best way to deliver instruction through a culturally competent approach. Many of the students in the project were members from diverse cultural populations. The university student teachers incorporated in their instruction elements that honored and celebrated the heritage of each student. Because music is a focus of many diverse cultures, instruction delivered by the university student teachers frequently deviated from traditional music materials and was developed with a focus on the performance level of the individual students, their interests in music, and music that reflected their backgrounds. Although the time required to develop relevant materials was substantial, highly individualized materials emphasized the importance of culturally relevant instruction to inspire and maintain success in creative activities.

Successes Celebrated and Challenges Resolved

Although success in this project was measured in a case-by-case subjective method, students, parents or caregivers, teachers, and others involved in the System of Care were included in frequent reviews. Data were gathered through structured personal interviews and by the administration of a written questionnaire that encouraged an open response to every item. A number of themes emerged that were common to the majority of students. The success of the project was confirmed at every phase. The data, however, were mostly anecdotal, and all were descriptive. None of the sample data was analyzed for statistical significance.

Successes Celebrated

1. Four themes provide a foundation for teaching and learning. The idea of using the four themes for learning (as described by Bruner, 1960), which include structure, readiness, motivation, and intuition, provided a consistent foundation for delivering musical instruction to students living in various outlying communities and to include culturally diverse students and special needs learners.

2. Instruction was organized to meet objectives. Success with students was based on organizing and focusing instruction on the following objectives: (1) acquiring knowledge, (2) developing skills, (3) fostering a positive attitude, and (4) acknowledging the importance of the aesthetic experience.

3. The ideal teaching ratio was one teacher to one student. Working with students in a one-to-one instructional setting proved to be an ideal teaching strategy. The music student was able to experience being center stage and the only person important during the private lesson. The music students consistently expressed surprise that so much effort had been devoted to their

musical instruction by their parents, university student teachers, the university professors, the public school teachers, and others within the System of Care. Although the instruction in larger groups and classes provided valuable musical experiences for public school students, the ability of the university student teacher to help the music student to develop, in terms of musical and personal achievements within the private instructional setting, cannot be underestimated.

4. Family-centered communication allowed learning from one another. Communication among parents or caregivers and the music students was enhanced substantially. Because the musical instruction was so different from typical school activities, parents and students often spoke about how they learned from one another. Because parents brought some students to the university, the time driving in the car, waiting for the lesson, and in some cases, sitting in the lesson became a valuable time for parent–child communication. Furthermore, as the achievement of the music students progressed, parents reacted by reinforcing the success through praise and encouragement. Parents rarely provided a negative critique. Infrequent conflicts between parents and music students were reported. The parents admired the music students for their accomplishments, and the students respected their parents because of the family's involvement in the student's musical learning. In instances where parents had little or no knowledge about operating a computer, the music student served in the role of the instructor to the parents. A number of responses indicated that the parents benefited substantially from learning to use the computer and, as in other areas, praised their son or daughter for the expertise that he or she had developed.

5. Success was transferred from music to other academic domains. Students who studied music did not drop out of school nor did they discontinue their interest in music performance and listening. Many students began to attend concerts and special musical events. Frequently, students who appeared initially to be uninterested in learning developed a more positive attitude toward school and homework. As observed by the public school teachers, many students were more dedicated to learning in classes other than music and were ultimately more successful. Several students assumed leadership roles in their school music

programs as well as in other school activities and organizations. Many of the more productive students ultimately enrolled in college, whereas others exhibited leadership skills in other areas.

6. Accommodation for special needs students provided opportunities for success. Special needs students were included in this project. All students had the opportunity for musical performance and creation expressions. Access to learning music required the learning environment to be tailored for learning modalities, learning disabilities, physiologic limitations, and other special needs. Whereas music instruction traditionally has been geared toward the elite, this project reinforced the fact that all students can receive the benefits from participation in creative experiences as long as instruction is understandable. Involvement in learning music does not only have to be restricted to listening, but also can involve students who have special needs in successful music performances. The project demonstrated that the successful accomplishments of special needs students cannot by underestimated.

7. Cultural competence was important. Delivering instruction through the use of a variety of materials that celebrate cultural diversity can be developed individually for students. Although traditional instructional materials are necessary, music and creative projects designed to enhance the student's cultural background can provide substantial motivation and promote self-worth. Although substantial time was required to develop individualized materials to meet the needs of special students, the university student teachers agreed that individualizing instruction was a primary factor in student success.

8. Technology was applied to musical instruction for special needs students. Although technology was not an initial component of the project, the integration of technology into the learning situation proved to be a foundation for student success. Not only were the musical objectives accomplished, but also skills, including writing effectiveness, reading comprehension, the ability to follow step-by-step instructions, and the capacity to maneuver within the complexities of the Internet and computer technology, were improved. Furthermore, parents and caregivers learned from the music students how to use the computer. The ability of the computer to provide a full range of accompaniments to musical performances allowed students to

demonstrate their progress in a satisfying musical presentation that could be experienced with peers, teachers, and family members. The successful music student performances that were reinforced and supported through the audience's responses appeared to have a sustaining effect on the student's progress.

9. Self-esteem and self-respect were enhanced. The study of music reinforced student independence, initiative, and personal achievement, which resulted in improved self-esteem. Students learned to organize and plan in a more effective manner. Many students demonstrated more of a focus on learning than had been observed previously. Furthermore, students experienced musical achievements that were replicated in other areas of learning, including academic studies, personal relationships, and family interactions.

10. Music education became a catalyst for growth and development. For many students in the project, the long-term nature of the instruction, the planning for accomplishments, and the realization of achievements proved to be a stimulus to maturity in their transition from adolescence into adulthood. Marginal academic students began to focus more on their studies and envision professional careers and prepare for their future. A sense of stability was generated among many of the music students because of music lessons that were consistent and predictable and that optimized their strengths. Using the values of the System of Care in teaching children with special needs fostered a positive attitude toward what they as individuals could achieve and fostered a feeling of importance and self-worth.

Challenges Addressed and Resolved

Although the successes in music instruction typically outweighed any difficulties encountered, specific challenges were addressed and resolved. The following areas at times impacted on the delivery of instruction.

1. Overcoming negative attitudes: Initial contact with students and parents did not elicit a positive reaction. Frequently, the parent and student assumed that the student was being identified because of some kind of failure at school. The fact that the musical instruction, some of the equipment, and teaching materials bore no costs or fees was viewed suspiciously and initially re-

jected by some of the parents or caregivers. Although students were less concerned with this aspect, parents were skeptical about enrolling in a project that was in essence a long-term contract. Both students and parents initially were reluctant to travel to the university, and in fact, many expressed their anxiety about going into the academic buildings. Both verbal and written communication methods were used to explain the project in an attempt to diminish the anxiety that both parents and students experienced. Students and parents always were greeted in a specific place, normally at the front entrance to the building. Detailed planning and attention by the university student teachers and faculty enabled the parents and students to feel comfortable in coming to the lessons that were held at the university. The instruction, always positive and nonconfrontational, was punctuated by follow-up and further reinforcement afterward.

2. Student attendance: One of the most difficult aspects of providing the instruction was ensuring that the students could or would actually attend. Initially, many students missed lessons and failed to notify the university student teachers. Telephone calls regarding an upcoming absence were rarely delivered to the university student teachers before the missed lesson. Issues of transportation were addressed in a variety of ways. To resolve this issue, some instruction was delivered at the student's school to avoid travel. Several transportation problems were addressed by moving the lesson time to a nontraditional hour that allowed both the parent and student to attend. A number of transportation issues were resolved through a combination of rearranging the teaching schedule and consulting public transportation alternatives. With the integration of technology and the implementation of the daily contact through e-mail, occurrences of a student missing a lesson without contact became rare.

3. Maintenance of the equipment: Although acquiring instruments, music materials, and computer/audio playback equipment was accomplished with support and enthusiasm, consistent attention was required to keep the systems functional. In fact, many home visits were required to solve technology or software issues. Some problems required the removal of the equipment for repair and, in some cases, replacement. The services of an instructional technology consultant were required on a consistent basis. The students, however, learned how the computer

functions and how to resolve basic kinds of issues. In some home situations, instruments, damaged by siblings and even the students themselves, required the services of a professional repair technician.

4. Scheduling conflicts: Schedule conflicts for university teachers because of their required curricular commitments had to be resolved. To assure week-to-week consistency, the university student teacher coordinated a long-range calendar with the student and parent. Special attention was devoted to consistent meetings with the music student for 13 to 16 weeks, roughly corresponding to an academic semester calendar. Contact during planned breaks was accomplished through only e-mail messages. Although ideally contact should have been continual, these periodic, planned interruptions in instruction did not appear to impede the student progress. The more significant factor, however, was the consistent weekly participation in lessons.

Summary

Music and the arts can be incorporated using a System of Care approach for educational interventions. Within the study of music, both performance and listening activities can be accomplished by individuals based on the System of Care core values. Individuals can become successful and productive through the study of arts and by participation in arts activities, which can build on the student's inherent strengths. Academic progress, personal relationships, family interactions, and other skills can all be impacted substantially through creative experiences in music and the arts. A teacher who is a specialist in the arts can present instruction to all students with special needs who may be participants in a System of Care program. An understanding of wraparound is essential, although knowledge about the specifics of each child's individual educational plans is not necessary. A teacher who has a basic idea of the themes in learning, structure, readiness, motivation, and intuition can design instructional sessions that can enable a student to succeed and feel successful. As well, structuring the learning experiences through the four objectives—acquisition of knowledge, development of skills, fostering a positive attitude, and enhancing aesthetic experiences—can be used in the instruction of music and other creative arts.

Activities to Extend Your Learning

■ Observe a music or arts class that includes a student within a System of Care.
  ■ Does the learner appear to be involved in the activities?
  ■ Does the individual appear to be confident with his or her artistic abilities?
  ■ Does the teacher provide instruction that involves the student and that is at the level of the learner?
  ■ Does the session involve observation or active participation, and to which does the learner respond best?
  ■ Can you envision yourself as the instructor in the class including individuals within the System of Care?
  ■ Identify some strategies that may be appropriate to the successful delivery of arts instruction in the class.
  ■ How would you convince others who work in the wraparound concept the value of arts instruction for students within the System of Care?

■ Observe an arts activities class that includess primarily students who have special needs.
  ■ How do the students respond to the artistic instruction or stimuli?
  ■ Does the instructor approach the special needs students any differently?
  ■ Are the students who have special needs involved and motivated?
  ■ Are there other approaches or activities that might be used to enhance the understanding and productivity of the students?
  ■ Discuss ways in which children with special needs can participate in arts activities.

■ Understand the four themes for learning
  ■ Discuss your understanding of how the four themes of learning can be used within the System of Care.
  ■ Observe students in a learning situation within an arts area to determine whether the four themes of learning are integrated into the instruction or activity.
  ■ Of the four themes, is there one that you believe is more appropriate for instruction in your particular area?

Suggested Reading

Abeles, H.F., Hoffer, C.R., & Klotman, R.H. (1994). *Foundations of music education* (2nd ed.). New York: McGraw Hill-Schirmer Books.

Anderson, W., & Campbell, P.S. (2001). *Multicultural perspectives in music education* (2nd ed.). Reston, VA: Music Educators National Conference.

Bruner, J.S. (1966). *Toward a theory of instruction.* Cambridge, MA: Harvard University Press.

Campbell, P.S. (2001). *Lessons from the world: A cross-cultural guide to teaching music and learning.* New York: McGraw Hill-Schirmer Books.

Campbell, P.S., & Scott-Kassner, C. (1995). *Music in childhood: From preschool through the elementary grades.* New York: McGraw Hill-Schirmer Books.

Durerksen, G.L., & Darrow, A. (1991). Music class for the at-risk: A music therapist's perspective. *Music Educators Journal, 78*(3), 46–50.

Ebie, B.D. (1998). Can music help? A qualitative investigation of two music educators' views on the role of music in the lives of at-risk children. *Contributions to Music Education, 2*(2), 63–78.

Ellis, P. (1996). Layered analysis: A video-based qualitative research tool to support the development of a new approach for children with special needs. *Bulletin of the Council for Research in Music Education, 30*(1), 65–74.

Erwin, J.H., Edwards, K.L., Kerchner, J.L., & Knight, J.W. (2003). *Prelude to music education.* Upper Saddle River, NJ: Prentice-Hall.

Gardner, H. (1985). *Frames of mind: Theory of multiple intelligences.* Boston: Basic Books.

Gorrasi, P. (1996). Talents for success. *Momentum, 27,* 36–37.

Hinckley, J. (1999). Best self forward. *Music Educators Journal, 86*(2), 6–7.

Kohut, D.L. (1973). *Instrumental music pedagogy.* Englewood Cliffs, NJ: Prentice-Hall.

Kuhn, T.L. (1975). The effect of teacher approval and disapproval on attentiveness, musical achievement, and attitude of fifth-grade students. In C.K. Madsen, R.D. Greer, & C.H. Madsen (Eds.), *Research in music behavior* (pp. 40–48). New York: Teachers College Press.

Mark, M.L. (1996). *Contemporary music education* (3rd ed.). New York: McGraw Hill-Schirmer Books.

Morado, D., Koenig, R., & Wilson, A. (1999). Miniperformances, many stars! Playing with stories. *The Reading Teacher, 53*(2), 116–123.

Rosenthal, J.S. (Ed.). (1978). *Ideas for kids: A multi-arts approach to fostering creativity.* New Haven, CT: Area Cooperative Educational Services/Connecticut State Department of Education.

Scripp, L., & Meyaard, J. (1991). Encouraging musical risks for learning success. *Music Educators Journal, 78*(3), 36–41.

Shuler, S.C. (1991). Music, at-risk students, and the missing piece. *Music Educators Journal, 78*(3), 21–29.

Smith, D.S., & Wilson, B.A. (1999). Effects of field experience on graduate music educators' attitude toward teaching students with disabilities. *Contributions to Music Education, 26*(1), 33–49.

Wiggins, J. (2001). *Teaching for musical understanding.* New York: McGraw Hill-Schirmer Books.

References

Bruner, J.S. (1960). *The process of education.* Cambridge, MA: Harvard University Press.

Huber, D.L. (2000). The diversity of case management models. *Lippincott's Case Management, 7*(6), 212–220.

Thomas, R.B. (n.d.). *Manhattanville music curriculum project synthesis.* Bardonia, NY: Media Materials, Inc.

Chapter 14

Professional Development Using a System of Care Framework: The Journey to Working with Families

Sarah Moore Shoffner

Objectives

- Identify one's own values, strengths, and professional skills to prepare to work with families.
- Develop skills in planning and preparation in job seeking in cross-cultural settings.
- Interpret core values and principles in the System of Care/wraparound process and how they may be applied in community service settings.
- Prepare for a supervised professional experience and secure an interdisciplinary internship.

Using System of Care principles and values to guide their education and practice, students as preprofessionals are beginning the journey to becoming professionals who will work with families in many settings in the human services arena. Three major aspects of preparation for the preprofessional's journey include professional orientation, development of an understanding of system of care concepts, and a supervised professional experience—preferably one that is interdisciplinary in focus. In preparing yourself as a professional, your goal is to focus on learning System of Care content, having skill development, and identifying your personal values and strengths as you prepare to work with families.

When planning for careers in human services as child- and family-serving professionals, you begin your journey by identifying your own values, strengths, and professional skills. During a period of professional orientation, you learn the philosophy and practice of the system of care process and continue to learn by applying the principles in interdisciplinary family-centered, strength-based internships. The ultimate goal is to learn the core values and principles of system of care. Before entering the workforce, you want to have enough experiences through case studies and internship experiences to understand an agency's ability to deliver services that are family-centered, community-based, and culturally competent. Using services for families/children at risk as examples, this approach will prepare professionals to work in partnerships with families and to participate in interdisciplinary teams in a variety of settings, serving children and their families.

Professional Orientation

Professional Analysis: Preparing Oneself

Professional preparation, in itself, is a process. Examining your own needs and your own value system is an important starting point if soon you are to work with families in determining their own values and needs. Also, your preparation will include identifying your interests and skills, learning about career opportunities in your field, developing professional commitment, and honing your job-seeking skills.

Needs, Wants, Values, and Goals

Begin your journey to becoming the professional of your dreams by examining your needs, wants, and goals. Examine important values in your personal and work lives and your work ethic. What are the core values that make you who you are? What describes your wants and how you might work as a professional? How many of these core values might describe you (Michelozzi, Surrell, & Cobez, 2004, p. 33)? (See Table 14-1.)

Table 14-1	Selecting Core and Career Values

Core Values—The Ones That Make You Who You Are

achievement	balance	belonging
commitment	contribution	environmental awareness
family	honesty	independence
integrity	knowledge	power
self-respect	spirituality	status

Values Important to You in Your Career

adventurousness	advocacy	aesthetically pleasing
analytical	autonomous	benefits
caring	challenging	competitive
conceptualizing	cooperation	creative
decision making	detailed	diversity
excitement	fast-paced	flexible
friendships	fun	harmony
helping	high earnings	individualism
initiating	leadership	leading edge
learning	loyalty	management
open communication	organizing	physical
predictable	problem solving	public contact
quiet	recognition	relaxed
research	risk taking	security
sense of community	structured	support
teamwork	time freedom	trust
variety		

Adapted from Michelozzi et al. (2004, pp. 33–34).

How many of the values in Table 14-1 are important to consider in your career (Michelozzi et al., 2004)? As a starter, choose your top 10.

What you may want to achieve as a professional is different from anyone else's career path. Your goal for learning to work with families is to prepare yourself to help them to achieve success. To succeed yourself is not enough—others whom you influence must be successful as well. That phrase can be your motto along your professional development journey.

Identification of Interests and Skills

Your goal will be to develop professionally so that you can motivate, enhance, and facilitate others' opportunities for success. Think about who you are and where you are going ("growing") in the career search process. Getting thoroughly involved in your career choice process will help you to experience new confidence and greater clarity in defining your goals. Begin the process by examining the interests and skills that you have developed through your lifetime of choices. These choices indicate a pattern of strong interests. Analyze your personality type and whether you prefer to work mainly with data, people, or things. Michelozzi et al. (2004) have identified a list of skills to help students to identify their own skills/strengths. Table 14-2 includes some that relate to a human services worker.

Identify the skills that have motivated you in the past, your competencies that you enjoy using—these are the skills that you will want as a major part of your work in the future.

Career Development: Opportunities/Alternatives

Studying about System of Care and how to work in interdisciplinary settings in the classroom is certainly valuable, but getting out into the work world and exploring career opportunities are also necessary components in career development. Reading and discussing with peers

Table 14-2	Skills for the Professional	
Professional Skills: Which Ones Are Your Strengths?		
act as liaison	analyze	communicate
coach	compare	compile
conceptualize	construct	coordinate
counsel	decide	direct
encourage	evaluate	explain
facilitate	illustrate	influence
innovate	interview	lead
learn	listen	manage
mediate	mentor	motivate
negotiate	organize	perform
persuade	plan	process
program	record	represent
research	schedule	set up
stimulate	supervise	teach
troubleshoot	visualize	write

Adapted from Michelozzi et al. (2004, p. 64).

take you to a basic level of learning. Interviewing and observing professionals on the job bring you the knowledge gained from real-life experiences and take you further along in your professional development—your journey to becoming a successful service provider.

The *informational interview* is an opportunity to spend time with a professional who is working in a career field that is of interest to you. By talking with someone already in the field, you will acquire practical career information and expand your professional network. Most professionals enjoy talking to students about their experiences. It also enhances your interviewing skills through the meeting and interviewing of a "stranger." However, remember that this activity is not an employment interview! Information interviews are just to receive information; however, they may provide you with possibilities for a future internship, part-time work, or volunteer experience. This activity is also a way to identify potential internship sites (see the Activities to Extend Your Learning section).

Once you have determined a job area that really piques your interest, you may want to explore it more in depth and find out more details than were evident in the informational interview. Doing a *career analysis* is one method for gaining even more information (Table 14-3).

Table 14-3   **Career Analysis: What to Explore**

- Job description, including responsibilities of a person in the position
- Desired personal characteristics
- Specific courses/training needed in addition to knowledge of System of Care values and principles
- Career possibility—chances for getting that job and location
- Related career opportunities within the agency or possibilities for transfer or use of skills in another business/agency
- Advantages—good points about the job
- Disadvantages
- Professional qualifications, including certifications such as CPR and behavior management techniques
- Professional enrichment opportunities—ways to stay involved in your profession through this career area
- Creating opportunities—ways to get a job in the area

Adapted from Shoffner (2004, Section 9).

Establishing *professional relationships with peers and practicing professionals* is yet another area of importance to your career development journey. Joining professional organizations and attending professional meetings are viable strategies to use in developing these relationships as you widen your knowledge of the "community context" of your potential work areas (Sweitzer & King, 2004). In human service delivery, professionals learn to focus on strengths of families in a community-based framework. Conducting a community inventory or analysis focusing not on deficits but on strengths, assets, or human capital is a way to "get to know something about the people in the community, their social and emotional needs, and their strengths" (Sweitzer & King, p. 160). Everything that you learn about a community will be valuable to you professionally and in your work in helping families solve their problems.

Professional Development and Commitment

As a professional (and personally for you as an individual), you will need to *develop the habit and skills of reflection*. As a professional, reflection becomes a fundamental concept in your experiential education. Sweitzer and King (2004, p. 9) supported the importance of reflection in this statement: "In order to turn your experience into learning you need to stop, recall events, analyze and process them." Furthermore, they stated that "reflection is what connects and integrates the service, or the work in the field, to the learning." Without reflection, theories learned in class may not necessarily be integrated with the field or real-world experience. Likewise, at the other extreme, the practical experiences are left to stand on their own. Reflection, then, is "a powerful key to your success, your growth, your learning, and even your transformation" (Sweitzer & King).

Actually, we reflect all of the time in informal ways. You are reflecting when you mull over a conversation that you had with someone, try to figure out what happened in a particular situation, or analyze how you could have handled an interaction differently. These are instances of spontaneous reflection. However, reflection should be deliberate and become a habit for professionals.

Keeping a journal is a powerful tool for reflection. Even if you are not required to keep a journal in a class or in an internship program, it is strongly recommended that you do so. Journal keeping is a way to see yourself grow and change. It is also a structured way for you to take time on a regular basis to reflect on your experiences. In the long run, a journal could become a part of your portfolio that presents your professional experiences and skills as well as a record of your journey. For journaling, Sweitzer and King (2004) suggested that it "may be helpful to divide what you learn at an internship into four categories: (a) knowledge, (b) skills, (c) personal growth, and (d) career development" (p. 11). Although at times you may think writing is difficult, considering some key questions may stimulate your thoughts (see the Activities to Extend Your Learning section).

Job-seeking Skills

After you have assessed your needs, wants, values, and interests as a process of self-understanding, you will be ready to identify some strategies and tactics to enhance the internship- and job-seeking processes. *Networking* is talking to people to get information and to broaden your circle of contacts and acquaintances. It is not asking for a job. However, networking "implies that you are using various contacts, including those acquired while information hunting, to find out about job openings" (Michelozzi et al., 2004, p. 213). What can you gain by networking? Here are some outcomes: increased visibility, information about an agency/company, advice about "fit," educational and certification requirements, feedback on a resume, names of referrals, interview practice, clarified goals and focus, and momentum and enthusiasm. The "who should you contact" list includes anyone you know who has some relationship to what you want to do. Other than professionals actually working in your chosen area, it could be family, friends, neighbors, faculty, and alumni. (See the Activities to Extend Your Learning section.)

Resume development is another job-seeking skill. You will want your resume to create a positive image highlighting the important things that you have done in your academic and professional experiences. It is a summary of your information and serves as a source for questions that may be asked during an interview. Invest time in preparing your resume, remembering that several revisions will be needed. Invite feedback from friends and professionals and ask them to critique it. Next, edit the resume to ensure that it is easy to read and best represents you. (Refer to the Activities to Extend Your Learning for resume guidelines section.)

Many professionals would advise you to prepare an answer to the most frequently asked question in interview situations, "Tell me something about yourself" (Michelozzi et al., 2004, p. 251). Seldom will you have a better opportunity than this to talk about yourself and your preparations for working in a System of Care setting. Having thought about these areas in a clear, concrete, and concise way will prepare you for the "big question." Include reasons why your background, attitudes, skills, and experiences would be suitable for a particular job area and how you see your future with a particular agency. These statements, sometimes called the *30-second commercial*, need to be well planned and concise. Rarely would one have to respond in such a short time, but having planned a succinct response may mean that you will give the important information without rambling. This in itself will make a good impression. (See the 30-second commercial in the Activities to Extend Your Learning section.)

System of Care Content

Beginning with a comparison of traditional service delivery versus wraparound services or System of Care can provide you with a framework for studying basic System of Care content. You can then focus on your professional competence in developing the skills to provide services and apply System of Care concepts in your work with children and families. Several key elements that provide a background for your study of the System of Care basic principles are outlined in Table 14-4 (see Chapters 1 and 2 for a review). While considering these elements, remember that change is often slow and difficult, and we know that adopting these principles into service delivery has been challenging in traditional service delivery agencies. This approach may seem like the common sense way, but families and service providers have to learn new ways of solving problems and change their behaviors accordingly. Your challenge will be to learn the System of Care/ Wraparound process so that you can become the "change agent" for and with families. (Review Chapter 2.)

Although learning System of Care content can be approached in several ways, there are basic principles that every professional must know and be able to apply in working with families. These three core values are the basis for all systems of care: Services are family-centered, community-based, and culturally competent.

Services Are Family Centered

"The System of Care should be child-centered and family-focused, with the needs of the child and family being of primary importance and dictating the types and mix of services provided" (adapted from Stroul, 1996). (Refer to Chapters 1 and 2 for a more in-depth review.)

Table 14-4	Comparison of Traditional and Wraparound Services

Traditional (Categorical)	*vs.*	*Wraparound (System of Care)*
Families are passive recipients of services.	vs.	Families have a "voice" in what happens to them.
Services are not individualized to the child's needs; they are aimed only at children.	vs.	Specific services are tailored to meet the specific needs of children and families.
If the child has multiple needs, he or she is moved from service to service; services are not coordinated with each other.	vs.	Services are based in the community and are coordinated with each other; no overlap and no gaps exist in service.
Focus is on problems of child/ family and blame; professionals treat patients as "clients."	vs.	Focus is on the strengths of the child/family, empowerment, family-centered collaborative partnership, interdisciplinary team (not clients), and cultural sensitivity.

Adapted from Stroul (1996) and VanDenBerg and Grealish (1996).

Professionals need to acquire skills to invite family members to take an active role in deciding how needs are to be met. As allies, they become partners in the change process with the professional, or change agent. Professionals plan with the families to identify their own strengths, goals, needs, and strategies. The professional should make a strong effort on identifying and building on strengths for a positive outcome, rather than focusing on how to fix problems. The professional must make a commitment to unconditional care; therefore, when things do not go as planned and plans need to be altered, services are not stopped, but they are changed, facilitated by the professional who remains by the family's side through thick and thin.

Why should professionals partner with families? There are benefits for the child/family as well as for the professionals in the delivery system. Parents (Douglas & Jones, 2001) said that "everyone wins" in this system, and they listed several benefits for the child/family (explained previously in Chapters 1 and 2), along with the benefits that they perceived as important for the professional and others working in a delivery system (Table 14-5).

"Families want to be partners with the system . . . not advisers" (Douglas & Jones, 2001). They believe that both parents and professionals are experts who work together. As these working relationships develop, parents feel that they have power with the system rather than professionals having power over the families.

Services Are Community Based

The System of Care should be community-based, with the locus of services as well as management and decision-making responsibility resting at the community level (adapted from Stroul, 1996). Professionals need to become familiar with the community. Communities provide less structure for the professional than do large institutions, and thus, the professional must be self-directed, creative, and resourceful to use the community resources to meet the complex needs of children and families. Whenever possible, families need to be surrounded with the supports that they need so that children can be kept in their own homes, in school, and out of trouble. One of the values of System of Care is to use family and community strengths, and thus, it is important to include neighbors, family friends, and other informal resources in the treatment process as well as social workers, teach-

Table 14-5	Benefits from System of Care for the Professional/Service Providers

- It helps to make services better—family-centered and family-friendly.
- It improves the quality of services.
- The child and family have better outcomes when involved.
- Families' involvement increases professionals' appreciation for diversity.
- Professionals gain perspective from families about service design and delivery as well as gaps and barriers in service.
- It develops an avenue for positive working partnerships and a continued effort to make system changes.
- Professionals gain new ideas about solutions.

Adapted from Douglas and Jones, 2001.

ers, and mental health professionals, all of whom can serve as advocates for the child and family.

Services Are Culturally Competent

Being culturally competent refers to the professional and all other entities involved in the process. "The system of care should be culturally competent, with agencies, programs, and services that are responsive to the cultural, racial, and ethnic differences of the population they serve" (adapted from Stroul, 1996). What is culture? Although the answer can start with a simple definition, becoming cultural competent is more complex because it involves so many areas of culture. A definition of a culture can begin with the skills, behaviors, arts, habits, customs, and so forth, of a given people. Culture shapes how people experience their world and determines their way of thinking and of doing. It can also be defined as the shared values, traditions, norms, customs, arts, history, folklore, and institutions of a group of people. Culture is determined not only by ethnicity and race, but also by factors such as geography, age, religion, gender, sexual orientation, disability, and socioeconomic status. Decisions on quality of work, family life, and how one relates to others are determined in part by culture.

What, then, is cultural competence for the professional? The answer to this question is not simple, either. Acquiring cultural competence begins with a careful look inside yourself and moves to the acquisition of the skills necessary to work effectively in cross-cultural situations. It is the ability to "learn from and relate respectfully with people of your own culture as well as those from other cultures." It includes "adjusting your own and your organization's behaviors based on what you learn. Cultural competence is not something you master once and then forget. It is a lifelong journey" (Dean, 2000, p. 136).

A definition of cultural competence for the professional is about developing "the ability to think, feel, and act in ways that acknowledge, respect, and build upon ethnic, socio-cultural, and linguistic diversity" in order to work effectively with members of different groups. It does not mean changing others to become more like you. However, it does mean "exploring and honoring your own culture, while at the same time learning about and honoring other people's cultures" (Dean, 2000, p. 136).

As a professional, you will strive to accomplish the knowledge and skills that will enable you to accomplish these overall cultural competence objectives as you work with families:

- To feel comfortable and effective in the interactions and relationships with families whose culture and life experiences differ from those in your background
- To interact in ways that enable families from different cultures and life experiences to feel positive about the interactions and the providers who are working with them
- To accomplish the goals that each family and its provider establish

In addition to focusing on these objectives, you will strive to use techniques that will allow you to reach beyond traditional service delivery practices. Recognize differences in families' languages, backgrounds, and values. This information will be valuable in enhancing your effectiveness as a service provider.

One can learn many techniques; however, your perspective, as a service provider, is a key element in cultural competency. Two perspectives are often used to describe how professionals may perceive the persons with whom they work. The one-way mirror view is seeing everything from our own view of our experiences and our culture. The other perspective is described as getting to the other side of the glass, a position that allows you to see clearly and imagine, but not really know, what it is like for the other person. You may ask, "How can I get to the other side of the glass?" The process involves finding information and using techniques that will help you understand others (Table 14-6).

Achieving cultural competence can become more manageable if you look at the process in three steps: self-awareness, cultural-specific awareness and understanding, and differences in communication among cultures. The first step, self-awareness, may be the hardest but will move you toward competence in achieving the other steps and in working with families from different cultures.

Self-awareness begins with understanding and appreciating your own culture. To do so, begin by examining some of the values, behaviors, beliefs, and customs identified with your cultural heritage. As a part of self-awareness, it helps to recognize the dominant values that characterize your own culture as compared with those in other cultures. In doing so, remember that any one or the other is not right or wrong, only different. Eight values of the dominant American culture have been identified (Lynch, 1992, p. 38):

- Importance of individualism and privacy
- Belief in the equality of all individuals

Table 14-6	Striving for Cultural Competence: How Do You Get There?

- Research as much as you can find about cultural differences—read, study, and ask questions of people who are different from you.
- Imagine what it is like for others.
- Empathize—put yourself in another person's place. This is hard because you never really know, but it is much better than not trying at all. This quotation is offered as our guide: "We cannot put ourselves in someone else's shoes; or rather we can, but it's still our own feet we will feel" (J. Claes, personal communication, March 1, 2001).

- Informality in interactions with others
- Emphasis on the future, change, and progress
- Belief in the general good of humanity
- Emphasis on importance of time and punctuality
- High regard for achievement, action, work, and materialism
- Pride in interaction styles that are direct and assertive

Comparisons of these dominant values with values in other cultures lead one to a greater understanding of cultural competence. Comparing common values among groups is another way to understand yourself and others with whom you may work better. Table 14-7 shows a comparison of 22 common values between Anglo Americans and other ethnocultural groups.

The second step, *cultural-specific awareness and understanding*, is learning to explain values, beliefs, and behaviors of a given cultural group. You can choose among many activities in your attempt to be aware of others' choices and to understand their behavior. Read and study—learn through books, art, and technology. Have discussions—talk and work with individuals from the culture who can act as cultural guides or mediators. Get involved—participate in the daily lives of people from another culture. Learn a language. Probably this age-old wisdom will serve you well: "stop, look, and listen." You will need a range of skills in working with families: patience, compassion, and an understanding of the role culture plays in shaping families' decisions. Furthermore, if you are working with immigrant families, you will need the ability to speak or learn another language as well as having information about services available specific to immigrant populations (i.e., English as a second language and citizenship classes and job training).

Table 14-7   Comparison of Common Values

Anglo American	vs.	Other Ethnocultural Groups
Mastery over nature	vs.	Harmony with nature
Personal control over the environment	vs.	Fate
Doing . . . activity	vs.	Being
Time and punctuality dominate	vs.	Personal interaction dominates
Human equality	vs.	Hierarchy/rank/status
Individualism/privacy	vs.	Group welfare
Youth	vs.	Elders
Self-help	vs.	Birthright inheritance
Competition	vs.	Cooperation
Future orientation	vs.	Past or present orientation
Informality	vs.	Formality
Directness/openness/honesty	vs.	Indirectness/ritual/"face"
Practicality/Efficiency	vs.	Idealism
Materialism	vs.	Spiritualism/detachment
Small unit families with little reliance on extended family	vs.	Extended family and kinship networks
Individuality	vs.	Interdependence
Independence of young children	vs.	Nurturance of young children
Time is measured	vs.	Time is given
Emphasis on youth, future, and technology	vs.	Respect for age, ritual, and tradition
Ownership—individual and specific	vs.	Ownership defined in broad terms
Equal rights and responsibilities	vs.	Differentiated rights and responsibilities
Control	vs.	Harmony

Developed from various sources in the System of Care, cultural competence literature (Isaacs-Shockley, Cross, Bazron, Dennis, & Benjamin, 1996; Lynch, 1992).

Understanding *differences in communications among cultures* or acquiring *culturally competent communication skills* is the third step in the cultural competence process. It is recognizing that cultures differ in the amount of information explicitly transmitted through words and paying attention to what you hear and see through body language—again, "stop, look, and listen." Develop strategies to improve cross-cultural communication, including working with interpreters and translators. Also, a part of this process is to understand the potential for miscommunication by learning about high-context versus low-context cultures.

Communication in high-context cultures (such as Asian, Native American, African American, Latino, and Arab) tends to be less verbal than in low-context cultures. It is very important to understand nonverbal communication, particularly the meanings associated with eye contact, facial expressions, proximity, touching, body language, and gestures. Communications in these cultures are more formal, relying on hierarchies that are likely rooted in the past.

In low-context cultures, such as Anglo American, Swiss, German, and Scandinavian, verbal communication is precise, direct, and logical. Often people are impatient when others do not understand the point quickly. Also, communicators from low-context cultures may not process or correctly interpret gestures, environmental cues, and unarticulated moods, all of which are important to understand fully the messages in cross-cultural interactions.

As preprofessionals or new professionals, you can work toward becoming culturally competent communicators by developing cross-cultural communication strategies. Learn the differences in how people communicate in high- and low-context cultures. Look for the indicators of nonverbal communication: eye contact, proximity and touching, body language, and gestures. Listen to the family's perspective, always acknowledging the differences rather and minimizing them. You may find that working with interpreters and translators is an important step early in your learning process.

In your goal to develop effective overall behaviors to cultural competence, three overarching words—remember, listen, and respect— can serve as reminder guidelines. Also, they can be used to summarize one's overall behavior to cultural competence:

- Remember the core values (needs of child and family first, community-based services, and culturally competent services).
- Listen, listen to the family's perspective.
- Respect, respect, respect the family's cultural differences.

This segment of the poem *"On Caring"* by Milton Mayeroff (1971, pp. 30–31) explained cultural competence well in showing what we must be able to do if we are to work with others in culturally competent ways:

To care for another person
I must be able to understand
them and their world, as if I
were inside it.

I must be able to see, as it were,
with their eyes what their world
is like to them and how they
see themselves.
I must be able to be with them in
their world, going into their world
in order to sense from inside what
life is like for them,
what they are striving to be,
and what they require to grow.

Supervised Professional Experiences

Internships provide opportunities for students to "become" professionals (Shoffner, 2000). The internship, or supervised professional experience, is a critical stepping stone to your professional success. It is a vital learning experience in the journey to becoming a professional who will work on interdisciplinary teams in providing strength-based care. Good internships are prized by today's college students and offer an opportunity to test your interests, develop new strengths, and learn of opportunities and career paths. They are increasingly popular with employers, too. For many agencies, the internship is an effective source of new recruits.

The overall objectives of an internship are for the student (intern) to experience firsthand the scope of the job; to develop further communication skills, subject matter mastery, and problem solving; and to evaluate the needs relative to career aspirations. As an intern, you will want to understand how to create a quality internship and recognize its potential. It is essential that you have a learning plan that will translate your learning objectives into action. For you to make the most of the internship, it is recommended that this plan include objectives (written in behavioral terms), actions planned to achieve these objectives, indicators of achievement, and self-evaluations. Sweitzer and King (2004) encouraged a "balance between learning and contributing in a supervised setting" and noted that "interpersonal relationships, reflection, self-understanding, and feedback are essential factors in creating that balance" (p. xiii).

One student intern (Allen, 2004) described how the internship supported the application of skills and knowledge from the major field of study as well as how knowledge from System of Care was so important to serving an agency's clients.

Working within the human service field demands that one have an appreciation for diversity as we serve a diverse population of individuals. Having an appreciation for diversity also helps us to avoid judging others by the standards that we live by in our own lives. While similar in some respects, clients come from different walks of life and we, as human service workers, need to be cognizant of the differences that exist among the people we serve. While their troubles may be alike in some respects, it is important to consider each situation and make decisions accordingly. My work at the Women's Resource Center has required that I be empathetic and open-minded toward others, as well as accepting of others no matter what their problems or life experiences might be.

In addition, the work that I do has forced me to confront my own prejudices. Working with clients who come from backgrounds of poverty and unemployment has caused me to consider some of the attitudes or stereotypes that we, as a society, hold about individuals in these situations. What I have found, for the most part, is that these individuals want to overcome the challenges that they face in life and have an opportunity to live as self-sufficient people in society.

A large part of working with others revolves around the ability to be an effective communicator, and a team player. It also involves the ability to problem-solve and to use critical thinking. These are all skills which have been reinforced during my educational experience and these skills have helped me tremendously in the work that I have been doing at Women's Resource Center. Not only have I spent time talking with clients in order to determine the best way in which to meet their immediate needs, but a portion of my time has been spent communicating with other staff members, interns, or volunteers. Participating in the evaluation of programs has allowed me the opportunity to see firsthand the need for such programs in our community. In addition, it has given me the chance to consider additional ways in which to meet the needs of our clients. (Allen, 2004, pp. 5–6)

Interdisciplinary internships and seminars for the preprofessional are extremely valuable learning experiences in the overall journey to becoming service providers in a variety of settings operating within the System of Care process. The goal of the interdisciplinary field experience is to provide students with an opportunity to be active participants on an interdisciplinary team. Arbuckle et al. (2000) identified ways that students learn in such interdisciplinary settings (pp. 8–9). Interns have the opportunity to

- Learn the disciplinary perspective of other professionals on the team.

- Evaluate the effectiveness of contrasting practice theories of the various disciplines.
- Understand the methods and techniques for dealing with strengths and problems from the various disciplinary perspectives.
- Integrate research findings from interns' own and other disciplines with practice.
- Learn collaborative techniques with persons from other disciplines on behalf of children and families.
- Express findings and conclusions in an integrated statement that summarizes issues from the various disciplinary perspectives.
- Use the research findings of various disciplines to determine the utility of alternative intervention approaches.
- Learn how to work as a member of an interdisciplinary team.
- Evaluate participation in the interdisciplinary effort and the strengths and weaknesses of the effort.
- Understand the mandate, structure, and operation of the agencies, schools, or programs represented on the team, and their interorganizational relationships.
- Identify and assess strengths and problems based on their disciplinary perspective.
- Interpret the role of a team member to other professionals and members of the community.

An interdisciplinary field placement is an educational experience for students to gain understanding about how community support systems are changing to meet the needs of families through a System of Care approach (wraparound process) (VanDenBerg & Grealish, 1996). The program goal is to facilitate the training of child and family-serving professionals in the philosophy and practice of the System of Care model. Experiences with an interdisciplinary team of students, faculty, and agency personnel, cooperating in a semester-long effort, is shown in Table 14-8. (This interdisciplinary experience is described from the nursing perspective in Chapter 6.)

Furthermore, one might ask, "What is the value of being on an interdisciplinary team combined with team study/process groups and seminars with agency supervisors, faculty, and interns all participating in the effort?" Active interdisciplinary teams become professional support groups if they meet periodically, outside of the internship setting. The purpose of these meetings is to "provide an opportunity for students and [System of Care] field supervisors/preceptors and faculty liaisons to collectively reflect on the strengths and challenges

Table 14-8	Internship with a System of Care Interdisciplinary Field Team

Agency Setting—Long-term residential facility in the community for mothers who are recovering substance abusers and their children.

Participating Academic Departments—Human development and family studies, nursing, social work, public health, and therapeutic recreation.

Five Interns—Members of the interdisciplinary team, majors from the five participating departments, worked with the mothers and their children. Team members shared their objectives and special projects as they defined their roles.

Training/Process Groups—Training for the interdisciplinary placement began with participation in coursework in the respective student's department that included System of Care curriculum infusion in three areas: cultural competence, family participation, and interdisciplinary collaboration. Throughout the placement period, faculty members who supervised the students met with them in group seminars to discuss the agency-field experiences, interdisciplinary teams, individualized service plans, and assigned readings. Topics included individualized services and supports through the wraparound process (Betz, 1997; Lourie, Stroul, & Friedman, 1998), substance abuse/addiction from an interdisciplinary perspective, treatment issues for alcohol- and drug-dependent pregnant and parenting women (Finklestein, 1994; Wald, Harvey, & Hibbard, 1995), development of cross-cultural competence (McIntosh, 1990; Pinderhughes, 1996), strength-based assessment in another culture that may have different values, family–professional relationships (Adams, Bliss, Mohammad, Meyers, & Slaton, 1997), and success and barriers to working in teams (Anderson, 1993). Also, students learned the purpose, process, and interorganizational relationships for the child and family team meetings that included family members and a variety of community-based representatives, such as schools, agencies, or programs.

Outcomes—The interdisciplinary team approach was beneficial for both students and clients.
- The team provided clients (mothers/children) with a more structured environment and fostered better interpersonal communication than single-service models.
- Students benefited from the interaction and support of the representatives from each discipline and approached problems more holistically.
- Students practiced flexibility and learned that "my way" is not the "only way" when partnering with "all" of the team members, which resulted in serving these families more effectively.

Developed from Cohort of Interns (2000).

of the System of Care placement" (Arbuckle et al., 2000, p. 10). This group of participants collectively reflected on relevant readings and research findings, identified the strengths and barriers to interdisciplinary work, solved problems, and identified interdisciplinary strategies to address issues relating to interdisciplinary placements. A cohort of students who participated in this interdisciplinary experience described the value of the interdisciplinary experience (presented in Table 14-8). They shared their experiences in a written evaluation, as well as processing their ideas in a team meeting. Their comments (Cohort of Interns, 2000) provide many insights and points of wisdom for the student considering a potential internship in an interdisciplinary setting:

Interns' Voices

"I found the interdisciplinary internship experience to be invaluable. I was able to learn so much more than I ever could have by sitting in a classroom."

"One of the hardest, but best lessons for me was learning that everything does not come out the way you plan it, especially when working with people. This is particularly so with women in crisis situations."

"I had to learn to adapt with my environment."

"Working with the women at M's House was amazing. It was wonderful to see them grow and change over the few months I was there. I am grateful that they let me into their world and were willing to teach me about addiction."

"I also was grateful to have other students from different fields there with me. I learned much from them. They also provided me with support."

"I learned the value of a team as well as the various strengths that each person brings."

"I was able to use my understanding of child development to plan activities and interact with the children in ways that were appropriate and educational. I was also able to use my understanding of the theories behind parenting, relationships, and individual behaviors while at the agency to facilitate a positive working environment."

"I was able to integrate much of the knowledge I gained from the interdisciplinary faculty–student seminars into my experiences with the team. The faculty-led discussions about cultural competence and domestic violence were useful while working with the women and children at family service."

"Although I was able to apply system of care principles, in comparing my experiences at Family Service/C House with those of the interdisciplinary team at M's House, there was a difference in what I felt I could accomplish. Because C House only houses women and children during times of crisis, their stay at the shelter is very temporary. In contrast, the interns at M's House were able to build relationships with the women and children they worked with because M's House is a long-term residential facility. Although I understand that agency policy was appropriate in limiting my contact with clients in the crisis situation, in some ways, I wish I could have had more in-depth interaction with the clients. I appreciated hearing about the relationships other interns built with the women at M's House. That helped me further understand interdisciplinary work settings."

"I was able to gain insight into how the 'system of wraparound care' would benefit the clients."

"I was able to see how implementation of this type of system of care can be easy on a theoretical level, but difficult when considering specific populations and their needs."

"Being involved with this team was a positive experience. My only suggestion would be for this team to meet on a more frequent basis to further encourage the sharing of knowledge between professionals and students."

These students' comments convey how real these interdisciplinary team experiences can be and show how students are able to articulate the value received.

Summary

As the System of Care framework has been implemented in various communities to serve many different populations, the need for professionals to practice in family-centered, culturally competent, interdisciplinary teams has become increasingly important. Preprofessionals prepare to provide quality care through a journey of experiences throughout their undergraduate and graduate programs. They learn about System of Care core values and principles and its application in interdisciplinary, collaborative partnerships. The focus is on a family-centered approach, with community-based services delivered in culturally competent ways. Preprofessionals begin with a personal analysis—an examination of their own needs, wants, and goals—before moving on to an identification of interests and skills and an exploration of ways to develop career opportunities and alternatives. Preparing oneself to practice in an interdisciplinary, family-centered, System of Care setting is enhanced through a supervised professional experience in an interdisciplinary internship.

Activities to Extend Your Learning

- Writing Assignment to Reinforce Knowledge about Systems of Care
  - Learning to follow directions and write informative, succinct records, memos, and reports is important for the pre-professional because these skills are required in the work world. Write answers to questions to reinforce learning about Systems of Care in the following three areas:

    Unit 1: Wraparound Services/Family-Centered Services or Care

    1. What are some of the key elements of family-centered service?
    2. How does the concept of family-centered service coordination differ from traditional case management models of service delivery?

    Unit 2: Building Partnerships/Family-Professional Collaboration

    1. Describe ways that parents (families) may collaborate with professionals in a wraparound system of service delivery.

    Unit 3: Cultural Competence/Family-Centered Communication/Assessment

    1. What is cross-cultural competence, and what are some ways in which it can be obtained?
    2. What are some ways in which stress in the relationship between professionals and parents can be alleviated?

  - Based on the readings in each unit, answer questions in five to seven well-constructed, grammatically correct sentences, making them informative and including the most important ideas in the topic area. Follow these guidelines:
    - Write only one question per page and state the full question at the top of the page.
    - Write only one page (five to seven sentences) in answering the question. Type or key your responses using double spacing.

- Informational Interviews
  - Identify agencies and professionals that are known for practicing the wraparound process and implementing the principles of System of Care in delivering services. Acquire information about these career areas. Make 20- to 30-minute appointments with six professionals in the identified areas.
- Cultural Competence
  - Share the following with your classmates: Who are you? How did you grow up? What are your characteristics? What was it like to be in your family? What do you value? Describe yourself and what you believe.
- Keeping a Journal
  - Try keeping a journal of your experiences—an interdisciplinary internship, a family collaboration experience, shadowing a supervisor, learning about a new program for families in an agency. These questions may be helpful in guiding your thoughts as you make journal entries (especially when you do not know what to write):
    —What work did you perform?
    —What was the best thing that happened today at your site?
    —What experiences did you have?
    —What thing(s) did you like the best (or least)?
    —What knowledge and insights did you gain?
    —What kind of new skills have you learned since the beginning of your work?
    —What questions arose in your mind?
    —How do people you work with treat you, and how does it make you feel?
    —How have you changed or grown since you began your work at this site?
    —What have been your contributions to the programs at your site?
    Include observations and feelings regarding events that puzzle, surprise, frustrate, cause anxiety, and delight you. The journal approach is open-ended in that typical sentences might start as follows: A challenging idea that I heard today . . . ; Although I seriously questioned that activity, I . . . ; In working on this project, I learned . . . ; My management skills . . . ; I believe . . . ; I feel . . . ; I value . . . .

- 30-Second Commercial
  - Write your 30-second commercial in time to revise/refine/ practice it before you have to present it in class or use it in an interview situation. Practice. You want the words to be so much a part of you that they flow when you are in a tense situation. Remember that you want to show your best self when someone says, "Tell me about yourself!" Here are a few phrases to stimulate your thoughts about your own characteristics: Adaptable to a variety of work situations, resourceful in working collaboratively in teams, personable with others, considerate in dealing with others' feelings in culturally competent ways, logical thinker, and take time in making big decisions.
- Networking
  - Prepare for networking: Expand your 30-second commercial into a 1- to 2-minute version about yourself and your work with System of Care. Prepare a list of questions you would like to ask: How did you get into this type of work? Why do (don't) you like it? Would you be willing to review my resume? How could I enhance my credentials? What other people can you refer me to?
- Resume Guidelines
  Prepare a winning resume using these brief guidelines:
  - Use a word processing program to give the greatest flexibility in tailoring subsequent versions.
  - List name, address, phone, and e-mail address but no other personal information.
  - Keep it to one to two pages—no double-sided pages.
  - Use a clean, readable, serif font of 10 to 12 points (Times New Roman, Arial, etc.) and no elaborate graphics.
  - Gear the content to your objectives and be selective (do not list everything you have ever done).
  - Use approximately 1-inch margins on all sides.
  - Put your strongest selling points near the objective.
  - Use active verbs, not pronouns.
  - Check your spelling, grammar, and punctuation.
  - Consider a different version for different job types.
  - Be consistent with your format.
  - Use a laser-quality printer and light-colored resume paper (guidelines adapted from UNCG Career Services).
- Seek a Professional Development Experience to Meet Your Goals

Finding an internship or professional development experience to help you meet your professional career goals takes planning, lots of time and perseverance, and networking. However, in the long run, the benefits outweigh the time and commitment involved. Here are things to think about as you seek and complete such an experience.

- Conduct information interviews and use your network to find a placement or program that meets your career goals.
- Develop a learning plan or contract that includes these components: (1) learning goals/behavioral objectives, (2) activities to reach the goals/objectives, and (3) assessment measures.
- Plan and write clear learning goals/objectives because they will help you to focus your efforts throughout the internship/experience. In the helping professions, goals tend to be categorized in four areas: (1) knowledge; (2) skills—collaborative, team building, presentation, and technical; (3) development—personal, professional, etc.; and (4) self-assessment—to measure your progress and attainment of your objectives.
- Use action verbs to describe the outcomes you desire, and write objectives in these areas: (1) those related to your area of specialization, (2) those related to your internship field placement, and (3) those related to your own personal development.
- As you develop your learning plan, discuss it with your on-site supervisor. Use your own initiative first, seeking help when you need it.
- Use the plan as your guide when choosing appropriate activities to help you meet your objectives and in monitoring your progress throughout the experience.

- Evaluation Paper

Toward the end of your experience, write an evaluation (five- to seven-page paper) of your interdisciplinary internship experience for the professional audience, that is organized and easy to understand—be descriptive, yet concise. The following are helpful guidelines: Plan and organize the paper so that your ideas are clear, to the point, and easily understood by the reader. It may be written with the perspective of a future employer in mind. Think about things you would tell a prospective employer who might say, "Tell me about your internship experience, things you did, and what you learned."

Be serious about a good presentation, and do a good editing job! It is a mark of your professional competence! Organize your paper with the following sections:

1. Description of Agency/Placement Site/Overall Program
   This section should include the mission/purposes of the agency, the setting, the target population(s) served. You might name or include the description of programs, if that is part of the agency focus/structure. Think of this section as "setting the stage" for subsequent parts.

2. Internship Responsibilities
   Summarize your responsibilities in the internship placement. This gives a future intern an idea of what is available in this agency. It also sets the stage or establishes the context for the remainder of your paper. A synopsis of your involvement in the internship could include a description of your position and the nature of the work environment. Include the number of hours spent there, how many days a week you went to the work site, who your clients were, and the estimated time (percentage) that you spent in various activities (i.e., directly with clients, paperwork, meeting with supervisor, and any other information you think would give insight into the nature of your involvement in the internship).

3. Objectives and Accomplishments
   Include a discussion (maybe even a list) of your learning objectives and how you accomplished your objectives. Try to summarize your accomplishments by general ideas, major activities, programs, etc., rather than accounts of individual incidences.

4. Application of Skills and Knowledge from Your Major
   Describe the application of the skills developed in your major. Evaluate your strengths and areas that need improvement.

5. Relationship of Internship to Career Goals
   Relate your internship to your career goals. Indicate how your experiences have helped you clarify your future career path. Also, you may wish to address areas of leadership and/or professional development.

Suggested Reading

Sweitzer, H.F., & King, M.A. (2004). *The successful internship: Transformation and empowerment in experiential learning* (2nd ed.). Belmont, CA: Brooks/Cole.

References

Adams, J., Bliss, C., Mohammad, V.B., Meyers, J., & Slaton, E. (1997). *Family professional relationships: Moving forward together.* Washington, DC: National Peer Technical Assistance Network's Partnership for Children's Mental Health.

Allen, S.F. (2004). Internship evaluation paper (HDF 499 course). Unpublished manuscript, University of North Carolina at Greensboro, Department of Human Development and Family Studies.

Anderson, L.K. (1993). Teams: Group process, success, and barriers. *Journal of Nursing Administration, 23*(9), 15–19.

Arbuckle, M.B., Shoffner, S.M., Rummage, W.L., Bartlett, R., Stone, C., McCoy-Pulliam, R., Tyler, E.T., & Claes, J.A. (2000). *Interdisciplinary field education manual.* Unpublished manuscript, University of North Carolina at Greensboro.

Betz, C. (1997). Interdisciplinary practice and education. *Journal of Pediatric Nursing: Nursing Care of Children and Their Families, 12*(1), 1–2.

Cohort of Interns. (2000). Interns in interdisciplinary field placement. Unpublished paper, University of North Carolina at Greensboro, Department of Human Development and Family Studies.

Dean, C. (2000). *Empowerment skills for family workers.* Unpublished manuscript, Cornell University.

Douglas, F. and Jones, L. (2001). Personal communication, March 1, 2001.

Finklestein, N. (1994). Treatment issues for alcohol- and drug-dependent pregnant and parenting women. *Health & Social Work, 19*(1), 7–15.

Isaacs-Shockley, M., Cross, T., Bazron, B.J., Dennis, K., & Benjamin, M.P. (1996). Framework for a culturally competent system of care. In B.A. Stroul (Ed.), *Children's mental health: Creating systems of care in a changing society* (pp. 23–39). Baltimore: Paul H. Brookes Publishing.

Lourie, I.S., Stroul, B.A., & Friedman, R.M. (1998). Community-based systems of care: From advocacy to outcomes. In M. Epstein, K. Kutash, & A. Duchnowski (Eds.), *Outcomes for children and youth with emotional and behavioral disorders and their families* (pp. 3–19). Austin, TX: Pro-Ed.

Lynch, E.W. (1992). Developing cross-cultural competence. In E.W. Lynch & M.J. Hanson (Eds.), *Developing cross-cultural competence* (pp. 35–62). Baltimore: Paul H. Brookes.

Mayeroff, M. (1971). *On caring.* New York: Harper and Row.

McIntosh, P. (1990, Winter). White privilege. *Independent School, 50*, 1–6.

Michelozzi, B.N., Surrell, L.J., & Cobez, R.I. (2004). *Coming alive from nine to five in a 24/7 world: A career search handbook for the 21st century* (7th ed.). Boston: McGraw-Hill.

Pinderhughes, E. (1996). Difference and power in therapeutic practice. *Family Resource Coalition Report, 14*(3/4), 20–23.

Shoffner, S.M. (2000). *Internship field placement manual: Guidelines for supervised professional experiences* (5th ed.). Unpublished manuscript, Department of Human Development and Family Studies, University of North Carolina at Greensboro.

Shoffner, S.M. (2004). Class materials for HDF 477 professional orientation. Unpublished manuscript, Department of Human Development and Family Studies, University of North Carolina at Greensboro.

Stroul, B.A. (1996). *Children's mental health: Creating systems of care in a changing society.* Baltimore: Paul H. Brookes Publishing.

Sweitzer, H.F., & King, M.A. (2004). *The successful internship: Transformation and empowerment in experiential learning* (2nd ed.). Belmont, CA: Brooks/Cole.

UNCG Career Services. (2004). *Resumes.* Unpublished manuscript, University of North Carolina at Greensboro.

VanDenBerg, J.E., & Grealish, E.M. (1996). Individualized services and supports through the wraparound process: Philosophy and procedures. *Journal of Child and Family Studies, 5*(1), 7–21.

Wald, R., Harvey, M.S., & Hibbard, J. (1995). A treatment model for women substance abusers. *The International Journal of the Addictions, 30*(7), 881–888.

III

The Impact on Children, Families, and Communities

Chapter 15

Evaluation in the Implementation of System of Care in North Carolina

MARIA E. FERNANDEZ, MARK O'DONNELL, AND TERRI GRANT

Objectives

- Describe the history of the development of System of Care programs in North Carolina.
- Discuss the evaluation methodology used in the federal system of care grant sites.
- Identify the outcomes that resulted from the analysis of the data.

After implementation of three federal grants from the Center for Mental Health Services (CMHS) and long-time work within the state, the North Carolina Division of Mental Health, Developmental Disabilities, and Substance Abuse Services launched a statewide implementation of System of Care in March 2001. The opportunity was created when the Willie M. Program, having achieved positive outcomes for the youth under a class action suit, was officially terminated.

The end of the program allowed the allocation of state funding that had been previously restricted to youth in the lawsuit (youth with mental health diagnosis who behaved violently) to be applied to a more broadly defined target population of children and youth with severe emotional disturbances. Based on Willie M. Program achievements and other success from North Carolina's three federal System of Care demonstration projects, the division staff regarded the System of Care approach as an emerging best practice that should serve as the platform of the state child mental health delivery system.

A Brief History of System of Care in North Carolina

The first implementation of System of Care values and principles in North Carolina was the result of a class action lawsuit in 1980. A public official's outrage over how children with the most severe mental health problems were being relegated to locked juvenile justice facilities led to the lawsuit that, in turn, started what was probably the broadest program for that target population in the country at the time (Soler & Warboys, 1990). The lawsuit was filed on behalf of children (the youngest of the four lead plaintiffs being named Willie M.) who were suffering from serious emotional, mental, or neurologic handicaps, whose behaviors had been described as violent or assaultive, who were in or at risk of involuntary placement in an institution or in a residential program, and who were not receiving appropriate services. The stipulations that were agreed to in the 1980 lawsuit settlement guaranteed that children meeting the criteria of the class defined in the lawsuit had the right to individualized treatment based on their particular needs (rather than on those services that happened to be available) and that they had the right to be served in the least restrictive setting possible (North Carolina Department of Health and Human Services and North Carolina Department of Public Instruction, 1999). The terms of the settlement became a foundation for the many state and national child mental health initiatives that followed.

The second set of circumstances that influenced the movement to community-based services was the implementation of two projects, one in the eastern part of the state and the other in counties in the western part. In 1989, the Fort Bragg Project in Fayetteville (Behar, Bickman, Lane, Keeton, Schwartz & Brannock, 1996) and the Robert Wood Johnson Mental Health Services Program for Youth initiative in the 11 western-most counties served by the Blue Ridge and Smoky Mountain Area Mental Health Programs extended the comprehensive system of services to a broader band of children with serious mental disorders. Also contributing was a Medicaid waiver program in 1994—Carolina Alternatives—that was geared to reducing institutionalization in areas where hospital costs were highest by reinvesting dollars diverted from inpatient care to community-based options (Burns, Teagle, Schwartz, Angold, & Holtzman, 1999).

The systematic implementation of elements fundamental to a System of Care came through three projects that were funded by Center for Mental Health Services grants obtained in 1994, 1997, and 1999 under the Comprehensive Community Mental Health Services for Children and Their Families Program. The Pitt-Edgecombe-Nash Public Academic Liaison (PEN-PAL) served children with serious emotional disorders and their families in three counties in the eastern part of the state. The second project, Families and Communities Equals Success (FACES), served two sites in the central region of the state and five counties in the western region, whereas the third System of Care Network (SOC-Net) served one county in the eastern region, three counties in the central region, and seven counties in the western part of the state.

These System of Care projects included the following basic components: (1) consumer, family, and community involvement through local organizations called Community Collaboratives; (2) individualized service plans (known as child and family service plans) that maximize and integrate formal services from traditional service delivery systems and incorporate informal community supports; (3) the development and implementation of strategies that ensure that the local System of Care is culturally responsive to the families and communities it serves; (4) training and technical assistance supports for the local System of Care development; and (5) analysis of the service outcomes and the use of the data to improve continuously the local System of Care. The state division's System of Care team, communities, families, public agencies, local universities, and colleges worked as partners to coordinate the activities of these components in establishment of each local system of care. The SOC-Net grant also added a special emphasis on involving children and youth in policy and practice at both the local and state levels.

Evaluation in the System of Care Demonstration Projects

Integral to the Center for Mental Health Services (CMHS)-funded projects was an evaluation component in which caregivers and children 11 years old and older were interviewed at 6-month intervals over a 3-year period. Sites collected descriptive information on all children enrolled for grant services so as to constitute a cross-sectional sample. Baseline and follow-up interviews were conducted on a smaller, randomly selected longitudinal sample of which 100 were expected from each FACES site and 145 from each SOC-Net site (per CMHS guidelines). The evaluation protocol was determined by CMHS and the national evaluation contractor, ORC MACRO International. Each grant community in North Carolina had a data director who coordinated data collection, analyses, and presentation of findings to the community collaboratives—collective bodies of public and private multiagency decision makers that also included parents, family advocates, and other community representatives. The state office had a research director who oversaw program evaluation of the System of Care demonstration projects and was responsible for the analyses of and presentation on data merged across all North Carolina grant communities. Over time, a wealth of information was collected on demographic characteristics, risk factors, service use, family assets, and a range of outcomes that included caregiver burden, living arrangements, strengths of the child and family, the child's level of functioning, clinical symptoms, school performance, delinquency behavior, and satisfaction.

The System of Care demonstration projects made a conscious and deliberate effort to use evaluation for the improvement of the system and examined individual outcomes to determine needed changes in a child's individual service plan (known as a child and family plan). Thus, the evaluation team, with representation from each site, regularly analyzed data collected using the national evaluation protocol. The areas of enquiry generally focused on the basic goals of the System of Care demonstration projects that were to keep children with severe emotional disturbance in stable living arrangements in their community, in school, and out of jail. In addition, the System of Care demonstration projects assessed program implementation using an in-state–developed quality improvement protocol consisting of case file reviews, observations of child and family team meetings, and service testing (a comprehensive approach via interviews with individual children, family members, and system leaders that allowed a deeper analysis and perspective on system effectiveness).

Evaluation presentations were a routine item on the agenda of meetings of the community collaboratives and the state oversight committee (which included family, staff, and research representatives from each site) and provided information on the status of program implementation and individual outcomes. Early reports consisted of descriptions of the demographic characteristics, risk factors, and clinical diagnoses of the children and families enrolled in the program. Toward the end of the first year of data collection, outcomes began to be tracked. As more data were collected, analyses were conducted to identify factors that might be associated with the changes that occurred.

Presentations were made to larger audiences at in-state and national conferences. More sophisticated analyses were performed for articles submitted to academic journals and publications. One of the most important features of the evaluation was the collaboration between the research team and local family organizations at conference presentations and in the preparation of one-page, bulleted findings that family members could take to legislators and administrators of child-serving agencies in their education and advocacy function.

This chapter focuses on the use of evaluation to improve child and family outcomes and the service delivery system at the local level. The remainder of the chapter is divided into four sections. The first describes the demographic characteristics of the children served through the three grants. Outcomes on selected indicators based on merged data from two of the three projects are presented in the next section. Service testing is discussed in the third section. The last section discusses the findings relative to statewide System of Care implementation.

Section 1: Demographic Characteristics

Findings on demographic characteristics are drawn from the cross-sectional sample referred to earlier. As of the end of July 2004, the North Carolina System of Care demonstration projects had enrolled a total of 1,832 children with 273 in the phase 1 (PEN-PAL) sites and 697 in the phase 2 (FACES) sites. The phase 3 (SOC-Net) sites have already enrolled 862 as they approach the sixth and final year of the grant period.   More than two thirds of the children (68%) across the three phases were male. The mean age at intake was 12.1 years. Approximately 40% of the children were 14 years and older. Less than 1% (0.7) of the children in PEN-PAL were reported to be of Hispanic origin. The proportion in this category rose to approximately 4% (3.5%) in FACES and increased slightly in SOC-Net to approximately 5% (4.8%). Close to half of the total number of children enrolled belonged to minority groups. More detailed information on the distribution of children by race and gender is shown in Figure 15-1.

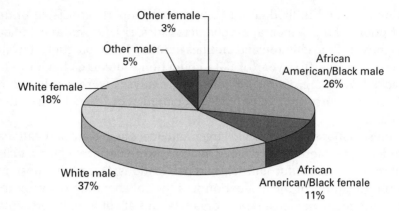

FIGURE 15-1 Children Enrolled in NC System of Care Demonstration Projects, by Race and Gender (N = 1746)*
*The sample size is lower than the total number enrolled because of missing information

Demographic characteristics varied by grant phases. PEN-PAL served a higher proportion of children in the younger age range than other sites. SOC-Net sites served older children. Table 15-1 shows variations among sites by age categories.

A composition by race and sex also varied by sites, as shown in Table 15-2.

African American or black males tended to be overrepresented among the children served through the grant, whereas females of both races tended to be underrepresented.

Section 2: Child Outcomes

The findings on outcomes are obtained from data collected for the sample of children who participated in the longitudinal study and had complete information at baseline, 6 months, and 12 months. The sample sizes vary because of missing information. Data from PEN-PAL are excluded because the evaluation for the first phase of CMHS-funded grantees (of which PEN-PAL was one) had a research protocol and outcome instruments that were different from those used in subsequent grant cycles.

Living Arrangements

Major mental health reform movements have been triggered by images of institutionalized individuals living in unfit and dehumanizing con-

Table 15-1	Age Categories by Grant Sites		
	PEN-PAL (%)	**FACES (%)**	**SOC-Net (%)**
10 years and younger	39.9	35.8	24.1
11–13 years	32.2	32.9	25.2
14 years and older	27.8	31.3	50.7

Table 15-2	Composition of Children, by Race and Sex, for the Three Grant Sites		
	PEN-PAL (%)	**FACES (%)**	**SOC-Net (%)**
African American male	41.0	27.5	19.8
African American female	22.3	12.2	6.2
White male	20.5	38.1	42.0
White female	13.9	15.4	21.2
Other male	1.5	5.1	6.2
Other female	0.7	4.6	1.8

ditions in cell blocks or in psychiatric facilities. Thus, federal System of Care projects have focused on keeping children with serious emotional disorders in the least restrictive setting possible—a perspective that has also found support in legal mandates. As children served in these projects tended to have many changes in living arrangements because of the complexity of their challenges, North Carolina also examined the data to determine whether multiple living arrangements were reduced over time.

Based on data from 315 children for whom information on living arrangements was available at baseline, 6 months, and 12 months, fewer children had more than one living arrangement in the follow-up periods. As shown in the Figure 15-2, 44% of the children enrolled in the program had more than one living arrangement in the 6 months preceding the baseline interview, with 3% living in four or more settings in the same interval. At 12 months, the proportion with two or more living arrangements had decreased to 30%. The number of children with only one living arrangement increased from baseline through the 12-month follow-up.

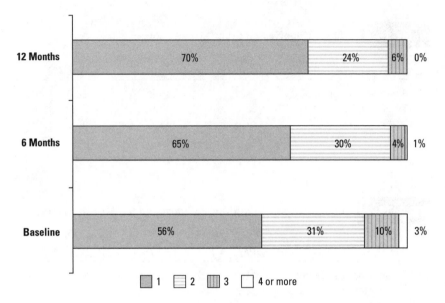

FIGURE 15-2   Number of Living Arrangements from Baseline through 12 Months (N = 315)

At one year after enrollment in the program, fewer children spent time in juvenile detention facilities or in jails (Figure 15-3). At baseline, 5.4% of children enrolled in FACES and SOC-Net were in correctional settings in the 6 months preceding their baseline interviews. The percentage decreased to approximately 3% at 6 months (3.2%) and 12 months (2.9%). Substantial reductions were observed in psychiatric placements. In the 6-month interval preceding the initial interview, 14% of children were admitted to psychiatric hospitals. The figure decreased to 4% at 12 months (Figure 15-3). However, the proportion of children in group homes or residential treatment facilities almost doubled from 11% at baseline to 20% at 12 months (Figure 15-3). At the same time, the proportion of children living with parents (including adoptive), relatives, or friends of the family or in foster care (including specialized and therapeutic foster care) declined (Figure 15-4).

The increase in the group home setting appears to be associated with gender, age of the child, custodial status, and year of enrollment in the System of Care project. The percentage of females was higher among group home residents compared with those living in nongroup home settings. More group home residents had Division of Social Service involvement. A marked increase in group home placements occurred around 2001, the year that the Comprehensive Treatment Services

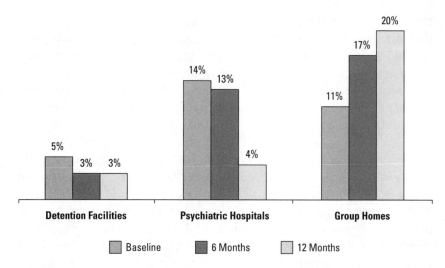

FIGURE 15-3   Out-of-Home Placements from Baseline through Twelve Months

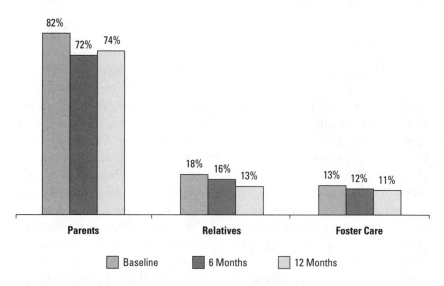

FIGURE 15-4   Living at Home or in Home-like Settings

Program (the successor to the Willie M. program) began. In response to these findings, the grant site where the increase was most apparent started a more rigorous tracking of the out-of-home placements of children enrolled in the local project. To do this, a review committee was established to screen potential residential placements to ensure that every formal service and informal support had been explored to keep the child from having to go into an out-of-home placement. Since then, that site has reduced out-of-home placements, particularly from more restrictive (level IV locked facilities) settings to less restrictive types.

These findings have implications at the policy level as well. Under the Comprehensive Treatment Services Program (Child Treatment Service Plan), state funding could be used to pay for room and board for children and youth with severe emotional disturbance who were in group homes. Recognizing the unintended consequences of this funding (i.e., more children were in out-of-home placement), the Division of Mental Health/Developmental Disabilities/Substance Abuse Services, as part of the new North Carolina Child Mental Health Plan (discussed later in the chapter), is carefully reviewing the residential service options of the state's child mental health service array to eliminate this incentive. The findings also highlight the need not only for more community-based services, but also for their remuneration at rates that will make them as financially viable for private providers as residential services.

School Indicators

Of all of the child outcomes tracked in the study, school performance was considered to be of the utmost importance. Parents and caregivers in their initial interviews reported academic problems as one of the five most frequently cited presenting problems. There was a common agreement among stakeholders that the school system needed to be a true and committed partner in System of Care to enable children served by the program to progress academically. The grant communities encouraged active involvement from the schools through school representation in the community collaborative meetings and on the collaborative's subcommittees. Schools participated more significantly at the individual child and family team level. School counselors, coaches, teachers, and even principals participated in many child and family team meetings. Grant communities also used flex funds and other community resources to support activities designed to keep children in school (e.g., tutoring). Children enrolled in FACES and SOC-Net showed positive outcomes in school attendance, average grades, and rates of suspension, detention, and expulsion.

School Attendance

The percentage of children attending school regularly (more than 75% of school days) increased, whereas the percentage of children attending school infrequently (less than 50% of school days) decreased (Figure 15-5). Excluded from the sample of 143 are 59 children who had either been suspended, detained, or expelled in the 6-month time-frame for each of the three interviews and for whom information on attendance was either "not applicable" or missing.

School Performance

Parents or caregivers were asked to describe which of five choices (*failing all or most, failing about half, D, C, B,* or *A*) described the child's grade or school performance in the past 6 months. Children enrolled in FACES and SOC-Net showed substantial improvements in school grades over the first 12 months of the project (Figure 15-6). The percentage receiving average grades of *C* or higher rose from 59% at baseline to 70% at 6 months to 73% at 12 months. Concomitantly, fewer children were getting failing grades. The percentage of children who failed half or all of their subjects decreased from 23% at baseline to 18% at 6 months to 16% at 12 months. The rate of improvement between baseline and 6 months was greater compared with the rate between 6 and 12 months.

Detentions, Suspensions, and Expulsions

Fewer children were removed from their classes or expelled from their school one year after enrollment in FACES and SOC-Net. The percentage of children detained or taken out of their classrooms for short periods of time declined between baseline and the two follow-up in-

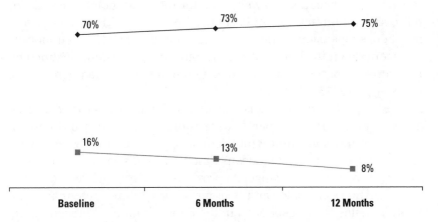

FIGURE 15-5 School Attendance from Baseline Through Twelve Months (N = 143)

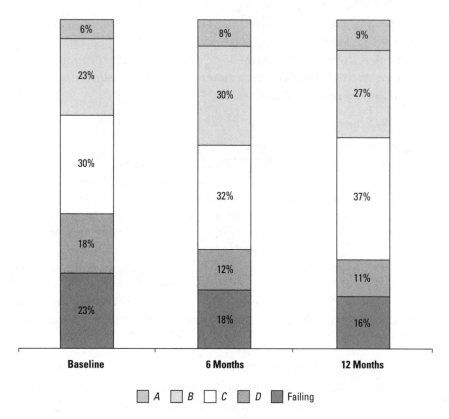

FIGURE 15-6   Average Grades from Baseline Through Twelve Months (N = 219)

tervals. Similar reductions were seen for more extended removals for more serious infractions. At baseline, 56% received in-school or out-of-school suspensions. The percentage decreased to 45% at 6 months and went down further, to 38% at 12 months. Expulsions declined by half between baseline and the specified follow-up periods (from 12% to 6%) (Figure 15-7).

The rates of detentions, suspensions, and expulsions varied by race and sex. Figure 15-8 compares suspensions among African American males, white males, and white females. Other groups were not included in the comparison because their sample sizes were too small to reflect meaningful change. Approximately three out of every four African American males and two out of every four white males and white females were suspended in the 6-month interval preceding the baseline interviews. All of the groups showed improvements at

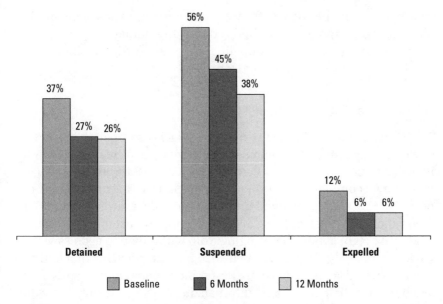

FIGURE 15-7 Children Suspended, Detained, and Expelled from Baseline Through Twelve Months (N: Detained = 253; Suspended = 256; Expelled = 252)

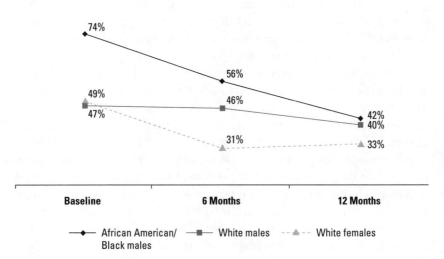

FIGURE 15-8 Percent Suspended among African American/Black Males, White Males, and White Females from Baseline Through Twelve Months (N: African American/Black Males = 78; White Males = 97; White Females = 49)

subsequent time periods, with African American males showing the most marked improvement, followed by white females. White males improved the least. These group differences are further elaborated in the discussion on problem behaviors.

Child Behavior Checklist Measures

The Child Behavior Checklist measures social competence and behavioral and emotional problems based on caregiver responses to 138 items (20 referring to social competence and 118 to problem behaviors). Raw scores are converted into normalized T-scores (based on percentiles of the normative samples) to provide a measurement that is common to all scales. The Child Behavior Checklist is also designed to identify eight syndromes ranging from withdrawn to aggressive behavior that may be further distinguished into internalizing problem behaviors (withdrawn), externalizing problem behaviors (aggressive), and behaviors that are neither internalizing or externalizing. Only the results for total competence, internalizing, and externalizing problem behaviors are reported here. The total competence scale measures participation in sports and nonsport activities, social relationships, and school performance. T-scores under 37 are considered to be in the clinical range for social competence. The internalizing problem behaviors subscale measures internal distress such as somatic complaints, anxiety, or depression, whereas the externalizing problem behaviors subscale measures delinquency and aggressive behaviors. T-scores of 67 and over are considered to be in the clinical range for the problem behaviors (Achenbach, 1991).

Improvements occurred in all areas measured by the child behavior checklist among children enrolled in FACES and SOC-Net. As shown in Figure 15-9, the percentage of children (total sample) in the clinical range for total competence decreased from 67% at baseline to 56% at 6 months and went down further to 49% at 12 months. Similar trends are seen for internalizing (Figure 15-10) and externalizing problem behaviors (Figure 15-11) for the total sample. The three figures also show changes over time for African American males, white males, and white females. African American males appear to have the smallest proportions in the clinical ranges at baseline for all of the scales. Where the percentages of white males and white females in the most severe range for social competence were above 70%, the percentage for African American males was 53%. White males had the highest percentage for internalizing problem behaviors. On the other hand,

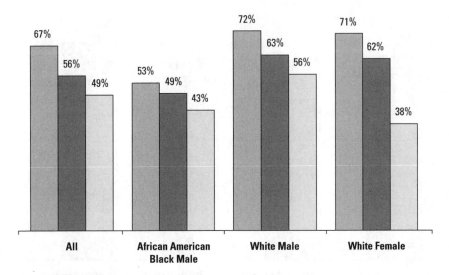

FIGURE 15-9 Percent of Social Competence T-Scores in the Clinical Range at Baseline, Six Months, and Twelve Months (N: All = 195; African American/Black Male = 49; White Male = 75; White Female = 42)

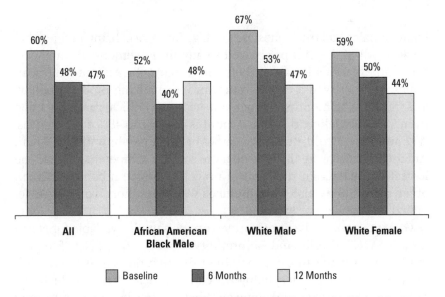

FIGURE 15-10 Percent of Internalizing Problem Behaviors in the Clinical Range at Baseline, Six Months, and Twelve Months (N: All = 303; African American/Black Male = 82; White Male = 119; White Female = 54)

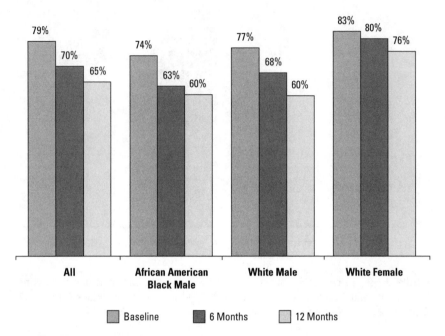

FIGURE 15-11   Percent of Externalizing Problem Behaviors T-Scores in the Clinical Range at Baseline, Six Months, and Twelve Months (N: All = 303; African American/ Black Male = 82; White Male = 119; White Female = 54)

white females had the highest percentage for externalizing problem behaviors. All of the groups showed steady improvements through the three time periods for all of the scales, except for African American males, who showed a deterioration in internalizing problem behaviors from 6 to 12 months; the percentage in the clinical range declined from 52% at baseline to 40% at 6 months but rose to 48% at 12 months. Although the Child Behavior Checklist results show that African American males were likely to be more socially competent and had the lowest percentage in the clinical range for problem behaviors than other groups, they also were the ones who were most likely to be detained, suspended, or expelled.

Growth curve analyses performed on the sample available for North Carolina (NC) Family and Community Equals Success (FACES) generally confirm the findings obtained through descriptive statistics. Length of time in service, being African American, being male, being 14 years of age or over, and being enrolled in a specific site significantly influenced increases in social competence T-scores and reductions in problem behaviors T-scores.

Summary of Findings

The findings presented in the chapter are summarized as follows:

- The majority of children enrolled in FACES and SOC-Net were male; African American males were overrepresented, whereas females were underrepresented in the group of children served through the two grant projects.
- Living arrangements became more stable in that fewer children had multiple living arrangements over time; fewer children spent time in correctional facilities or psychiatric institutions, but the number of children placed in group homes increased.
- The change trajectory varied by specific subgroups; for example, the decrease in suspension was most marked among African American males.
- Overall, children in FACES and SOC-Net showed consistent improvements on living arrangements, school indicators, and the child behavior checklist measures of competence and internalizing and externalizing problem behaviors through the first year of the program.

Implications

The findings shown here have implications for service delivery, policy formulation, and further empirical investigation. The demographic profile and findings on race and gender variations suggest the need for a more aggressive and concerted use of targeted intervention for groups that have greatest representation among the children served in the program. For instance, therapeutic approaches have been developed to address conduct disorders and reduce school problems among specific subgroups. For example, one-on-one mentoring may often be the most effective solution to a child's academic problems. However, there are times when simply having a school teacher or staff member as a participant in a child and family team may be all that the child needs to improve in school and turn his or her life around. Participation at this level obviously needs the support of school administrators from the school superintendent to the local school level, from the principals to the classroom teachers. Thus, having the school system as an active partner in the community collaborative is of the utmost importance in accomplishing the goal of keeping children in school until their graduation.

Females were underrepresented among the children served through FACES and SOC-Net but had the highest proportion in the clinical range for externalizing problem behaviors, indicating that females are not typically enrolled for services until their conditions worsen. This finding assumes particular significance when considered against the context of the recent increase of females in group homes based on FACES and SOC-Net data and a finding that more of them are now incarcerated in the nation's correctional facilities. Females also tend to improve noticeably after enrollment in the program, highlighting the need to increase their number among the children served through the program.

The finding that children improved one year after enrollment in System of Care leads to the basic question of "what changes were implemented at the service delivery level that had an impact on child outcomes?" Unfortunately, the national evaluation does not capture quantifiable data on system performance at the individual child and family level. However, the North Carolina System of Care Demonstration Projects did develop a protocol designed to collect data on System of Care implementation for quality monitoring and improvement that is further discussed in the next section.

Section 3: Service Testing

The quality improvement protocol for the North Carolina System of Care Demonstration projects consists of case reviews, observations of child and family team meetings, and service testing (sometimes known as coordinated practice reviews). The first two strategies are intended to be done monthly by the local evaluator and other members of the community collaborative to provide ongoing monitoring on the implementation of fundamental principles such as child and family participation, interagency collaboration, and cultural competence. The most intensive component of the protocol, service testing, is conducted at the beginning of the grant, at midpoint, and in the final year of the grant. Developed by Drs. Ivor Groves and Ray Foster (1995), service testing evolved in North Carolina into a 3-day process in which a team of 12 external raters and 12 local shadows (persons from the agencies in the service system) assesses the system of service delivery on the basis of outcomes observed in a stratified sample of 12 children receiving services through the local mental health program. On the first day, service testers (objective individuals who are external to the system being "tested," who are tasked with implementing the service testing protocol) and "shadows" (those locally based individuals who assist the service testers and lend local insight and knowledge) are given an orientation on System of Care principles and practices and trained on how to rate system performance indicators on a six-point scale (1 = grossly unacceptable; 6 = optimally acceptable) based on the service testing protocol. At the end of the orientation session and through the second day, service tester and shadow dyads collect information from case files and interviews conducted with parents or caregivers, the child if old enough, school teachers, therapists and other providers and sources of informal support. Each dyad then assigns scores on child outcomes and service performance indicators. Additionally, the service tester and shadow write a case report based on their observations. At the same time, as part of the service testing process, the project director and other staff members at the state level interview major stakeholders of the local grant project (e.g., agency directors, advocates, local law enforcement leaders, and members of the community collaborative) on their perceptions of the strengths, challenges, and opportunities that are presented by the local System of Care.

A unique feature of the service testing process is that the results are immediately (on the third day of the service testing event) provided to local sites so that modifications to System of Care implementation may be made where appropriate in a timely manner. Reports with recommendations are given for each case to local site administrators and providers before reviewers disperse. Findings from stakeholder interviews and aggregate results based on child indicators and service performance ratings are presented at a community meeting organized by the local community collaborative on the final day of service testing. Additionally, the reports may be presented at the next Community Collaborative meeting. The community meeting may also include a presentation of findings on outcomes collected through the national evaluation and education on System of Care values and principles and their implementation in the service system. Administrators and other representatives of child-serving agencies, local judges, police officers, university representatives, family members, legislators, and all of those interviewed in the course of the three days are invited to the presentation.

Table 15-3 shows the results based on the first and last service testing for the FACES sites, the only one of the three projects that has completed a first and final assessment. (Service Testing for PEN-PAL was conducted only for its final year. SOC-Net has yet to complete the final Service Testing process.) As shown in Table 15-3, improvements were observed in all but 3 of the 14 indicators of system performance in the service testing that was conducted in 2002 as compared with the one conducted in 1997. The changes were most substantial for successful transitions, service plan comprehensiveness, child and fam-

Table 15-3	Comparison of System Performance Indicators* Between 1997 and 2002		
Indicator	1997	FACES 2002	% Change
Child/family participation	52.0	83.0	60.0
Service team	65.0	62.0	−5.0
Functional assessment	45.0	64.0	42.0
Long-term view	33.0	34.0	3.0
Service plan	29.0	58.0	100.0
Resource availability	71.0	65.0	−8.0
Plan implementation	40.0	55.0	38.0
Mix, match, fit	50.0	67.0	34.0
Caregiver supports	66.0	69.0	5.0
Crisis planning	79.0	51.0	−35.0
Service coordination	47.0	68.0	45.0
Successful transitions	30.0	61.0	103.0
Effective results	56.0	57.0	2.0
Monitoring/modification	52.0	61.0	17.0

*Percentage of cases reviewed that were found acceptable (scored a 4 or higher)

ily participation, plan implementation, and service coordination. However, crisis planning and resource availability showed marked declines, possibly because of state budgetary constraints.

Section 4: The Future of System of Care in North Carolina

The State Plan 2001: Blueprint for Change (North Carolina Department of Health and Human Services, Division of Mental Health, Developmental Disabilities and Substance Abuse Services, 2004) launched the first major comprehensive reform of North Carolina's mental health, developmental disabilities, and substance abuse services in more than 30 years. The state plan was developed in response to the legislature's passage of Session Law 2001-437 that called for sweeping reforms in the service system over a 5-year period.

The primary objective of the reform is to improve service delivery by making it more consumer focused and to provide clear accountability for quality and effectiveness by making the local area programs (now referred to as local management entities, area authorities, county programs) *managers* instead of *providers* of the services.

The reform effort is being developed in stages. A new child mental health plan was released in October 2003 (North Carolina Department of Health and Human Services, North Carolina Division of Mental Health, Developmental Disabilities and Substance Abuse Services, 2003). The plan addresses services for all children who receive publicly funded mental health services, including those who are in residence at state facilities and in other out-of-home placements. This plan provides a framework to address structural, financing, and organizational issues encountered in serving children with mental health disorders and their families. Based on the positive outcomes for children and youth who were served in the System of Care sites and the recognition of System of Care's status as an emerging best practice nationally, the division established the comprehensive System of Care approach as the platform on which the North Carolina child mental health reform will be based. The reform's intent is to foster the development of a full range of formal and informal services and supports in communities across the state.

The System of Care project sites cover 22 of North Carolina's 100 counties. The 2001 Comprehensive Treatment Services Program legislation mandated that all mental health communities across the state adopt two core elements of System of Care. Each community must establish a community collaborative and use the child and family team process to create and support service plans for children with mental health needs and their families. The implementation of the Child Mental Health Plan focuses on strategies to support the development of other core elements as well, such as a broad service array, training and technical assistance, supportive financing, and administrative policies. The goal is to have well-functioning local Systems of Care operating across North Carolina by July 2007. This is a tremendous challenge, but a necessary one.

Change comes hard. System of Care recognizes and calls on the expertise of the families in supporting the child with whom all are concerned. In so doing, System of Care asks professionals to change how they work with and support children and families. It puts children and families in key roles in determining how the system will support them. This method of support and interaction is not how most professionals were or are trained. At one level, System of Care challenges their view of themselves as professionals and asks them to reach out to the families and into the community for resources that the "system" has itself only occasionally supplied. It asks them to track and evaluate their actions, to analyze what works and what does not, and then to apply those lessons learned in support of an ever evolving and increasingly effective System of Care. It asks all of this while providing little training, support, or recognition for this very different way of doing business.

So why do it? The simple answer, supported by evaluation data, is because it works.

The old system has allowed the burning out of professionals by supporting their working with outdated methods that, if they ever worked well, do not now. It is time to look at the data and, based on a critical analysis of our successes and failures, adjust how we all do business with families and with each other. The prize is this: children who are mentally healthy and successful. System of Care is the method by which we keep our eyes on the prize. This is both a worthy goal and one that makes sense. System of Care points the way toward our future success and toward mentally healthy children, families, and professionals. It is time to change.

References

Achenbach, T.M. (1991). *Manual for the child behavior checklist/4-18 and 1991 profile.* Burlington, VT: University of Vermont Department of Psychiatry.

Behar, L., Bickman, L., Lane, T., Keeton, W.P., Schwartz, M., & Brannock, J.E. (1996). The Fort Bragg and Adolescent Mental Health Demonstration Project. In M.C. Roberts & the Task Force on Model Programs in Service Delivery (Eds.), *Model programs in child and family mental health* (pp. 351–372). Mahwah, NJ: Lawrence Erlbaum Associates.

Burns, B.J., Teagle, S.E., Schwartz, M.S., Angold, A., & Holtzman, A. (1999). Managed behavioral care: A Medicaid carve-out for youth. *Health Affairs, 18*(5), 214–225.

Groves, I.D., & Foster, R.E. (1995). *Service testing: Assessing the quality and outcomes of systems of care performance through interaction with individual children served.* Unpublished manuscript.

North Carolina Department of Health and Human Services and North Carolina Department of Public Instruction. (1999). *Report to the Governor and the General Assembly 1998–1999.* Raleigh, NC: North Carolina Department of Health and Human Services.

North Carolina Department of Health and Human Services, Division of Mental Health, Developmental Disabilities and Substance Abuse Services. (2004). *Child Mental Health Plan: September 2003,* updated March 2004. Raleigh, NC: Author.

North Carolina Department of Health and Human Services, North Carolina Division of Mental Health, Developmental Disabilities and Substance Abuse Services. (2003). *State plan 2001: Blueprint for change: July 1, 2003.* Raleigh, NC: Author.

Soler, M., & Warboys, L. (1990). Services for violent and severely disturbed children: The Willie M. litigation. In S. Dicker (Ed.), *Stepping stones: Successful advocacy for children* (pp. 61–112). New York, NY: The Foundation for Child Development.

Chapter 16

Where Are We? Creating a Bow from the Threads of System of Care: A Philosophical Framework

Where Are We Going? Calls from Across the Nation: Implementing System of Care Concepts to Improve the Mental Health and Health Care Systems

Where Do We Go from Here? Keeping the Vision Alive and Sustaining the Momentum: Recommendations for the Future

CHARLOTTE A. HERRICK AND MARGARET B. ARBUCKLE

Objectives

- Describe the similarities and differences of multiple professional perspectives in applying System of Care to practice, professional training or education, and research.
- Discuss the national call to implement System of Care principles and values in health care, education, and human services, as described in these reports:
  - Annie E. Casey Foundation: Preparing Human Service Workers for Interdisciplinary Practice
  - The Surgeon General's Report on Mental Health
  - *Healthy People 2010*, published by the Department of Health and Human Services
  - The Institute of Medicine Report on Health Professions Education
  - The President's New Freedom Commission on Mental Health
- Identify strategies to maintain the national momentum for implementing System of Care principles and values in practice, professional training or education, and research.

This book has addressed the multiple needs of children and families in various settings that can be met by many professional disciplines using the core values and principles inherent in a System of Care philosophical framework. These needs can be met by working with children and families in a medical setting or a residential program, with those who need child welfare or psychological services, with students in schools, including the arts and music, or in recreational programs, with youth in the juvenile justice systems, or with adolescents who need substance abuse interventions demands family/ professional partnerships that are respectful, that honor people's humanity and cultural differences, and that build on the strengths provided by the collaborative efforts of professionals, families, and other support persons.

During the last several years, a number of national organizations have addressed the health care crisis in this country. The crises in mental health care may be best illustrated by a United States Senator in July of 2004 who tearfully introduced to Congress a "youth suicide prevention" bill in honor of his son, who had suffered from learning disabilities and a bipolar disorder, which led to his taking his own life. For a few moments, the only sounds in the US Senate chamber were those of a grieving father (Kenen, 2004).

Crises that families with emotionally disturbed children face are illustrated in Chapter 4, "Parents' Voices." The authors explain how they felt when their children were invisible. The children went unnoticed until their behavior demanded the attention of other people. Then the children were seen as bad, and the parents were considered inept.

Professionals must work together to address the needs of children who have an emotional disturbance and students who require special education. Child advocates need to monitor continually the quality of mental health care and special education in order to meet the needs of children who are the resources for this country's future. Without adequate mental health care, the ability of children to grow and develop normally may be severely hampered.

Care for the needs of persons with developmental disabilities, both children and adults, or those who may be handicapped must be coordinated to meet their needs across the health care continuum. Society cannot neglect the growing population of older people, whose risks for mental health problems and other medical and social problems increase each decade of their lives, as they live past 65 years, and those who are chronically and persistently mentally ill, as well as those who are homeless and need attention. Each person who is mentally ill is someone's loved one, a mother, a father, a son, or a daughter.

The purpose of this chapter is to (1) tie together the themes addressed in previous chapters; (2) focus on the reports summarizing the national concerns for the health and mental health care of the nation's citizens; and (3) recommend strategies to sustain the national momentum that supports the System of Care, as a framework for programs that address the complex needs of the most vulnerable in this society. This chapter is about sharing the vision.

Where Are We? System of Care: A Philosophical Framework: Summary of Themes in Previous Chapters

The System of Care values and principles are the threads that tie the chapters in this text together into a multicolored bow. Each chapter is unique, but all address system of care concepts, values, and principles that are applicable to the authors' professional practice.

The values and principles that Stroul and Friedman (1986) identified supported a shift from the traditional medical model of service delivery to a collaborative model among professionals and family members. This model has become the paradigm for the delivery of mental health services to children with severe emotional disturbances and their families. Research has demonstrated the effectiveness of programs based on a System of Care framework that is now considered as "best practice" or thought of as "evidenced based practice" (Hoagwood, Burns, Kiser, Ringeisen, & Schoenwald, 2001, p. 1179).

The contributors to this textbook are educators, social workers, psychologists, nurses, psychiatrists and program administrators, and parents of children with serious emotional disturbances who identified the prevailing themes: *comprehensive care*, coordinated and delivered by a collaborative health care team; *family-centered care*, which builds on individual strengths with the focus on both the child and the family; and *culturally competent* services that are delivered in the least restrictive environment, preferably in the community. The overall goals are to improve the quality of care and to achieve the best outcomes for children and their families. These principles and values should be applied to other populations with complex needs who require multiple services from across the health care continuum.

A Comprehensive Service Delivery System Based on a Collaborative Model

Children with serious emotional disturbances or special educational needs, developmental problems, and other disabilities require a comprehensive array of services that cannot be provided by one profession or a single intervention. A constant theme in this book is the need for a model of a collaborative service delivery system for professionals to work with families and children. Achieving collaboration is a challenge and usually moves through stages from cooperation to coordination to collaboration. To work together as collaborative partners is essential for children to receive adequate services to meet their complex needs.

Professionals need to gain collaborative skills and to develop an understanding of the language of other professions and their skills and expertise. As described in Chapter 6, on Nursing, and Chapter 14, on Professional Development, an educational opportunity for pre-professionals to learn to work together as a focused team promoted understanding of the other's professional perspectives. Although interprofessional clinical experiences are rare today, interprofessional education must be seriously considered in the future. True collaboration, as noted in Chapter 2 on Wraparound, can make a difference in reaching successful outcomes. It is essential to recognize that no "one" professional perspective is the right one and that jointly addressing solutions to problems and sharing the perspectives of multiple disciplines, to include the family's perspectives, will invariably lead to better outcomes.

Building Family/Professional Partnerships: Family-Centered Care

Another theme in this book is building partnerships with parents. Rather than collaboration with families, the relationship is best described as "partnering" with families. When System of Care is adopted as a framework for practice, partnerships between professionals and family members are essential. The relationship evolves into one that is deeply personal, empathetic, and "in relationship." When people have a connected relationship, a bond develops between the partners. The partnership between parent/child and the professional is mutual, inclusive, supportive, and caring—a connection between one human being and another.

The relationship between the professional and the client and family in a System of Care framework is different from relationships in the past—when the professional was "in charge." Client and family/professional partnerships are described in this book as family-centered care and are addressed in chapters by social workers, educators, psychologists, physicians, and nurses. The emphasis is on respect, equality, and mutuality, acknowledging the strengths of each of the partners. The partnership between the professional and the client or the consumer is no longer hierarchical but one of equality and mutual respect.

Because parents are equal partners in this "new" relationship, they must shift their expectations. Instead of the parent coming to the professional expecting that the child will be "fixed," parents now come to the relationship knowing that their own participation will be required to plan and implement their child's care. This shift has promoted the development of parent support and advocacy groups, providing parents the opportunity to learn a different paradigm in order to be equal partners with the professional team. This new role for parents can be challenging (see Chapter 4 "Parents' Voices"). Parental empowerment that results from increased knowledge and newly acquired skills, as well as an enhanced sense of self-confidence, provides the opportunity for success and an improved quality of care for the child and quality of life for the parents.

Cultural Competence

A third theme that is throughout this text is cultural competence, which is not just an understanding of the differences among people.

Achieving a culturally competent service delivery system requires an understanding of the multitude of influences on families, including nationality, religion, language, education, and socioeconomic status, as well as the client and family's perceptions of their health and mental health status. All of these influences lead to values, beliefs, traditions, and practices that define a specific person's cultural perspective. Cultural competence not only requires an understanding the culture of others, but also requires self-understanding. Professional and personal insights into one's own biases and prejudices, beliefs, and values are as important as understanding others. Self-assessment assists professionals to understand how their values, beliefs, and cultural norms influence their interactions with others.

Professionals need to recognize and understand that each professional discipline has its own culture. "Professional socialization teaches the student a set of beliefs, practices, habits, likes, dislikes, norms and rituals" (Spector, 2000, p. 91). Each profession has its own language. The language that is unique to each profession may lead to misunderstandings among the various disciplines, and because families rarely understand the language that is unique to each profession, they too may not understand the intended message. Therefore, each person must make certain that all of the others on the child/family team understand what is being said.

Community-Based Care

Professionals should advocate for children to remain at home, in school, and in their own communities. Keeping children and families together in the community as they face the crisis of mental illness enables each member to draw on each other's strengths, supporting their abilities to provide each other with loving care that promotes healing. Community-based care is central to the System of Care philosophy, which is to provide care in the least restrictive environment so that the child and family can have the most normal, safe, and therapeutic experiences possible. A network of community services should be developed that fosters community-based care.

Another theme that is addressed in this book is that System of Care principles and values can be applied to other vulnerable populations, not just children with emotional disturbances. The System of Care principles and values should guide care for those who are homeless or chemically dependent, the older population, foster children, children and adults with chronic or complex illnesses, such as asthma or AIDS, and children or adults with mental retardation. (See Chapter 11 on healthy lifestyles through inclusive recreation.) The challenge is to integrate these values throughout the medical and human service systems and into educational settings. This text provides an interdisciplinary perspective on how the values and principles of System of Care can be threaded throughout education, human services, health, and mental health practices to provide quality, holistic care.

The reports by national leaders (summarized later here) have incorporated the principles of family-centered, community-based care in a collaborative interprofessional model that focuses on individual and family strengths in a culturally competent service delivery. Stroul and Friedman (1986) identified these values and principles many years ago. However, only recently have they been viewed as best practice. These principles are considered necessary to achieve successful outcomes, not only for children with severe emotional disturbances but also for others in need of multiple professional services.

Where Are We Going? Calls from Across the Nation to Implement System of Care Values and Principles to Improve the Mental Health/Health Care System

The ability of our nation to foster our children's mental health care is of primary importance to the future of the country. At the same time, humane care, addressing the mind, body, and spirit, is important for all citizens. Access to health care for everyone must be a national priority. Several institutions have proclaimed a need to address mental illness in America. They have recommended that the mental health service delivery system be reformed and the educational curriculum of mental health professionals be redesigned. The Annie E. Casey Foundation and the Institute of Medicine were the two organizations that specifically addressed the need to develop programs for interdisciplinary education for human services, the health and mental health professions. The reports by national leaders promote the development of quality health and mental health care, as well as a social welfare system that supports children and families.

The Annie E. Casey Foundation examined the preparation of human service workers for interprofessional practice in *Myths and Opportunities*, written in 1999. The Surgeon General's Report, *Mental Health: A Report of the Surgeon General*, published by US Department of Health and Human Services in 1999, examined the status of the nation's mental health care. *Healthy People 2010*, written by the Office of Disease Prevention and Health Promotion, the U.S. Department of Health and Human Services in 2000, addressed the state of the union's general health. The Institute of Medicine report, *Health Professions Education: A Bridge to Quality: Executive Summary* (edited by Griener & Knebel, 2003), examined the education of health professionals across the nation. The most recent report was the President's New Freedom Commission on Mental Health (2003), *Achieving the Promise: Transforming Mental Health Care in America, Executive Summary*, the U.S. Department of Health and Human Services, which calls for a transformed mental health system in order to improve the quality of mental health care and to improve access to mental health.

All of the reports addressed System of Care values and principles, using different language in different contexts. The national reports that support System of Care values and principles are briefly summarized here and are introduced in the order in which the reports were published, starting with *Myths and Opportunities* by the Annie E. Casey Foundation, and ending with *Achieving the Promise: Transforming Mental Health Care in America, The Executive Summary* by the president's New Freedom Commission on Mental Health.

The National Reports

The Annie E. Casey Foundation

The primary mission of the Annie E. Casey Foundation (1999) is to promote public policies that support the welfare of children and families. In 1998, the foundation funded an interdisciplinary project to examine interprofessional education and to identify the barriers that must be overcome to develop interdisciplinary professional training programs in colleges or universities and service organizations. The participants were from the Council on Social Work Education, the School of Social Work and the School of Nursing at the University of Southern California, and the Center for Collaboration for Children at California State University, Fullerton. They joined forces to participate in the project.

The foundation was concerned about the quality of care in today's mental health and welfare systems. One of the concerns was the need to provide care holistically to meet the needs of children and families; another concern was the current barriers to implementing interprofessional education and training programs. The project members examined the impact of accreditation, licensing, certification, and credentialing issues (and other factors) related to interdisciplinary practice and education. In its 1999 report, *Myths and Opportunities*, The Council on Social Work Education recommended strategies to effect changes in the way professionals are educated in collegiate and professional training programs today and in the future.

The report pointed to the need for professional competence over and above each discipline's specialized skills, including competence in collaborative skills, as well as competence in cultural diversity and community-based practice. Interprofessional collaborative skills are defined as a composite of the following: "team-building, case management, conflict resolution, self-reflection, outcome measurement, organizational behavior and inter organizational structures" (Annie E. Casey Foundation, 1999, p. 5). The report also said that interprofessional education is more successful if implemented early in a student's educational experience as part of the professional socialization process. The foundation report's executive summary indicated reforms that need to be addressed now (Table 16-1).

Several other national organizations have also called for reforms in professional education to develop interprofessional clinical programs (Greiner & Knebel, 2003; Pew Health Professions, 1995). According to the foundation, the sustainability of interprofessional training and education will depend on the successful outcomes for children and families, as professionals put what they have learned in interdisciplinary education into practice. In *Myths and Opportunities,* the Council on Social Work (1999) has called for continuing dialogue among clinicians, educators, and members of accrediting organizations to overcome the barriers to the development of interprofessional education.

Mental Health: A Report of the Surgeon General

The 1999 White House Conference on Mental Health called for a national campaign to address the stigma associated with mental disorders and challenged the nation to improve the quality of mental health care and to address suicide prevention. However, mental health care is a system that is "plagued by disparities in availability and access to its services. These disparities may be viewed through the lenses of racial and cultural diversity, age, and gender . . . [and] often hinge on a person's financial status . . . whether one has health insurance with inadequate mental health benefits or is one of the 44 million Americans who lack any insurance" (preface by David Satcher, Surgeon General, in *Mental Health: The Report of the Surgeon General*, US Department of Health and Human Services, 1999) . The health of the nation

Table 16-1	Why Now? Issues Facing Professionals Today: Identified by the Annie E. Casey Foundation Report (1999):

- More children and families have multiple problems. Professionals need to understand the interplay among factors leading to poor health and poor mental health. Co-existing diagnoses or co-morbidities are more prevalent today.
- Because of the complexity of today's health care environments, no one profession has sole jurisdiction over health or mental health care. Traditional disciplinary boundaries must be crossed to provide holistic, culturally competent, family-centered care by an interdisciplinary team.
- Resources for schools, health care, and social services are shrinking. Therefore, collaboration may provide opportunities to share resources and decrease the fragmentation and duplication of services.
- There is increased understanding among policy makers, families, and professionals that there is a need for effective profamily interventions that will require integration across the child welfare, mental health, health, education, and juvenile justice systems.
- Public policies that address child and family welfare, health, and mental health care issues will require lobbying efforts by a team of professionals rather than by one professional group.
- Current funding mechanisms impede the delivery of quality care by interagency groups and also hinder the development of interprofessional collaborative teams.

Accreditation, credentialing, licensing, and certification issues are roadblocks to interprofessional education and practice. The 1999 project has placed the issues on the table for crediting bodies, professional groups, educators, and others to examine trends in professional practice and education.

Adapted from the Annie E. Casey Foundation (1999) *Myths and Opportunities,* Alexandria, VA, Council on Social Work Education.

depends on improving mental health care as well as improving care for the physically ill or disabled. The stigma associated with mental health prevents access to care.

The Surgeon General's report examined the mental health/illness continuum from both epidemiologic and public health perspectives. It addressed mental health promotion, illness prevention, access to care, and mental health care for citizens across the life span and evaluated the quality of services. Recent trends have led to the improvement of mental health services, but more must be done to improve the mental health care delivery system. Because System of Care was conceived originally as a philosophy to develop a better mental health care model to serve children with severe emotional disturbances, the children's chapter in the report was the focus of this review.

According to the Surgeon General's report, a myriad of therapeutic services are available, ranging from psychosocial to pharmacologic interventions. This book concentrates on psychosocial and educational interventions provided by an array of disciplines. It includes the psychiatrists' perspectives in the child and adolescent psychiatry and substance use chapters (Chapters 7 and 9). However, neither chapter addresses pharmacological interventions. Studies have shown that a multimodal approach to treat children and adults who are mentally ill is generally more effective than using either medications or psychosocial and educational interventions alone (Birmaher, 2004).

Early identification is essential to prevent chronic emotional problems. However, few educators are trained to identify children in need of mental health care, and often, if they do identify these children, the options for appropriate referral are limited, especially in rural areas (US Department of Health and Human Services, 1999). Early identification is a major reason for mental health and education to collaborate, and collaboration is an underpinning of the System of Care philosophy. (See Chapter 12 on Education and Special Education.)

According to the Surgeon General's report, the multiple problems associated with a serious emotional disturbance are best addressed with a systems approach in which multiple services work together. Current research on the effectiveness of system of care programs has demonstrated "positive results" (p. 18). (The array of services across the health care continuum is discussed in Chapter 6, System of Care in Nursing, in detail and is addressed in many of the chapters.)

The report took the position that children's services must be provided within the context of the family and community. Another important component of the System of Care framework is the role of the care coordinator or case manager, which was described as essential to the delivery of mental health services to children and their families, especially if multiple services from many different providers are required (US Department of Health and Human Services, 1999). (See Chapter 1, System of Care Principles and Practices, and Chapter 6, System of Care in Nursing.)

In the Surgeon General's report, the importance of the family advocacy movement was recognized, which evolved because so many parents experienced conflicting requirements for services, conflicting information and expectations, and felt blamed for their child's plight. Some parents were forced to give up custody of their children in order to obtain mental health services for them. (Review Chapter 1, System of Care Principles and Practices, and Chapter 4 on Parents' Voices.) Outcome studies have documented the importance of the family's role to enhance the quality of mental health services for children. The report acknowledged that the development of an integrated systems model of culturally competent wraparound services, emphasizing interagency collaboration, grew from the awareness that many children were being served in delivery systems other than just mental health (see Chapter 2 on Wraparound and Partnerships). Families of children with severe emotional disturbances were receiving services in juvenile justice, education, and social services, as well as mental health. It was clear that a concerted effort to coordinate these different services was needed (US Department of Health and Human Services, 1999). In 1984, the Child Adolescent Service System Program was launched to address the fragmentation of public services for children. (Review Chapter 1, System of Care Principles and Practices.) "When implemented well, wraparound programs [developed under the guidance of System of Care principles] can harness the strengths of families and communities and curtail the use of costly and overly restrictive institutional forms of care" (Furman & Jackson, 2002, p. 130). Findings from current research have demonstrated "positive results" (US Department of Health & Human Services 1999, p. 18) and supported the effectiveness of programs based on System of Care.

Although service providers now can identify, treat, and in some cases prevent mental disorders, we still do not have an adequate mental health service delivery system. Inadequate funding by insurance companies continues. The lack of federal and state legislation to address the needs of the mentally ill must be addressed. The Surgeon General attributed these deficits to the stigma associated with mental illness. Unfortunately, in 2001, the House of Representatives allowed the bill for parity in insurance coverage to die in the conference committee (Killeen, 2002). There are continuing concerns about a lack of resources for mental health care. The development of multidisciplinary programs that focus on health and mental health care must be a national priority in order to provide all Americans with quality holistic care.

Healthy People 2010

This report was written in 2000 in order to develop national health goals for 2010. Ten leading health indicators reflecting the general health of the nation were used to measure the nation's health with targeted goals for improvement. The leading health indicators are "designed to reflect the major public health issues in the nation" (Clark,

2003, p. 11). Seven of the leading health indicators are related to mental health and lifestyles. However, many insurance payers deny payments for the care or cure of the very diseases that have been identified as national public health indicators. Starred in Table 16-2 are those identified as either mental health or lifestyle indicators. It is important to recognize that "mental health is fundamental to [a person's] overall health and well-being" (Bush, 2001, p. 94).

The health indicators that are starred are the focus of many of the chapters in this book, such as children who are severely emotionally disturbed, foster children whose medical care, including immunizations, may have been neglected, and adolescents who participate in all sorts of risky behaviors, including alcohol and substance abuse and sexual promiscuity, or who have been adjudicated by the juvenile justice system for violent or other high risk behaviors.

In *Healthy People 2000*, the goal was to achieve equality in the delivery of health care to all population groups. However, in the 2010 report, the goal is no longer aimed at equity; rather, the goal for the next decade is to eliminate "health disparities" (Spector, 2004, p. 56).

System of Care is a philosophic framework that can be a guide toward achieving national goals for high-quality care for all Americans and for developing education, recreation, health care, and mental health care programs to address all of the care needs of every American within the context of the school, the community, and the culture.

Table 16-2	**Healthy People 2010**

The leading health indicators related to mental health issues are as follows:

- Physical activity
- Overweight and obesity*
- Tobacco use*
- Substance abuse*
- Responsible sexual behavior*
- Mental Health*
- Injury and violence*
- Environmental quality
- Immunizations
- Access to care* (www.health.gov/healthypeople/LHI/thiwhat.html)

*These indicators are considered by many experts as addictive behaviors.

The Institute of Medicine: *Health Professions Education: A Bridge to Quality: The Executive Summary*

The Institute of Medicine convened a summit of health care professionals to develop a blueprint for reforming the training and education of health care providers to build on the findings of an earlier meeting of professionals who had met to explore ways to fix a broken health care system. The initial report, *Crossing the Quality Chasm: A New Health System for the 21st Century* (Institute of Medicine, 2002), was then followed by a second report, *Health Professions Education: A Bridge to Quality* (Greiner & Knebel, 2003). A group of health care professionals developed a set of core competencies for all of the professions (Greiner & Knebel). The committee consisted of health care professions, both educators and students from across the health care continuum, and others from certifying organizations, consumers, policy makers, and members of various practice settings, all of whom contributed to the set of recommendations for reforming the education of health care professionals. They addressed (1) the lack of skills on the part of health care professionals that are important to the delivery of quality health care and (2) the strategies that might improve the education of health care professionals. The second summit focused on the redesign of educational curricula and the necessary reforms.

Today's health care system involves patients with complex needs and care that is delivered in complicated environments, which involves a variety of disciplines and health care systems and agencies. The participants concluded that health care delivery must be changed from the inside out by revamping education, rather than from the outside in (i.e., reorganizing the health care system) in order to improve the quality of American health care.

However, it may be necessary to make changes from both the inside out and the outside in so as to improve the quality of care. System of Care experts have approached the quality of mental health care for children from both inside and outside by changing the paradigm for health care providers through education and by building partnerships with families and community agencies.

As listed in the Table 16-3, the Institute of Medicine reports have identified some of the barriers to changing the health care system, but these may also be motivators for health care professionals to effect change. Many of these same concerns can also be found in the System of Care literature. The Institute of Medicine's concerns are briefly summarized in Table 16-3.

| Table 16-3 | Key Findings and Concerns Identified by the Institute of Medicine That Have Also Been Addressed in the System of Care Literature |

- Poor systems design has led to errors, poor quality of care, and dissatisfaction among patients and health professionals.
- Health care professionals are not adequately prepared to address the shifts in the nation's patient population: Americans are more diverse. More people are aging, and more patients have one or more chronic illnesses.
- Health care employers and recent graduates cite gaps between how they are prepared and what they are called upon to do in practice.
- Once in practice, health care professionals work in interdisciplinary teams, but they are not educated together or trained in team-based skills.
- Clinicians must be skilled in responding to varying expectations and values; providing ongoing patient management; delivering and coordinating care across teams, settings, and time frames; and supporting patients' endeavors to change behaviors and lifestyles (i.e., providing case management services).
- The needs of the chronically ill are not being adequately met. Addressing those needs requires system reforms and greater coordination and collaboration among health care professionals. (The chronically mentally ill should be included among the chronically ill.)
- Patients and consumers are not informed about their health. As a result, there is a need for shared decision-making between patient and health care providers, which considers the patient's values, preferences, and cultural background.
- A serious mismatch exists between good quality care and the care that is actually delivered.

Adapted from Greiner and Knebel (2003, pp. 2, 38).

A New Vision for Health Professions Education

The report quoted the group's vision:

> "All health professionals should be educated to deliver patient-centered care as members of an interdisciplinary team, emphasizing evidence-based practice, quality improvement approaches, and informatics" (Greiner and Knebel, p. 3).

The Bridge to Quality

The summit participants proposed a set of core competencies that all health professionals must have in order to ensure quality health care systems during the 21st century. In Table 16-4, the core competencies that were identified as applicable to all health care professionals are compared with System of Care values and principles.

The last two competencies were addressed in the System of Care literature by Woodbridge and Huang (2000), who claimed that "a supportive evaluation culture is the foundation, as well as the result, of producing effective data reports that have an impact at multiple levels" (p. xiii). All System of Care projects that have received federal funding have established evaluation procedures and have developed sophisticated information systems to measure outcomes on several levels, including the child, family, professionals, systems, and the community (see Chapter 15 on evaluation). Systematic monitoring for quality improvement is necessary in program evaluation (Winters, Marx, & Pumariega, 2003).

Common Language Necessary to Adopt the Core Competencies

Before integrating the core competencies, terms need to be defined by an interdisciplinary group to achieve consensus about the meaning of the terms. Educational reform in professional training must begin by developing a shared language. The lack of consensus among the professions around terminology may be a factor that limits interdisciplinary practice and inhibits the development of interdisciplinary educational programs.

Interprofessional Education

The participants attending the summit concluded that education for health care professionals should be redesigned. The skills identified as deficits, besides a lack of interdisciplinary skills, included "technical and computer skills, critical thinking, communication, management, delegation and supervision skills, and a [narrow] systems perspective" (Greiner & Knebel, 2003, p. 38).

Recommendations from the Institute of Medicine Report: Steps to Implementing Educational Reforms

After achieving consensus about the definitions of terms, the next step will be for professional educational programs to incorporate the competencies into training. Oversight processes must be in place, such as accreditation, certification, and licensure boards, in order to ensure that the competencies are integrated into the curricula. The subsequent step is to establish financial incentives for interdisciplinary practice and education. Medicare and Medicaid should provide leadership among third-party payers by funding collaborative clinical projects in

Table 16-4	Core Competencies Compared with System of Care Values and Principles

- *Patient-centered care:* Differences, values, preferences, and expressed needs should be respected. Health care professionals should relieve pain and suffering, coordinate continuous care, listen to, clearly inform, communicate, and educate patients. Decision-making should be shared. Health care professionals should continually advocate disease prevention, wellness, and the promotion of healthy lifestyles, with a focus on the health of specific populations.

  System of care principles and values: The clinician should provide client- and family-centered care that is culturally competent, community based, and coordinated across the health care continuum from prevention to chronic long-term care. Family–professional decision-making is necessary to promote and enhance the inherent strengths of the client and family in order to improve the quality of life and to encourage healthy lifestyles and self-care (see Chapters 1 and 2).

- *Work in interdisciplinary teams:* To cooperate, collaborate, communicate, and integrate care in teams is essential to ensure that care is continuous and reliable.

  System of Care framework: Interdisciplinary teams are established for each child that incorporate all disciplines, which are part of the family's system of care, as well as all people who are significant to the child, including family, friends, and extended family members. A team of collaborative partners who are professionals and community members of natural support systems plans and provides the interventions (review Chapters 1 and 2).

- *Employ evidence-based practice:* It is essential to integrate the best research with clinical expertise and patient values for optimum care, to participate in learning and research activities, and to design and test interventions to change processes and systems of care with the objective of improving quality (see Chapter 5 on Psychology).

  System of Care: These programs address evidenced-based practice continually, which implies that scientific study has been applied to clinical services for children and adolescent mental health problems (Rogers, 2003) (review Chapter 7 on Child and Adolescent Psychiatry).

- *Apply quality improvement:* It is important to identify errors and hazards in care; understand and implement basic safety measures, such as standardization and simplifications; use informatics to communicate and manage knowledge, support decision making and to mitigate errors; evaluate the quality of care in terms of structure, process, and outcomes in relationship to patient and community needs and determine ways to improve the quality of the program.

continues

Table 16-4	Continued

System of Care has the goals of providing quality care to children and adolescents, who have mental health concerns, and continually monitoring and evaluating programs. System of Care addresses quality by measuring outcomes related to structure, process, and the efficacy of therapeutic interventions. Measures include both client and systems outcomes. Winters, Marx, and Pumariega (2003) compared the development of System of Care to tending a garden: "One needs to continually adjust system goals and expectations to social and political influences (the weather) and community demographics (the soil) (pp. 389, 390) (review Chapter 15 on evaluation).

Adapted from Greiner and Knebel (2003); Rogers (2003); Stroul (1996); Winters et al. (2003); and Woodbridge and Huang (2000).

order to demonstrate the cost-effectiveness of interdisciplinary approaches. If time to attend meetings is not reimbursable, then meetings to collaborate will not occur. Changes in the policies for reimbursement are key to implementing interdisciplinary practice successfully. Finally, state-of-the-art demonstration centers funded by foundations should be established to provide leadership in developing innovative strategies to educate professionals in the five competencies.

Competency-based education makes learning outcomes explicit and enables evaluators to assess whether students have mastered the competencies (Greiner & Knebel, 2003). Research will be necessary to examine the efficacy of the competencies. Development of a set of measures reflecting the core competencies along with the nation's goals for improving the health care system will be needed. Summit meetings of health care leaders, practitioners, educators, and others must be ongoing to oversee the changes needed in education and practice in order to ensure that the nation meets the goals for health care reform: "safety, effectiveness, patient-centeredness, timeliness, efficiency, [and] equity" (Greiner & Knebel, p. 3).

Achieving the Promise: Transforming Mental Health Care in America: The Executive Summary of the President's New Freedom Commission on Mental Health (2003)

President Bush launched the President's New Freedom Commission in 2001 to address the problems in the national mental health system that inhibits American citizens from having full access to needed mental health care. The president challenged the commission to address the fragmentation of mental health services. In a letter to President Bush, as the chairman of the President's Freedom Commission, Hogan (2003) wrote, "Today's mental health system is a patchwork relic—the result of disjointed reforms and policies." Recognizing that mental health is central to the overall health of the nation, the president's commission examined strategies to incorporate research findings into service delivery. Issues of access to care and elimination of disparities in the quality of care for the mentally ill were addressed.

The interim report by the Freedom Commission acknowledged that there is fragmentation in service delivery and that there are serious gaps in mental health care for children and adults. Currently, research findings are not being used to improve mental health services in a timely manner. The commission recommended transforming the current system in order to redirect the focus from institutional care to community-based care, with the hope of promoting recovery and reducing chronicity. According to the commission, recovery means the ability of the person diagnosed with a mental illness to live, work, learn, and participate fully in the community (community-based care is addressed in most of the chapters).

In the final report issued in 2003, system of care language can be found throughout the report. For example, one of the recommended goals is that mental health care should be "Consumer and Family Driven" (The President's New Freedom Commission, *Achieving the Promise: Transforming Mental Health Care in America, Executive Summary,* 2004, p. 8), which includes developing individualized care plans, improving access to care that is culturally competent, and providing support services so that persons can function successfully while living at home. Recommendations related to children's services included support for early screening and detection through routine assessments and referrals in order to provide early intervention services and prevent the likelihood of an emotional disorder from becoming more severe. One of the recommendations is to expand school mental health programs and to include screening for co-occurring mental health and substance use disorders.

The President's New Freedom Commission Report, *Achieving the Promise: Transforming Mental Health Care in America, Executive Summary* (2003) clearly encompasses the values and principles of system of care. According to the report, persons at high risk for a mental illness must be identified early so that appropriate comprehensive plans can be put into place to meet the individual needs of the client, the child, and the family and to eliminate the possibility of a chronic disorder. Disparities in mental health services must be eliminated so that the overall goal of a healthy nation can be achieved.

Where Do We Go from Here?
Keeping the Vision Alive: Sustaining the Momentum

Professionals, educators, families, and national organizations such as the President's Freedom Commission must continue to support changes in the health care delivery system to promote access to holistic care, including health and mental health care within the context of the family, culture, and community. The following is a list of potential strategies that may be implemented by service providers, educators, legislators, and citizens to sustain System of Care, as a framework for program development in mental health care (Table 16-5).

The move toward community-based care has been progressing slowly since the early days of the community mental health movement (review Chapters 6 and 7, the Nursing and Child and Adolescent Psychiatry chapters.). Cultural diversity training for professionals to learn to be culturally competent has been instituted in many academic and clinical settings (see Chapter 14 on Professional Development). Family participation in decision making has also gained support nationally, and in some settings and educational institutions, it is now integrated into education and practice (see Chapter 4 on Family Voices). Integrating interdisciplinary practice into professional education will pose the greatest challenge.

The barriers to implementing interprofessinal education were identified by the Institute of Medicine in its report, *Health Professions Education: A Bridge to Quality, Executive Summary* (Griener & Knebel, 2003), and were similar to those of the Annie E. Casey Foundation, documented by the Council of Education in Social Work in *Myths and Opportunities*, 1999, whose focus was on welfare rather health care. The *Executive Report, Health Professions Education: A Bridge to Quality* by the Institute of Medicine (2003), edited by Greiner and Knebel, and the other national organizations addressed the barriers that need to be overcome (Table 16-6).

The Benefits of Interprofessional Education

In interprofessional courses, students learn to deal with complicated situations as they learn collaborative and negotiating skills, as well as

Table 16-5	Strategies to Keep the Vision Alive in the World of Health, Education, Human Services, and Mental Health

- *Disseminate information* about the System of Care principles and values at every opportunity. Information about models for interprofessional education from pilot projects should be infused into curriculum in professional schools.
- *Leadership* at all levels requires that the leader be someone who has staying power. This person not only needs to be visionary, but also flexible and creative. The leader must have good facilitation skills to work with diverse groups of people and good communication skills, including writing skills and good public speaking skills to convey clearly the need to adopt System of Care values and principles. The leader should be a community activist who is prepared to lobby legislators. He or she must be able to write grants to fund System of Care programs. This same leader should publish in national journals and the print media to disseminate the System of Care values and principles. In other words, the leader needs to be a person of many talents. Co-leadership, especially in an interdisciplinary world, should be encouraged.
- *Strong interagency collaboration* is needed among community agencies with the ability to pool resources so that System of Care programs remain accessible to the community when state or national funding no longer exists. Develop university/community partnerships. Build consensus among stake holders around the importance of interprofessional education.
- *Strong parent groups* are needed to support program development and research and to be advocates to ensure quality mental health care.
- *Data* that support System of Care principles and values must be collected systematically. Outcomes must be broadly disseminated. Data must be applied to continually address quality improvement.
- *Professional organizations* should work together on a national level to develop collaborative projects that will improve the quality of care. Many are already doing so, but more will be needed in the future. These same organizations need to lobby as advocates for quality health and mental health care.
- *Community organizations* that may be natural resources for clients, families, and agencies should be a part of the process of program development and maintenance.
- *The business community* is important to program development and can help program developers write a business plan to identify and reach short- and long-term goals.
- *Universities* should establish interdisciplinary task forces to establish centers for the study of collaborative interprofessional practice to address issues related to rewards and incentives for the development of interprofessional courses and projects and to acquire funding to support collaborative projects, as well as to examine curriculum development and study issues of accreditation, licensure, and certification.

Adapted from the Reports of the Annie E. Casey Foundation *Myths and Opportunities*, 1999, the Surgeon General's Report *Mental Health: A Report of the Surgeon General*, US Department of Health and Human Services, 1999, *Healthy People 2010*, Office of Disease Prevention, The US Department of Health and Human Services, 2000, the Institute of Medicine, *Health Professions Education: A bridge to quality, Executive Summmary* written by Greiner & Knebel, 2003and the President's New Freedom Commission on Mental Health *Achieving the Promise: Transforming Mental Health Care in America, Executive Summary*, US Department of Health and Human Services, 2003.

Table 16-6	Challenges to Effect Potential Professional Educational Reforms

- Fiscal Structures
  - Funding to review curriculum and teaching methods, a requirement before changes can be implemented.
  - The fiscal structures of universities inhibit interprofessional education.
  - There is an emphasis on research and patient care in many academic settings, with little reward for teaching. Patient care and research bring in money to departments, but teaching does not. Because of the demands for research and practice, educators experience time constraints that inhibit interdisciplinary program development and management.
  - The health care financing system is a deterrent to quality care. For example, third-party payers tend not to reimburse health care providers for educating clients about their health care needs nor do they reimburse for interdisciplinary program development, unless it can be billed as direct patient care.
- Faculty
  - There is a lack of faculty development on the principles of interdisciplinary education and practice and other competencies listed by the Institute of Medicine (2003), edited by Greiner and Knebel. The result is there may not be enough faculty available at training sites to teach the new competencies.
  - Faculty are resistant to change.
  - There is a lack of trust among professionals from different disciplines.
  - Faculty is not available to assume responsibilities for program development because of other responsibilities.

Different orientations and perspectives hinder consensus.
- Oversight: Accreditation, licensure, and certification
  - No coordinated oversight exists across the educational continuum from undergraduate to graduate education or across health care and human service professional education.
  - Accreditation and supervision issues exist.
  - There are oversight restrictions by crediting bodies.
  - There is no integration across oversight processes, including accreditation, licensing, and certification.
- A shortage of visionary leaders
  - Political will is lacking.
- Silo structures
  - Turf issues and long-standing disciplinary boundaries exist between the professions.
  - There is a lack of flexibility among disciplines.

- It is difficult to change educational programs and professional practices because the initial training of a health professional leaves a lasting and powerful impression that leads to reluctance to change.
- Cultural norms in each of the professional disciplines may have conflicting values that do not support interprofessional education.
- The resistance of traditional educational structures makes setting up interdisciplinary programs difficult.
- Curricular requirements
  - Overly crowded curricula and competing demands are a deterrent to change.
  - Fieldwork or clinical requirements differ among professional groups
  - Highly prescribed curricular requirements make for a lack of flexibility.
  - Requirements for supervision differ.
  - The supervisor is often required to be from the same discipline as the student's major.
- Insufficient channels for sharing information
  - Best practice may never be achieved if information is not shared among colleagues working on the same or similar projects. A lack of shared information often has to do with assumed issues of confidentiality.

Adapted from Annie E. Casey Foundation (1999) and Greiner and Knebel (2003, pp. 36, 38).

conflict resolution skills. Students learn team building skills and how to be a leader or follower. The students become knowledgeable about group dynamics. When an interdisciplinary team is role modeled in a clinical setting, students identify with that model of care and then can transfer it from education to practice (see Chapter 14 on Professional Development).

Clients, children, and families benefit from a team of experts providing coordinated care, which also makes the transition from one service system to another easier to maneuver and more effective. Therefore, interdisciplinary practice improves the quality of care.

Interprofessional education will not happen overnight. The challenge will be to not only overcome obstacles, but also to clarify the contributions of each of the disciplines to the welfare of society. Fortunately, with the number of national organizations calling for reforms in professional education and practice based on system of care principles and values, progress should be made.

Conclusions and Recommendations

Family voices and the voices from the national institutions that oversee the nation's state of public health, mental health, and human services, all speak to similar issues. Table 16-7 is a summary of the national "call."

Table 16-7   **Health Care Professionals, Educators, and Human Service Providers Champion the Cause**

Professionals from all of the health and service disciplines must do the following:

- Educate professionals in service delivery systems differently to address adequately the needs of children, adults, families, and others who are at risk for educational, physical, and emotional difficulties.
- Teach professionals the art of establishing interpersonal relationships so that all of the professionals can work together in partnerships with clients, children and families, and each other.
- Assist in the development of family organizations that support families experiencing complex problems.
- Establish training programs for families so that they can become strong advocates for their children and other family members.
- Build a consensus in terms of goals and to establish a common language.
- Make concerted efforts to build interdisciplinary teams that are responsive to people's needs that are complex, acute, and/or chronic.
- Include in professional training and education both interdisciplinary practice and multiculturalism.
- Become more person and family centered in order to deliver health care that is holistic, addressing the mind/body/spirit and emotional connections.
- Change from looking at problems and solutions to identifying strengths and building on them to empower people to solve their own problems and determine their own destinies.
- Aim to preserve the family's and the client's integrity and dignity by conveying respect.
- Build interagency collaborative partnerships to provide a network of community services.
- Elicit the participation of clients and families in decision making about improving the health and mental health of individuals, groups, and communities.
- Improve access to care for all population groups to eliminate health care and mental health disparities. Lobbying efforts for parity must be continued on behalf of the mentally ill.

Challenges for the Future

The greatest challenges will be for professionals, educators, family members, and other stake holders to reach a consensus so that they can advocate for those who cannot advocate for themselves with *one voice* and to ensure that all members in our society receive quality care.

Overcoming the stigma of mental illness and the lack of funds for mental health care will continue to be a challenge. These will be monumental barriers, as the politicians promise both guns and butter, while not having the political will to pass a bill on parity of health insurance for mental health care. Professionals must continue to overcome the barriers to caring for the mentally ill. Supporting System of Care must be a national priority. In an era of "quick fixes" for the least cost, quality care must be a national goal, especially for the nation's children who are our resources for the future. Health care professionals practicing today and tomorrow should examine what needs to be done to ensure the implementation of System of Care values and principles. Programs based on these principles and values must survive financial cuts and remain the focus of national, state, and local legislative agendas. More System of Care programs need to be developed, especially in rural America. We must continue the call for quality health and mental health care for all Americans.

References

Annie E. Casey Foundation. (1999). *Myths and opportunities: An examination of the impact of discipline-specific accreditation on interprofessional education: Executive summary: A report from preparing human service workers for interprofessional practice: Accreditation strategies for effective interprofessional education project.* Alexandria, VA: Council on Social Work Education. Available from: http://ww.cswe.org.org.

Birmaher, B. (2004). TADS findings presented at the American Academy of Child and Adolescent Psychiatry Annual Meeting, Washington, DC: Treatment for Adolescent with Depression Study Team (TADS): Stage I outcomes. *The Journal of the American Medical Association (JAMA) 292,* 807–820.

Bush, C.T. (2001). Eye on Washington: Excerpts from the report of the Surgeon General's conference on children's mental health: A national action agenda. *Journal of Child and Adolescent Psychiatric Nursing, 14*(2), 94–95.

Clark, M.J. (2003). The population context. In M.J. Clark (Eds.), *Community health nursing* (4th ed., pp. 3–14). Upper Saddle River, NJ: Prentice Hall.

Furman, R., & Jackson, R. (2002). Wrap-around services: An analysis of community-based mental health services for children. *The Journal of Child and Adolescent Psychiatric Nursing, 15*(3), 124–130.

Greiner, A.C., & Knebel, E. (Eds.). (2003). *Health professions education: A bridge to quality.* The Executive Summary. The Committee on Health Professions Education Summit Board on Health Services. Institute of Medicine of the National Academies. Washington, DC: The National Academies Press. Available from: www.nap.edu.

Hogan, M.F. (2003). Letter to President Bush, as Chairman of the President's New Freedom Commission on Mental Health. Preface to the Final Report: *Achieving the Promise: Transforming Mental Health Care in America, Executive Summary.* Rockville, MD: The Department of Health and Human Services (DHHS Publication No. SMA-0303831). Available at www.mentalhealth commission.gov; www mental health.samsha.gov.

Hoagwood, K., Burns, B., Kiser, L., Ringeisen, H., & Schoenwald, S. (2001). Evidence-based practice in child and adolescent mental health services. *Psychiatric Services, 52*(9), 1179–1189.

Institute of Medicine. (2002). *Crossing the quality chasm: A new health system for the 21st century.* Washington, DC: National Academy Press.

Kenen, J. (2004). A senator's tearful plea helps pass suicide bill. Washington, DC: Reuters. Retrieved July 13, 2004, from: http://news.yahoo.com/news?tmpl=story&cid=594&u=20040709/hl_nm/congress_sui.

Killeen, M.R. (2002). Eye on Washington: Mental health parity: Just an illusion? *Journal of Child and Adolescent Psychiatric Nursing, 15*(1), 37–38.

Office of Disease Prevention and Health Promotion, The US Department of Health and Human Services. (2000). *Healthy People 2010.* Retrieved September 24, 2004, from: www.health.gov;healthypeople/LHI/thi what. html.

Pew Health Professions (1995). *Critical challenges: Revitalizing the health profession for the 21st century.* San Francisco: University of California San Francisco Center for the Health Professions.

Rogers, K. (2003). Evidenced-based community-based interventions. In A.J. Pumariega & N.C. Winters (Eds.), *The handbook for child and adolescents systems of care: The new community psychiatry* (pp. 149–170). San Francisco: Jossey-Bass.

Satcher, D. (2003). Preface by the Surgeon General, *Mental health: A report of the Surgeon General.* Rockville, MD: The US Department of Health and Human Services Substance Abuse and Mental Health Services Administration, Center for Mental Health Services. National Institute of Mental Health.

Spector, R.E. (2000). *Cultural diversity in health and illness* (5th ed.). Upper Saddle River, NJ: Prentice Hall.

Spector, R.E. (2004). *Cultural diversity in health and illness* (6th ed.). Upper Saddle River, NJ: Prentice Hall.

Stroul, B.A. (1996). *Children's mental health: Creating systems of care in a changing society.* Baltimore, MD: Paul H. Brookes.

Stroul, B.A., & Friedman, R.M. (1986). *A system of care for children and youth with severe emotional disturbances* (rev. ed.). Washington, DC: Georgetown

University Child Development Center, National Technical Assistance Center for Children's Mental Health.

The President's New Freedom Commission on Mental Health. (2003). *Achieving the promise: Transforming mental health care in America. Executive summary.* Rockville, MD: The US Department of Health and Human Services. (DHHS Pub. No SMA-03-3831). Available from: www.mentalhealthcommission.gov; www.mental health.samsha.gov.

US Department of Health and Human Services. (1999). *Mental health: A Report of the Surgeon General.* Rockville, MD: US Department of Health and Human Services, Substance Abuse and Mental Health Services Administration, Center for Mental Health Services, National Institutes of Health, National Institute of Mental Health.

Winters, N.C., Marx, L.S., & Pumariega, A.J. (2003). Systems of care and managed care: Are they compatible? In A.J. Pumariega & N.C. Winters (Eds.), *The handbook of child and adolescent systems of care: The new community psychiatry* (pp. 380–413). San Francisco: Jossey-Bass.

Woodbridge, M., & Huang, L. (2000). Using evaluation data to manage, improve, market, and sustain children's services. *System of care: Promising practices in children's mental health* (2000 series, Vol. II). Washington, DC: Center for Effective Collaboration and Practice, American Institutes for Research.

Index

Italicized page locators indicate a figure: italicized *t* indicates a table.